MRI of the Knee

Nicolae V. Bolog · Gustav Andreisek
Erika J. Ulbrich

MRI of the Knee

A Guide to Evaluation and Reporting

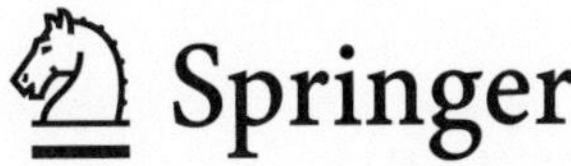 Springer

Nicolae V. Bolog, MD, PhD, MS
Phoenix Diagnostic Clinic
Cluj-Napoca
Romania

Gustav Andreisek, MD, MBA
Institute of Diagnostic and
Interventional Radiology
University Hospital Zürich
Zürich
Switzerland

Erika J. Ulbrich, MD
Institute of Diagnostic and
Interventional Radiology
University Hospital Zürich
Zürich
Switzerland

ISBN 978-3-319-35253-4   ISBN 978-3-319-08165-6   (eBook)
DOI 10.1007/978-3-319-08165-6
Springer Cham Heidelberg New York Dordrecht London

Foreword I

MRI of the Knee – A Guide to Evaluation and Reporting covers one of the most common and most relevant topics in any imaging practice. The authors are a senior staff radiologist and a junior staff radiologist from a university hospital, both specializing in musculoskeletal imaging, and a radiologist working in private practice with close contacts with academic radiology and a keen interest in teaching. All of them have worked in several institutions in different countries. This guarantees a broad view on the topic and adds details not covered by other textbooks. This includes a discussion of nerves and vessels about the knee. The authors' background also guarantees practical relevance of the covered topics. An emphasis on postoperative imaging is another interesting aspect of this book which is not as widely covered in literature as anatomy, variants, acute and chronic trauma or cartilage abnormalities. The book is characterized by a very systematic approach to disease, which is relevant for teaching, reliable reporting, quality initiatives and research purposes.

MRI of the Knee – A Guide to Evaluation and Reporting is a carefully edited book covering all relevant aspects of MR imaging of the knee, which will find its way to the bookshelves of many radiologists and clinicians interested in the knee.

Zurich, Switzerland   Jürg Hodler

Foreword II

MRI of the Knee – A Guide to Evaluation and Reporting focuses on providing a strong platform for learning and understanding the standard evaluation and accurate reporting of knee MR imaging.

The authors, experienced in the field of musculoskeletal imaging, have foreseen the practical fit of the thorough approach depicted in this textbook for both radiologists – in assessing MR images of the knee systematically – and referring specialists, who will become more familiar with the terminology used in the reports covering various conditions.

The book is structured into 11 chapters, with each chapter covering the normal anatomy and normal MR imaging findings, followed by a detailed description of abnormal and postoperative findings well supported by relevant case images.

Each chapter ends with a summary written in the form of a paragraph that readers are encouraged to use as a standardized MR report.

MRI of the Knee – A Guide to Evaluation and Reporting is bringing a unique and distinctive approach to knee imaging, with practical application related to day-to-day reporting, educational purposes such as teaching and further research into this part of the musculoskeletal system mostly benefiting from the state-of-the-art MR imaging evaluation.

New York, USA   John A. Carrino, MD, MPH

Preface

In the past few years, magnetic resonance (MR) imaging of the knee has become the current state-of-the-art imaging modality to evaluate knee disorders. Decreasing costs and the noninvasive nature of MR examinations made them widely accepted for the evaluation of meniscal and ligamentous as well as bone marrow and soft tissue injuries or abnormalities. In current medical practice, MR examination is essential not only in the preoperative setting but in general for the first-line diagnosis of most knee derangements. Theoretically, patient history and the course of an accident are often strongly suggestive of certain knee injuries and could be examined clinically. Practically, the relatively low sensitivity of clinical examination and the fact that clinical examination is often hampered by pain make diagnostic imaging indispensable. In the past, diagnostic arthroscopy has played an important role. However, since the introduction of MR imaging of the knee, this rather invasive diagnostic tool has also widely been replaced by MRI. Moreover, MR imaging has been increasingly used for detailed preoperative planning.

Today's importance of MR imaging of the knee is also illustrated by the fact that apart from the spine, more musculoskeletal MRI examinations are performed on the knee than on any other region of the body.

With the widespread use of an imaging technique, several challenges in terms of quality arise. Firstly, image acquisition must follow current standards, and image quality has to be provided on a high diagnostic level. Secondly, image storage and transfer need to be guaranteed to supply referring physicians with the original source information of the examination. Lastly, image evaluation and reporting of findings have to meet the referring physician's need and must answer the medical question. Therefore, standardized evaluation and reporting were suggested by several imaging societies and were proposed as a potential solution.

This background led PD Dr. Gustav Andreisek and Dr. Nicolae Bolog to aim for a book project, which was dedicated to the idea to provide the educational basis for standardized evaluation and reporting of knee MR imaging. The book was created as a classic textbook, with several chapters ordered by anatomical structures. Each chapter contains a detailed description of the normal anatomy, normal and abnormal MR imaging findings as well as postoperative findings. At the end of each chapter, a summary is provided in the form of a paragraph that can be used for a standardized radiological report.

The following two chapters provide an overview of the normal anatomy of the knee, in particular of the anterior and posterior cruciate ligaments, as well as the most common knee disorders concerning the two ligaments. A special emphasis was laid on postoperative imaging, and thus both chapters discuss postoperative findings in detail. The authors consider this discussion as very important as the respective chapters in current textbooks are rather short and these topics are otherwise in general not widely discussed in original literature.

The systematic approach of the textbook as well as the following chapters should help novice as well as senior doctors get through the book easily and quickly find what they are looking for. The well-organized structure helps radiologists, giving them a guideline of how to assess MR images of the knee systematically, hence reducing the risk of leaving a relevant finding aside. On the other hand, the book should also serve as a field manual of how to effectively report imaging findings to clinicians. Using a clear and structured order for reporting as proposed here, the book helps create a comprehensive report, which minimizes the peril of forgetting relevant results.

Finally, this textbook is addressed to referring clinicians as they will much better understand a radiological report and what is meant by a specific terminology. Ultimately, the patient will benefit from a much better education and communication between different medical specialists.

Cluj-Napoca, Romania   Nicolae V. Bolog, MD, PhD, MS
Zürich, Switzerland   Gustav Andreisek, MD, MBA
Zürich, Switzerland   Erika J. Ulbrich, MD

Contributors

The authors thank Dr. Brian M. Devitt for his constant professional advice as well as his comments and edits for several chapters of the book.

Brian M. Devitt, MD, FRCS
Consultant Orthopaedic Surgeon
Sports Surgery Clinic Dublin
Ireland

The authors thank Mr. Rene Roth for his help in image postprocessing and his contribution for several chapters of the book.

René Roth
Medical student
University Hospital Zurich
Switzerland

Contents

1 Anterior Cruciate Ligament (ACL) 1
1.1 Anatomy and Normal MRI Appearance 1
1.2 MRI Pathological Findings 1
    1.2.1 Congenital Absence (Agenesia)................ 1
    1.2.2 Acute Tear 3
    1.2.3 Chronic Tear.............................. 8
    1.2.4 Ganglion Cyst............................. 8
    1.2.5 Mucoid Degeneration of ACL 9
1.3 Postoperative Anterior Cruciate Ligament (ACL)........ 11
    1.3.1 Normal Postoperative ACL Graft
        and MRI Appearance 11
    1.3.2 MRI Pathological Postoperative Findings 12
1.4 MRI Impression................................. 17
    1.4.1 Nonsurgical ACL 17
    1.4.2 Postoperative ACL 17
References.. 18

**2 Posterior Cruciate Ligament (PCL)
and Meniscofemoral Ligaments........................** 21
2.1 Anatomy and Normal MRI Appearance 21
    2.1.1 Posterior Cruciate Ligament (PCL) 21
    2.1.2 Meniscofemoral Ligaments 21
    2.1.3 Retrocruciate Fat Pad....................... 24
2.2 MRI Pathological Findings 24
    2.2.1 Acute Tear 24
    2.2.2 Posterior Cruciate Ligament Avulsion Fracture.... 26
    2.2.3 Chronic Tear and Mucoid Degeneration 28
    2.2.4 Ganglion Cyst............................. 28
    2.2.5 Retrocruciate Fat Pad Impingement............. 28
2.3 Postoperative Posterior Cruciate Ligament (PCL)........ 29
    2.3.1 Normal Postoperative PCL Graft
        and MRI Appearance 30
    2.3.2 MRI Pathological Postoperative Findings 32
2.4 MRI Impression................................. 33
    2.4.1 Nonsurgical PCL 33
    2.4.2 Postoperative PCL 33
References.. 33

**3 Medial Collateral Ligament (MCL)
and Medial Supporting Structures** 35
   3.1   Anatomy and Normal MRI Appearance 35
   3.2   MRI Pathological Findings 38
       3.2.1   Acute Tear 38
       3.2.2   Chronic Injury of MCL 41
       3.2.3   Healing Stages of MCL 42
   3.3   MRI Postoperative Findings 44
   3.4   MRI Impression................................... 46
       3.4.1   Nonoperative MCL 46
       3.4.2   Post-Injury Nonoperative MCL................. 46
       3.4.3   Postoperative MCL 46
   References... 47

**4 Lateral Collateral Ligament (LCL)
and Posterolateral Corner (PLC)** 49
   4.1   Anatomy and Normal MRI Appearance 49
       4.1.1   Lateral Collateral Ligament (LCL)
              and the Anterior Oblique Band (AOB) 49
       4.1.2   Popliteal Tendon (PT), Anterolateral
             Ligament (ALL), Popliteomeniscal Fascicles
             (PMF), and Popliteofibular Ligament (PFL) 49
       4.1.3   Arcuate Ligament (AL) and Fabellofibular
             Ligament (FFL) 51
   4.2   MRI Pathological Findings 53
       4.2.1   Sprain and Partial Tears 53
       4.2.2   Complete Tears............................. 55
       4.2.3   The "Arcuate" Sign and the Segond Fracture 59
   4.3   Role of Preoperative MRI 60
   4.4   MRI Postoperative Findings 61
       4.4.1   Indications for Posterolateral Corner
             Repair/Reconstruction 61
       4.4.2   Operative Versus Nonoperative Management 61
       4.4.3   Posterolateral Corner Structures Typically
             Repaired/Reconstructed...................... 62
       4.4.4   Role of Postoperative MRI.................... 62
   4.5   MRI Impression................................... 63
       4.5.1   Nonoperative Lateral Collateral Ligament
             and Posterolateral Corner.................... 63
       4.5.2   Postoperative Lateral Collateral Ligament
             and Posterolateral Corner.................... 63
   References... 63

5 Meniscus.. 65
   5.1   Anatomy and Normal MRI Appearance 65
       5.1.1   Medial Meniscus 65
       5.1.2   Lateral Meniscus 69
       5.1.3   Normal Variants – Meniscal Flounce............ 71

5.2   MRI Pathological Findings   72
        5.2.1   Discoid Meniscus...........................   72
        5.2.2   Meniscal Avulsion   73
        5.2.3   Meniscal Extrusion.........................   75
        5.2.4   Meniscocapsular Separation....................   76
        5.2.5   Degenerative Changes   77
        5.2.6   Meniscal Contusion   77
        5.2.7   Meniscal Tears   78
        5.2.8   Meniscal Cysts............................   85
        5.2.9   Meniscal Calcifications   87
5.3   MRI Postoperative Findings   89
        5.3.1   Meniscectomy and Meniscal Repair   90
        5.3.2   Transplantation...........................   92
        5.3.3   Complications After Surgery   92
5.4   MRI Impression................................   92
        5.4.1   Nonoperative Meniscus   92
        5.4.2   Postoperative Meniscus   92
References......................................   93

6   Articular Cartilage and Subchondral Bone   95
6.1   Anatomy and Normal MRI Appearance   95
6.2   MRI Pathological Findings   97
        6.2.1   Nontraumatic Cartilage Changes and Subsequently
                Subchondral Lesions   97
        6.2.2   Osteonecrosis of the Subchondral Bone   102
        6.2.3   Traumatic Osteochondral Lesions   104
6.3   MRI Postoperative Findings   107
6.4   MRI Impression................................   110
        6.4.1   Nonoperative Cartilage and Subchondral Bone....   110
        6.4.2   Postoperative Osteochondral Findings...........   111
References......................................   111

7   Patella, Femoropatellar Joint, and Infrapatellar Fat Pad....   113
7.1   Anatomy and Normal MRI Appearance   113
        7.1.1   Patella and Patellar Retinaculum   113
        7.1.2   Femoropatellar Joint........................   114
        7.1.3   Infrapatellar Fat Pad and Suprapatellar Fat Pad....   116
        7.1.4   Patellar Calcar   116
7.2   MRI Pathological Findings   117
        7.2.1   Patellar Dysplasia.........................   117
        7.2.2   Patella Alta and Patella Baja   118
        7.2.3   Patellar Instability   120
        7.2.4   Patellar Dislocation   122
        7.2.5   Pathological Findings of the Patellar Tendon   125
        7.2.6   Pathological Findings of the Infrapatellar Fat Pad. .   129
7.3   MRI Postoperative Findings   132
7.4   MRI Impression................................   134
        7.4.1   Nonoperative Findings.......................   134
        7.4.2   Postoperative Findings (Intervention for Instability
                and Dislocation)..........................   134
References......................................   134

8   Synovium and Capsule 137
  8.1   Anatomy and Normal MRI Appearance 137
      8.1.1   Capsule and Synovial Compartments 137
      8.1.2   Synovial Bursae and Synovial Recesses 137
      8.1.3   Synovial Plicae 139
  8.2   MRI Pathological Findings 139
      8.2.1   Joint Effusions 139
      8.2.2   Intra-articular Bodies 143
      8.2.3   Synovitis 145
      8.2.4   Bursitis 153
      8.2.5   Synovial Cysts 155
      8.2.6   Ganglion Cysts 155
      8.2.7   Synovial Plica Syndrome 159
      8.2.8   Synovial Tumor-Like Lesions
                and Synovial Tumors 160
  8.3   MRI Impression 164
  References 165

9   Muscles and Tendons 169
  9.1   Anatomy and Normal MRI Appearance 169
      9.1.1   The Anterior Muscle Group 169
      9.1.2   The Posteromedial Muscle Group 170
      9.1.3   The Posterolateral Muscle Group 172
      9.1.4   Anomalous Knee Muscles 173
  9.2   MRI Pathological Findings 176
      9.2.1   Traumatic Injuries: General Findings 176
      9.2.2   Traumatic Injuries: Clinical and Imaging Findings
                of Specific Muscles Around the Knee 180
      9.2.3   Intratendinous and Peritendinous Ganglion Cyst ... 184
  9.3   MRI Impression 186
  References 187

10   Arteries and Nerves 189
  10.1   Anatomy and Normal MRI Appearance 189
      10.1.1   Arteries 189
      10.1.2   Veins 191
      10.1.3   Nerves 192
  10.2   MRI Pathological Findings: Arteries 193
      10.2.1   Atherosclerosis, Thrombosis, and Embolism 194
      10.2.2   Aneurysms 194
      10.2.3   Traumatic and Iatrogenic Injuries 196
      10.2.4   Artery Entrapment Syndrome 196
      10.2.5   Hemangiomas 196
      10.2.6   Vascular Malformations 198
  10.3   MRI Pathological Findings: Nerves 198
      10.3.1   Habitual, Traumatic, and Iatrogenic
                Nerve Disorders 201
      10.3.2   Entrapment Neuropathies 201

10.3.3 Tumors and Tumorlike Lesions 201
10.3.4 Systemic Diseases That Involve
the Peripheral Nerves 201
10.4 MRI Impression 202
10.4.1 Arteries and Veins 202
10.4.2 Nerves 203
References 203

11 Bones 205
11.1 Anatomy and Normal MRI Appearance 205
11.2 MRI Pathological Findings 206
11.2.1 Transient Bone Marrow Edema 207
11.2.2 Disuse Osteopenia and Epiphyseal
Growth Arrest Lines 207
11.2.3 Avascular Necrosis and Bone Marrow Infarction . . 209
11.2.4 Subchondral Bone Contusions (Bone Bruises) 210
11.2.5 Trauma to Synchondroses 214
11.2.6 Avulsion Fractures 214
11.2.7 Stress Injuries/Fractures 215
11.2.8 Bone Tumors Around the Knee 219
11.3 MRI Impression 221
References 226

Index 229

MRI Protocol: Routine Examination

Native MRI sequences:

Sequence	Plane	FOV (mm)	Slice thickness (mm)
PD FSE	Sagittal	135–180	3
T2 FSE fat suppression/STIR	Sagittal	135–180	3
T1 FSE	Coronal	160	3
PD FSE fat suppression/STIR	Coronal	160	3
PD FSE fat suppression	Axial	160	3

Additional sequences after contrast administration (indicated in postoperative knee, arthritis, tumors)

Postcontrast MRI sequences:

Sequence	Plane	FOV (mm)	Slice thickness (mm)
T1 FSE fat suppression	Sagittal/ axial/ coronal	135–180	3

MRI Protocol – Direct artrography (e.g. used for intra-articular bodies, osteochondritis dissecans, and meniscal retears)

Sequence	Plane	FOV (mm)	Slice thickness (mm)
T1 FSE fat suppression	Sagittal	140–160	3
PD FSE	Sagittal	140–160	3
T2 FSE fat suppression/STIR	Coronal	160–180	3
T1 FSE fat suppression	Coronal	160–180	3
T2 FSE fat suppression/STIR	Axial	140–160	3

MRI Report of Normal Knee

Patient: Doe, John	**Referring physician**: Dr. ………
ID:	**Fax**:
Date of birth:	**Telephone**:
Examination date:	**E-mail**:

Indication: Pain of the left knee without traumatic history

MRI of the right/left knee without contrast (iv or intra-articular)

MRI protocol: standard (sagittal PD and T2 fat suppression, coronal T1 and PD fat suppression, axial PD or T2 fat suppression)

MRI findings:

Ligaments

Anterior and posterior cruciate ligament normal in appearance.

Medial and lateral collateral ligaments are intact without signal changes noted. No pathological changes of the posterolateral corner of the knee. Meniscofemoral ligaments present normal.

Menisci

The medial and lateral meniscus with normal dimensions and structure (normal contour and thickness). No acute meniscal tears, no degenerative changes. No perimeniscal cysts. The transverse geniculate ligament is indistinct/normal.

Cartilage

The femorotibial and retropatellar cartilage is preserved without remarkable changes.

Patella

Patella in normal position and the extensor mechanism (quadricipital tendon and patellar tendon) as well as the patellar retinacula are intact without signal changes or thickening.

Synovium

There is no joint effusion, sign for synovitis, or bursitis. There are no intra- or extra-articular cysts noted. No pathological synovial plica noted.

Muscles

Muscles and tendons are normal in appearance. No anomalous muscles are noted.

Arteries and nerves

No pathological changes of the neurovascular structures are noted. There are no signs of compression.

Bones

There are no signs of fractures or tumors. The bone marrow is unremarkable.

Impression:

Normal MRI appearance of the knee.

Anterior Cruciate Ligament (ACL)

Nicolae Bolog, Gustav Andreisek, Erika Ulbrich, and René Roth

1.1 Anatomy and Normal MRI Appearance

The ACL extends from the posterior part of the medial aspect of the femoral condyle to the anteromedial tibial plateau. The normal sagittal angle between ACL and the tibial plateau depends on patient's age and gender. The mean sagittal angle between ACL and the tibial plateau in adults is between $54°$ and $55.5°$ with a cutoff angle smaller than $45°$ suggestive of an ACL tear in adults [1, 2].

The ligament is intra-articular but extrasynovial being enveloped by a fold of synovium.

It consists of two bundles named according to their tibial insertion: a small anteromedial bundle and a larger posterolateral bundle. The posterolateral bundle is shorter (18.4–22.9 mm) than the anteromedial bundle (34.1–39.7 mm) [3]. The anteromedial bundle limits anterior-posterior translation, while the posterolateral bundle limits anterior tibial translation and knee rotation [4].

On MR images, the ACL is seen as a band of low signal intensity in all sequences (Fig. 1.1). The different bundles can however be well appreciated on MR images. The anteromedial bundle can be seen on MRI in the sagittal and coronal planes as oblique fibers inserting at the anterior border of the ACL on the tibia and the proximal aspect of the femoral insertion on the lateral femoral condyle (Fig. 1.1). The posterolateral bundle is represented by oblique fibers inserting posteriorly on the tibia and on the distal aspect of the femoral insertion just below the anteromedial bundle (Fig. 1.1). As a consequence, in general the low signal intensity of the ACL is separated by several lines of increased signal intensity on T1- or intermediate-weighted images, most prominently near the tibial attachment. These lines are consistent with stripes of fat and synovium of high signal intensity at the tibial attachment (Fig. 1.1).

1.2 MRI Pathological Findings

1.2.1 Congenital Absence (Agenesia)

Unilateral or bilateral agenesia of ACL is a very rare condition and may be accompanied by other knee abnormalities such as hypoplasia of the medial tibial plateau and/or the lateral femoral condyle, patellar hypoplasia, an abnormal shape of the intercondylar notch, hypoplasia of the lateral part of the tibial spine, or fibular hypoplasia [5]. Only half of the patients present clinical signs of instability, and compared with posttrauma cases, ACL agenesia has a better prognosis regarding the progression to osteoarthritis [5].

On MR imaging, the anterior cruciate ligament is absent and cannot be identified on any of the examination planes (Fig. 1.2).

N.V. Bolog et al., *MRI of the Knee: A Guide to Evaluation and Reporting*,
DOI 10.1007/978-3-319-08165-6_1, © Springer International Publishing Switzerland 2015

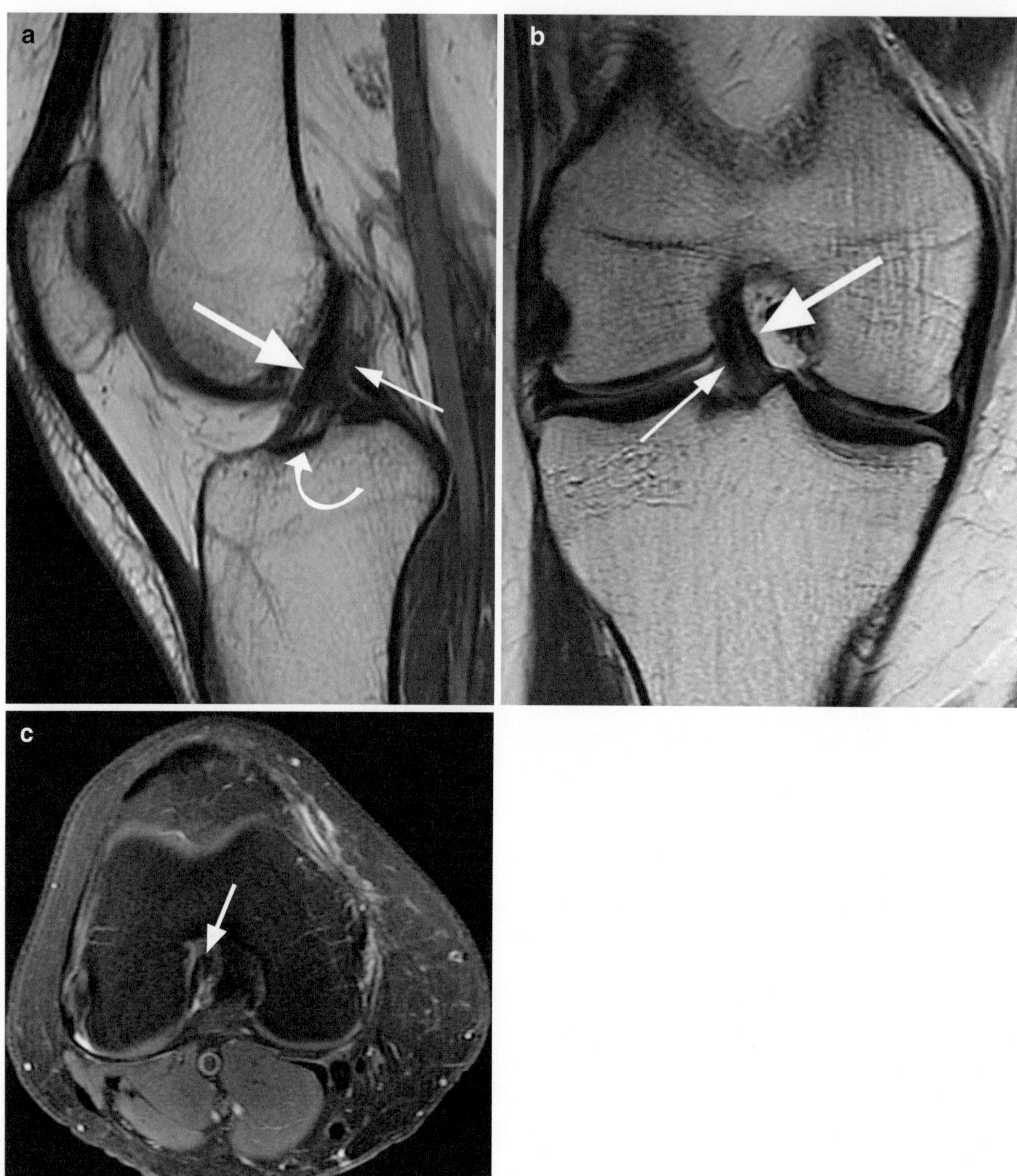

Fig. 1.1 Normal anterior cruciate ligament (ACL) in a 33 year old female. Sagittal proton-density (PD) FSE image (**a**), coronal proton-density (PD) FSE MR image (**b**), and axial proton-density (PD) FSE fat-suppressed image (**c**) show the anteromedial bundle of ACL inserting at the anterior border of the ACL on the tibia (*large arrow*) and the posterolateral bundle which is shorter and thicker (*small arrow*). Notice the several lines of increased signal intensity on sagittal intermediate-weighted image (*curved arrow* in **a**) representing stripes of fat and synovium between the two bundles at the tibial insertion

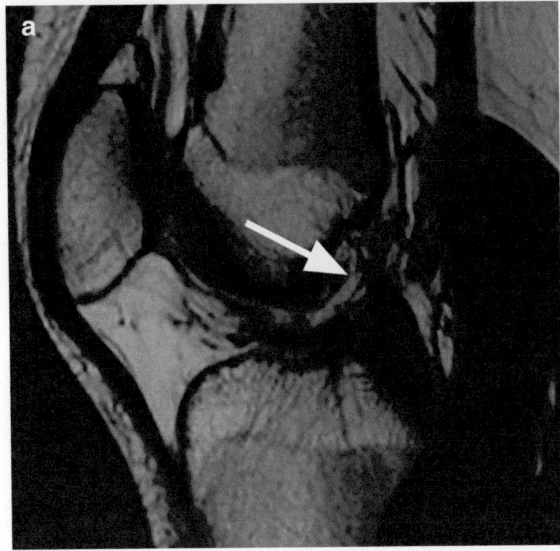

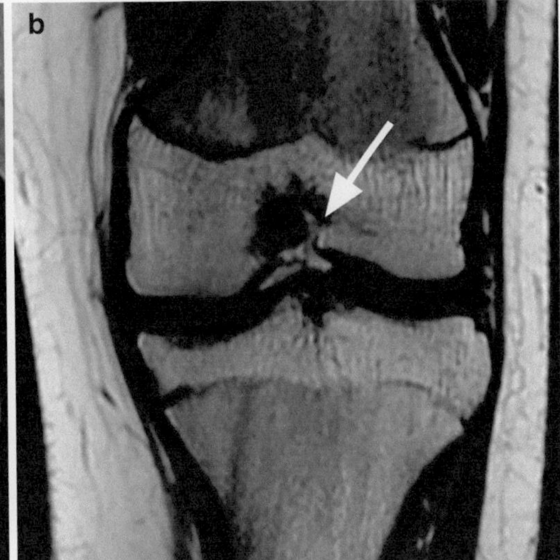

Fig. 1.2 Unilateral congenital absence of anterior cruciate ligament (ACL) in a 13 year old female tennis player without trauma or clinical instability. Sagittal proton-density (PD) FSE image (**a**) and coronal T1-weighted FSE MR image (**b**) show the absence of ACL with fatty tissue where the ligament should have been present (*arrow*)

1.2.2 Acute Tear

Complete Tear: Primary Signs

Ligament discontinuity and an abnormal high signal intensity with no depiction of the ACL are direct signs of ligament tear (Figs. 1.3 and 1.4). The presence of fluid or high signal intensity between ACL and the lateral femoral condyle on axial images indicates a proximal tear (Fig. 1.5).

An ACL acute tear may present with a mechanical block caused by an ACL stump between femoral condyle and tibial plateau (Fig. 1.6). The stump may also appear as a nodular mass with heterogeneous signal on T2-weighted images reflecting fibrosis or an inflammatory response (Fig. 1.7) [6].

Complete Tear: Secondary Signs

In addition to direct visualization of the torn ACL, MR images can be evaluated for indirect signs known to be typically associated with ACL tears. The secondary signs may appear in more than 90 % of the acute ACL tears and the mostly used secondary signs for diagnosis of ACL tears are as follows: the femoral and tibial contusion in the lateral compartment (indicated by an acute traumatic bone marrow edema) (Fig. 1.8), altered

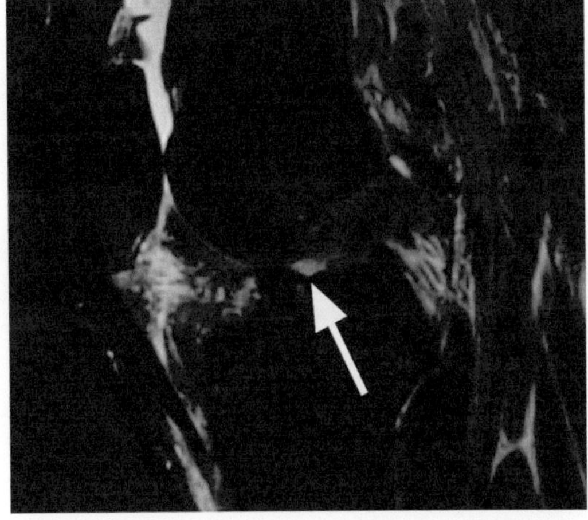

Fig. 1.3 Acute complete tear of anterior cruciate ligament (ACL) in a 26 year old male. Sagittal T2-weighted FSE fat-suppressed image shows complete discontinuity of the ligament adjacent to the tibial insertion (*arrow*)

angle between lateral tibial plateau and ACL (less than 45°) (Fig. 1.9), altered posterior cruciate ligament angle (less than 107°) (Fig. 1.10), abnormal (buckled) course of the PCL (Fig. 1.11), and the anterior displacement of tibia (Fig. 1.12) [7]. These secondary signs have high specificity and their presence corroborates with the diagnosis

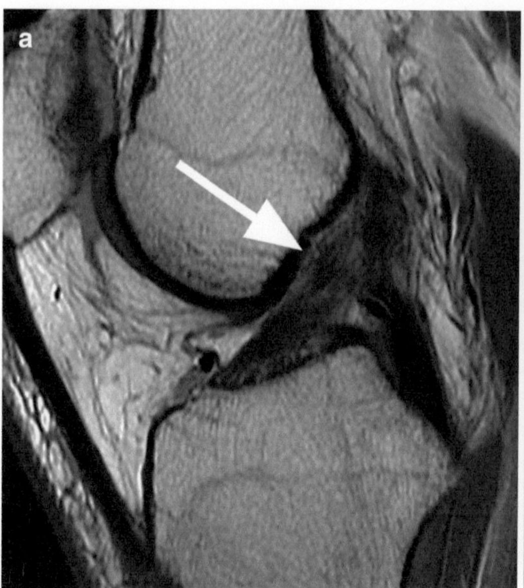

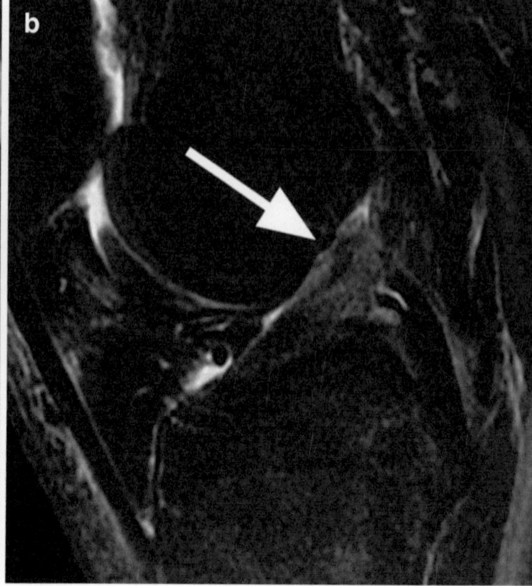

Fig. 1.4 Midsubstance acute complete tear of anterior cruciate ligament (ACL) in a 36 year old female with knee trauma. *S*agittal proton-density (PD) FSE image (**a**) and sagittal T2-weighted FSE fat-suppressed image (**b**) show an abnormal high signal intensity with no depiction of the ACL representing direct signs of a complete tear (*arrow*)

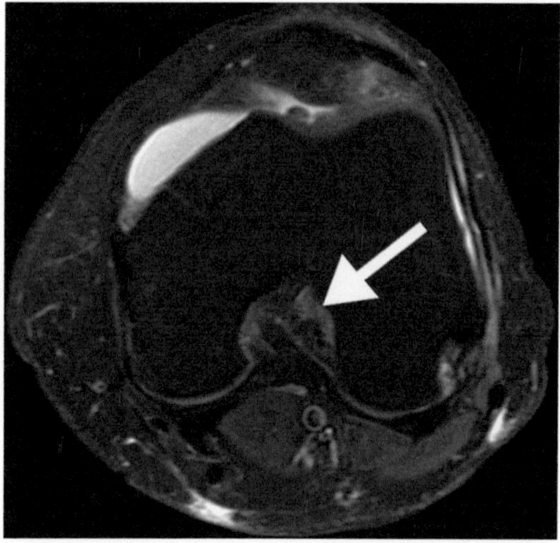

Fig. 1.5 Complete acute tear of the anterior cruciate ligament (ACL) at the femoral insertion in a 36 year old female. Axial proton-density (PD) FSE fat-suppressed image shows high-signal-intensity changes due to hematoma at the femoral insertion of ACL (*arrow*)

of ACL tear. However, sensitivity is generally low and the absence of these signs does not exclude the presence of an ACL tear [1].

Partial Tear

The partial tears represent 10–28 % of all ACL tears. The criteria of diagnosis include the absence of primary signs of complete ACL tear in conjunction with discrete focuses of high signal intensity within the midsubstance of the ACL or high-signal-intensity changes at the insertions with a normal ACL course (Fig. 1.13). The nonvisualization of the ACL on one MRI sequence with visualization of the fibers on other sequences or the bowing or undulating course of otherwise intact ACL also indicates a partial ACL tear (Fig. 1.14) [4].

Partial tearing may affect one or both bundles of the ACL which means that one bundle can be torn completely with the other bundle being partially torn at the same time (Fig. 1.15). In partial ACL tears, the involved fibers and bundles can often be well seen, and the percentage of torn fibers should be reported (e.g., "75 % of the substance of the ACL is torn") (Figs. 1.14 and 1.15).

Diffuse high-signal-intensity changes of one of the bundles at the tibial insertion with the nonvisualization of the linear high-intensity distal stripes indicate a partial distal tear of one of the bundles.

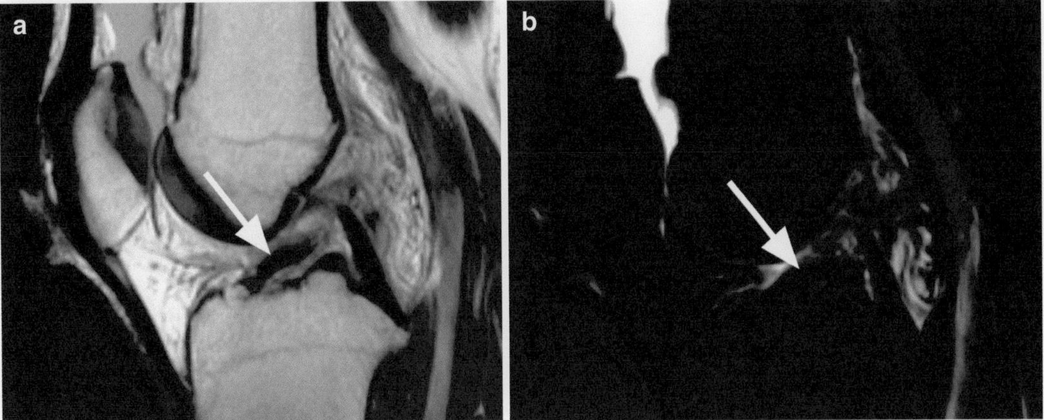

Fig. 1.6 Complete tear of the anterior cruciate ligament (ACL) in a 35 year old male with mechanical block. *S*agittal proton-density (PD) FSE image (**a**) and sagittal T2-weighted FSE fat-suppressed image (**b**) show an ACL stump (*arrow*) anteriorly between femoral condyle and tibial plateau

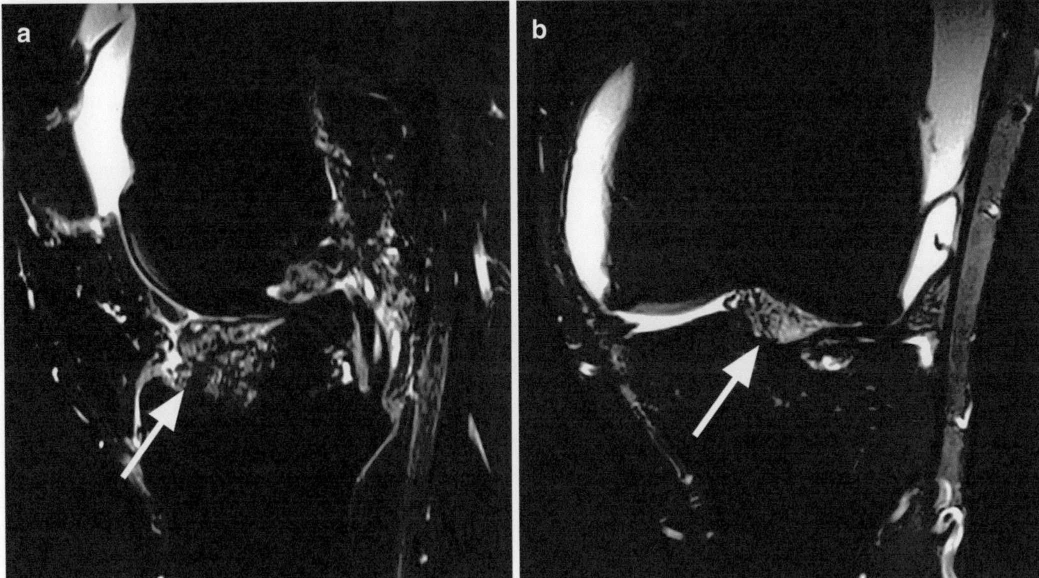

Fig. 1.7 Anterior cruciate ligament (ACL) stump after complete tear in a 30 year old male with mechanical block. Sagittal T2-weighted FSE fat-suppressed image (**a**) and coronal proton-density (PD) FSE fat-suppressed image (**b**) show a high-signal-intensity nodular mass (*arrow*) as a result of fibrosis and inflammatory response around the ACL stump

Widening of the entire ligament is associated with interstitial or intrasubstance partial tear.

Avulsion Fracture of the Intercondylar Eminence

Excessive tension on ACL may result in an inter-articular avulsion fracture of the intercondylar eminence of the tibia. This type of fracture occurs more frequently in children than adults, and the mechanism varies between children and adults. In adults, the fracture most commonly occurs secondary to an extreme hyperextension. The role of MRI is to confirm the fracture and to evaluate the ACL since partial or complete tear

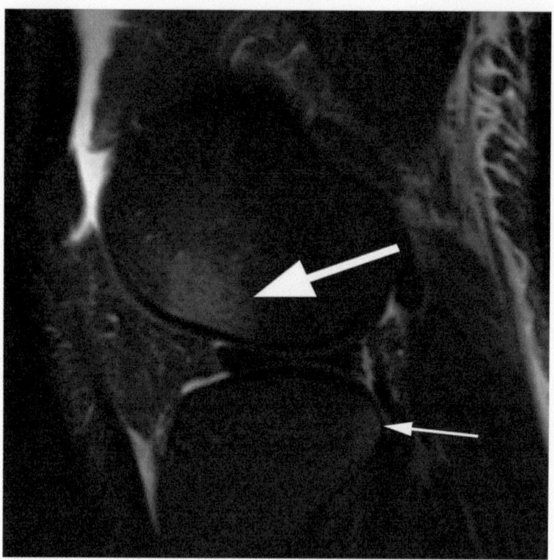

Fig. 1.8 Bone marrow contusions as indirect sign of anterior cruciate ligament (ACL) tear in a 27 year old male. Sagittal T2-weighted FSE fat-suppressed image shows high-signal-intensity contusions of the lateral femoral condyle (*large arrow*) and posterolateral tibial plateau (*small arrow*)

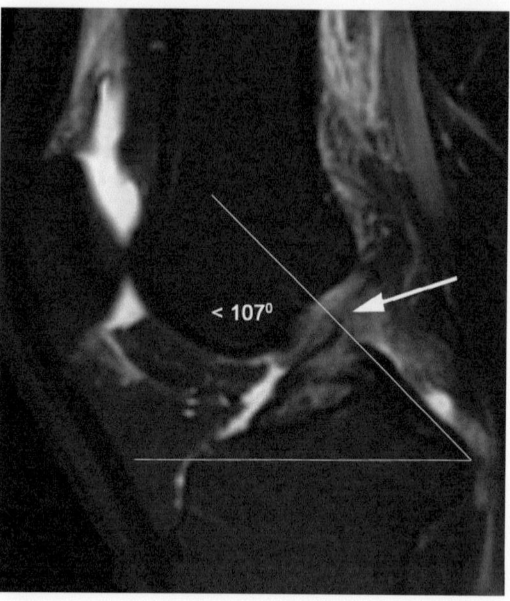

Fig. 1.10 Anterior cruciate ligament (ACL) tear in a 27 year old male (*arrow*). Sagittal T2-weighted FSE fat-suppressed image shows the angle between the posterior cruciate ligament and the plane of the tibial plateau less than 107°

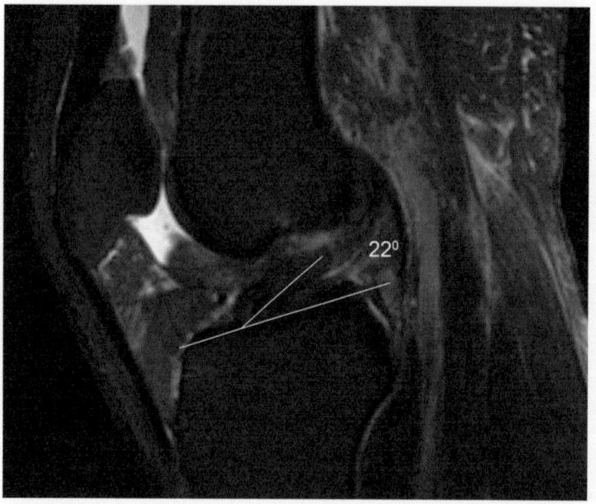

Fig. 1.9 Altered angle (22°) between lateral tibial plateau and anterior cruciate ligament (ACL) (normal value 45° or more) as an indirect sign of complete ACL tear in a 27 year old male. Sagittal T2-weighted FSE fat-suppressed image

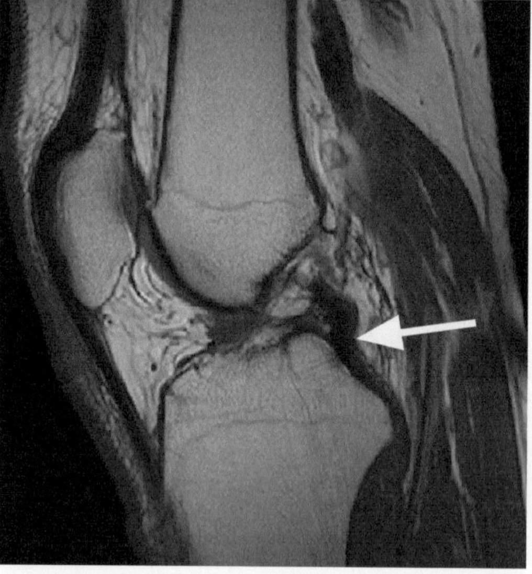

Fig. 1.11 Buckled course of the posterior cruciate ligament (PCL) as an indirect sign of complete anterior cruciate ligament (ACL) in a 26 year old male. Sagittal proton-density (PD) FSE image shows an indentation of the distal part of the PCL (*arrow*) resulting from tibial anterior translation

of ACL is often associated with this type of fracture (Figs. 1.16 and 1.17). There are three types of tibial avulsion fractures that describe a minimally or partial displaced fragment (type I and type II) (Fig. 1.16) or a complete separation of the fragment from the adjacent bone (type III) (Fig. 1.17) [8]. For type III fractures, surgical therapy is needed.

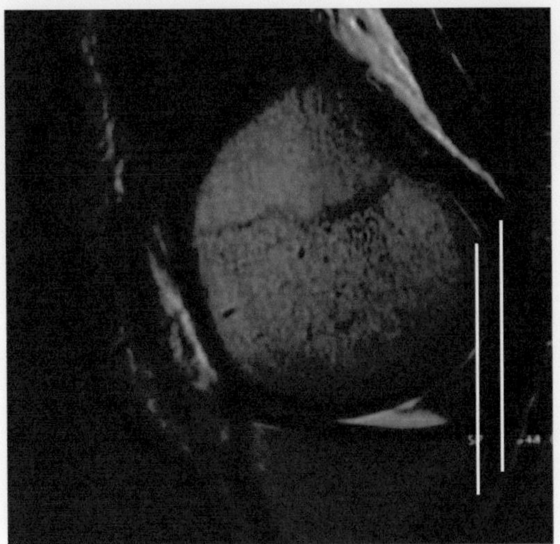

Fig. 1.12 Abnormal femorotibial relationship in a 35 year old male with complete tear of anterior cruciate ligament. The absence of the main restraint of anterior tibial translation represented by the anterior cruciate ligament (ACL) is visualized on sagittal MR images as an abnormal femorotibial relationship. *S*agittal proton-density (PD) FSE image shows an increased distance between the tibial posterior margin (*line 1*) and femoral posterior margin (*line 2*). A distance more than 5 mm is suggestive for ACL tear

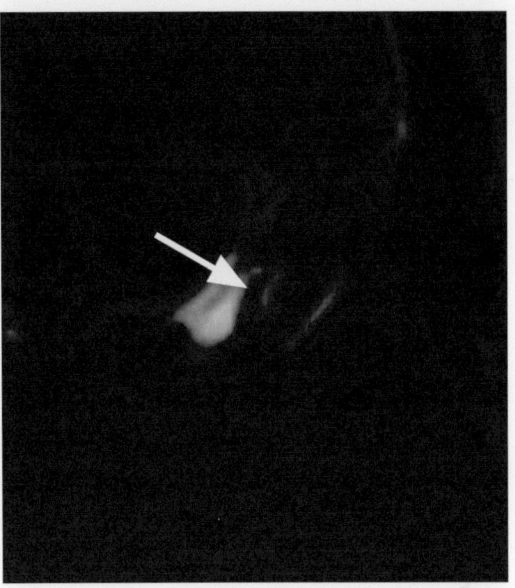

Fig. 1.14 Typical partial tear of anterior cruciate ligament (ACL) involving 50 % of the ligament thickness in a 29 year old female with knee injury. Sagittal T2-weighted FSE fat-suppressed image shows a complete tear of the distal anteromedial bundle demonstrated by discontinuity of the bundle with a focal high-signal-intensity intrasubstance lesion (*arrow*) and an undulating course of the ligament

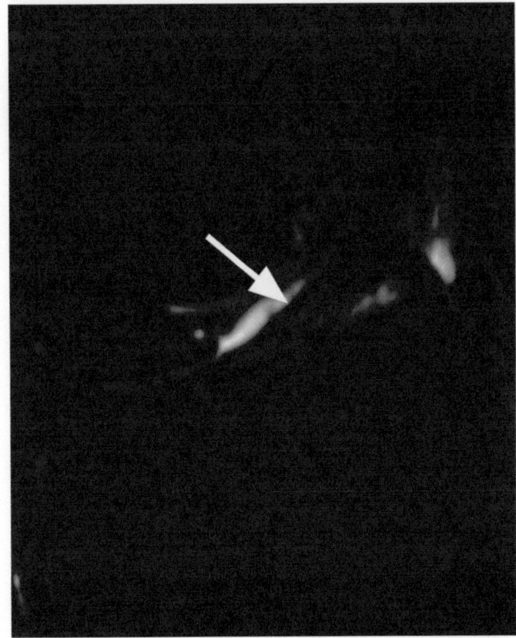

Fig. 1.13 Partial anterior cruciate ligament (ACL) tear in a 28 year old female. Sagittal T2-weighted FSE fat-suppressed image shows diffuse intrasubstance high-signal-intensity changes of the distal portion of ACL (*arrow*). Note that there are no pathological changes of the normal ACL course

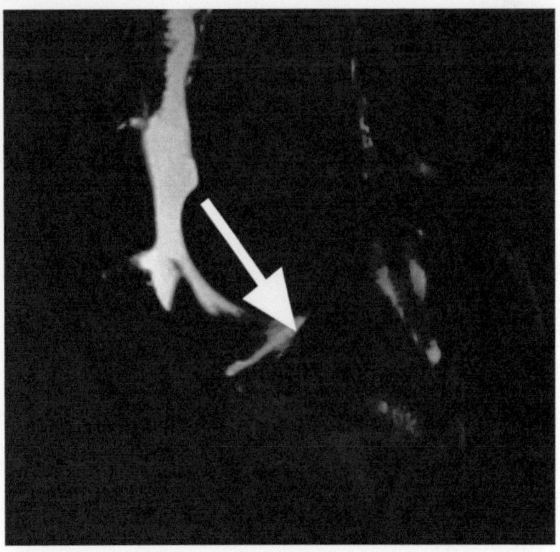

Fig. 1.15 Partial tear of the anterior cruciate ligament (ACL) involving more than 75 % of the distal ligament thickness in a 19 year old male. Sagittal T2-weighted FSE fat-suppressed image shows diffuse high-intensity changes (*arrow*) which involve the entire posterolateral bundle and partially the anteromedial bundle at the tibial insertion of the ligament

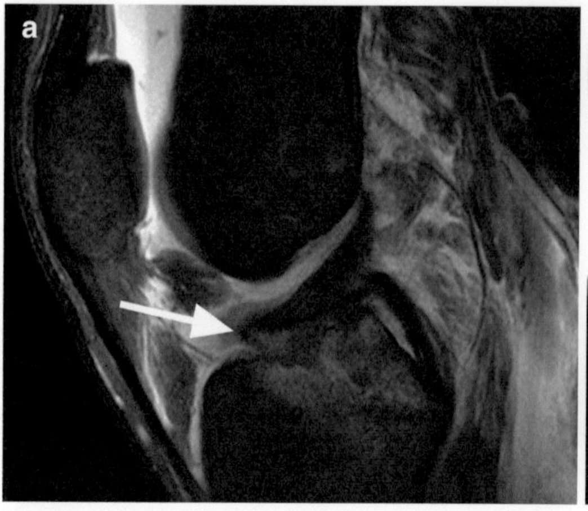

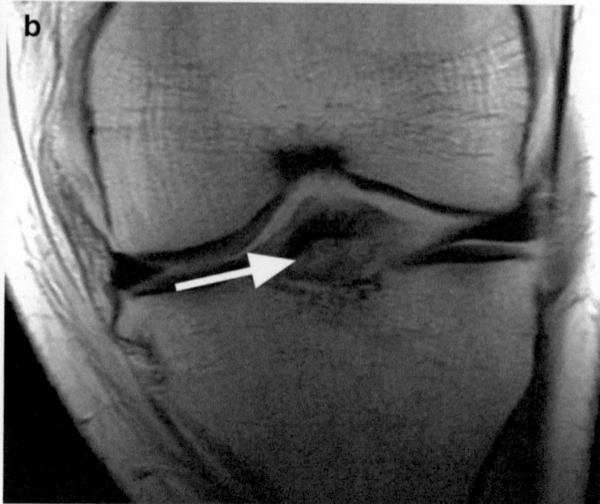

Fig. 1.16 Avulsion fracture type II of the intercondylar eminence of the tibia at the insertion of anterior cruciate ligament (ACL) in a 27 year old male with severe knee injury. Sagittal T2-weighted FSE fat-suppressed image (**a**) and coronal proton-density (PD) FSE MR image (**b**) show a bone fragment (*arrow*) from the intercondylar eminence with anterior elevation of the fragment without complete separation

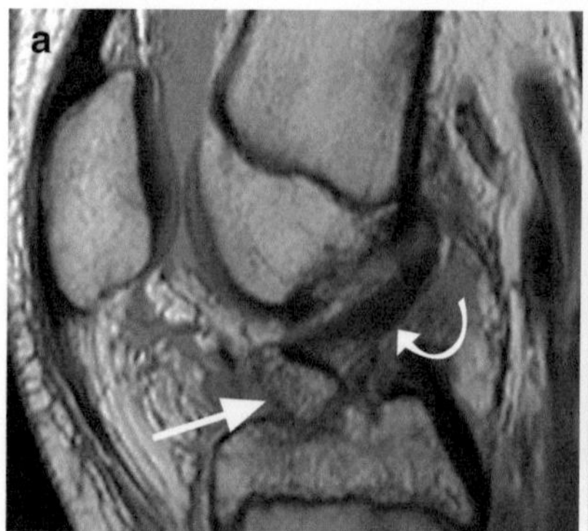

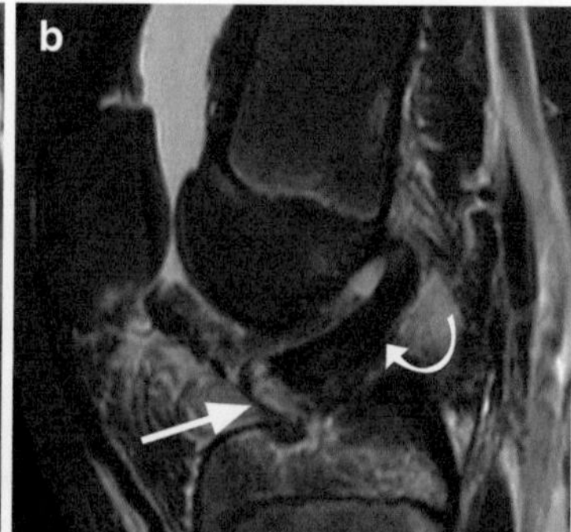

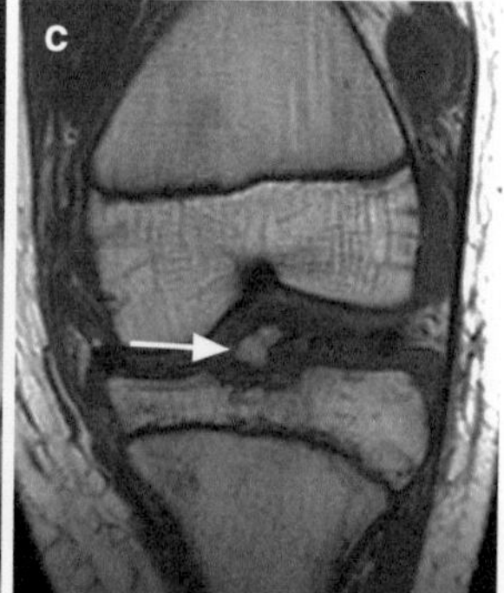

Fig. 1.17 Avulsion fracture type III of the intercondylar eminence of the tibia at the insertion of anterior cruciate ligament (ACL) in a 17 year old female with acute trauma. *S*agittal proton-density (PD) FSE image (**a**), sagittal T2-weighted FSE fat-suppressed image (**b**), and coronal T1-weighted FSE MR image (**c**) show a completely detached bone fragment from the intercondylar eminence (*arrow*). Note the partial tear of the posterolateral bundle of anterior cruciate ligament (*curved arrow* in **a** and **b**)

1.2.3 Chronic Tear

Diffuse or focal midsubstance low or intermediate signal changes of the ACL without visualization of the fibers are signs of chronic ACL tears (Fig. 1.18).

Other signs of chronic ACL tear are the focal fibrotic changes of low signal intensity at the insertions in the case of ACL healed on the notch (Fig. 1.19) or a normal ACL course without a clear delineation of the fibers in the case of chronic ACL tear healed on the posterior cruciate ligament (Fig. 1.20).

1.2.4 Ganglion Cyst

The incidence of ganglion cyst related to the ACL represents 20 % of all intra-articular ganglion cysts in the knee [9]. Knee pain at the medial joint

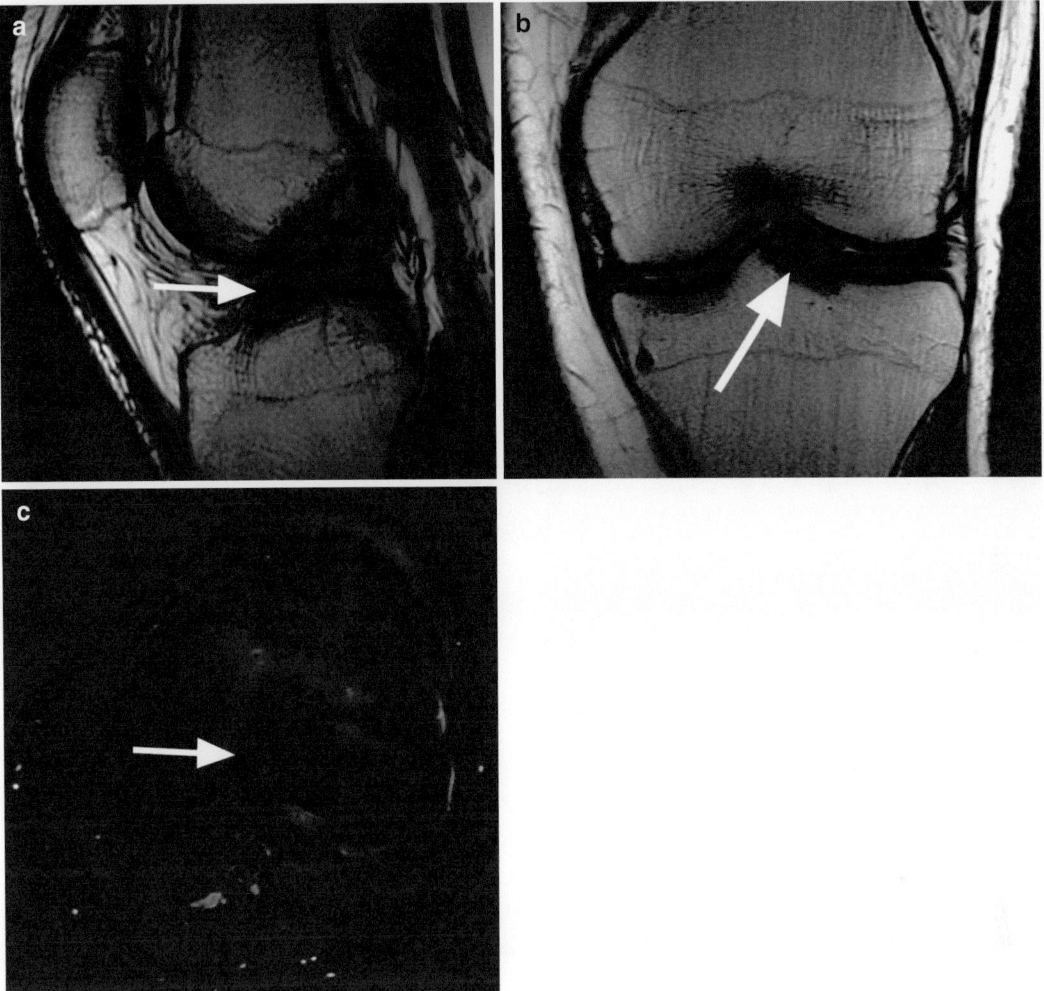

Fig. 1.18 Chronic distal tear of anterior cruciate liga-ment (ACL) healed on the notch in a 28 year old male with old knee trauma. *S*agittal proton-density (PD) FSE image (**a**), coronal proton-density (PD) FSE MR image (**b**), and axial proton-density (PD) FSE fat-suppressed image (**c**) show thickening of the ligament with diffuse intermediate signal changes at the tibial insertion (*arrow*). The absence of a clear delineation of the fibers is also an indicator of chronic tear

line, mechanical locking, clicking, and swelling are the most common symptoms of these patients. The etiology is unknown, but some authors attri-bute the cyst formation to a product of mucinous degeneration or a herniation of synovial tissue. In MR images ganglion cysts appears as a lobu-lated fluid-filled structures with internal septation having a similar signal intensity to that of joint fluid on T2-weighted images (Fig. 1.21) [10]. On T1-weighted images after contrast administration the cyst often displays diffuse enhancement, larger ganglion cysts may show only peripheral enhance-ment. ACL ganglion cyst and mucoid degenera-tion commonly coexist on MRI [11].

1.2.5 Mucoid Degeneration of ACL

The mucoid degeneration of ACL is a rare cause of knee pain which predominantly affects elderly

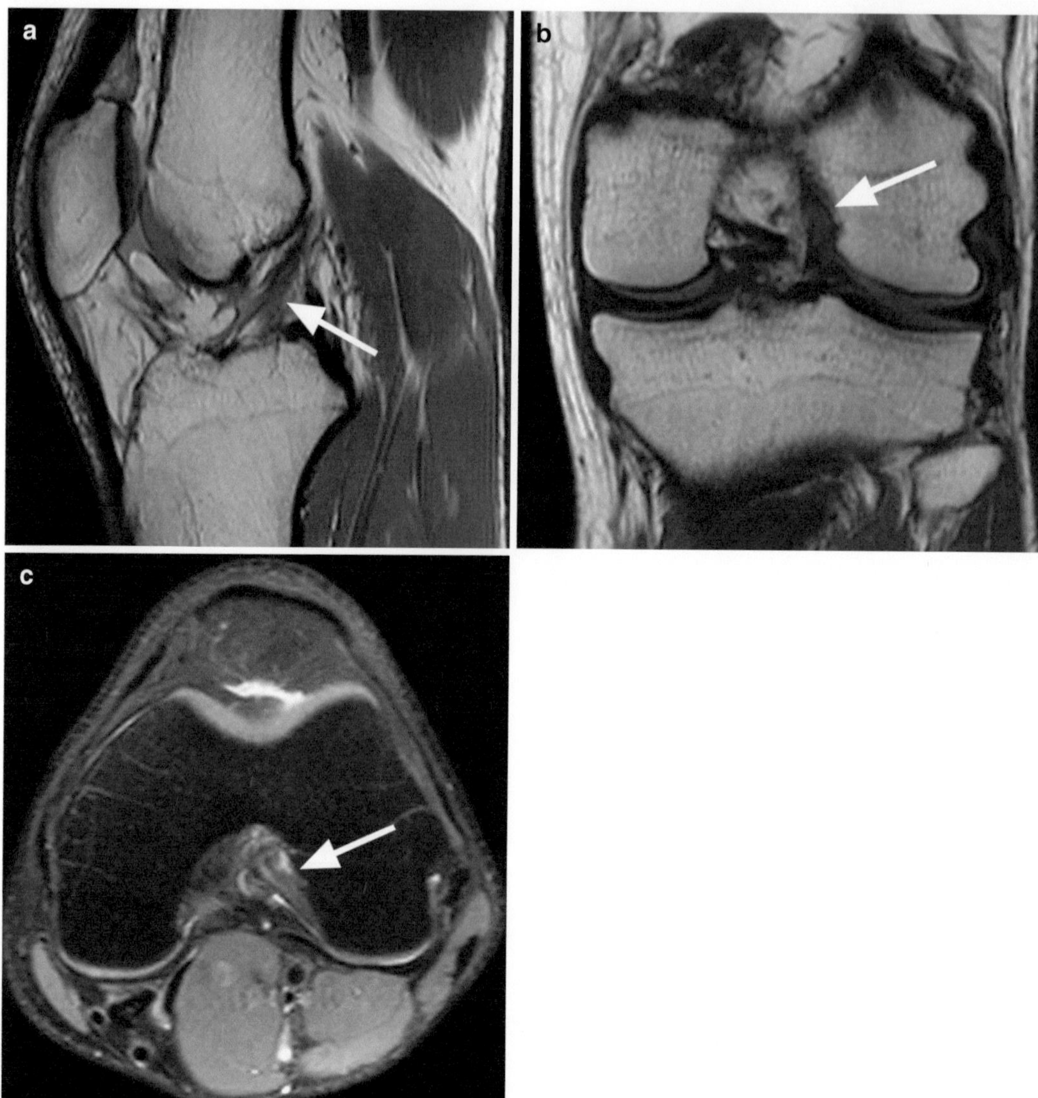

Fig. 1.19 Chronic anterior cruciate ligament (ACL) tear healed on the notch in a 21 year old patient with old knee trauma. *Sagittal* proton-density (PD) FSE image (**a**) shows a thin ACL with intermediate-signal-intensity changes (*arrow*). However, the ligament does not display disconti-nuity and the course is linear. Coronal T1-weighted FSE MR image (**b**) and axial proton-density (PD) FSE fat-suppressed image (**c**) show fibrotic changes at the femoral insertion of the ACL with no visualization of the normal fibers (*arrow* in **b** and **c**)

women. The ACL appears hypertrophied with diffuse high signal with subtle appearance of some linear, low-signal-intensity fibers parallel to the long axis of the ligament ("celery stalk" sign) (Fig. 1.22) [12]. Mucoid degeneration may coexist with ACL ganglia, as well as with intraosseous cysts at the femoral and tibial attachments. The latter location is the most frequently affected [11].

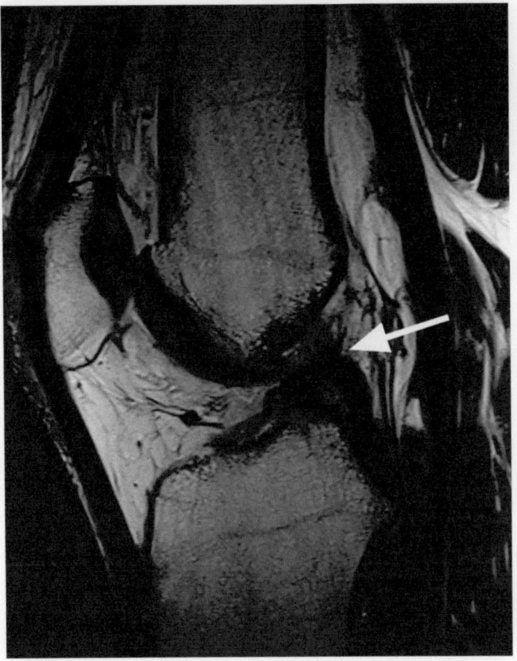

Fig. 1.20 Chronic anterior cruciate ligament (ACL) tear in a 42 year old patient with knee instability and without recent trauma. *S*agittal proton-density (PD) FSE image shows an abnormal undulating ACL course with the ligament attached to the posterior cruciate ligament (*arrow*). Note that ACL has an inhomogeneous signal intensity without a clear delineation of the fibers distally to the attachment

1.3 Postoperative Anterior Cruciate Ligament (ACL)

1.3.1 Normal Postoperative ACL Graft and MRI Appearance

Femoral and Tibial Tunnels

The correct location of the femoral tunnel is important for obtaining isometry, and the correct location of tibial tunnel is important for avoidance of impingement [13]. On sagittal images, the femoral tunnel should be located posterior to the intersection of the Blumensaat's line and a line parallel to the posterior femoral cortex (Fig. 1.23), and on coronal images the femoral tunnel should be located at 11 o'clock for the right knee and 1 o'clock for the left knee (Fig. 1.23) [13]. The slope of the ACL graft should be less than 75° measured as the angle between the long axis of the ACL graft and the plane of the articular surface [14].

The anterior border of the tibial tunnel should be located posterior to the Blumensaat's line but not posterior to the midpoint of tibial plateau (Fig. 1.23) [13].

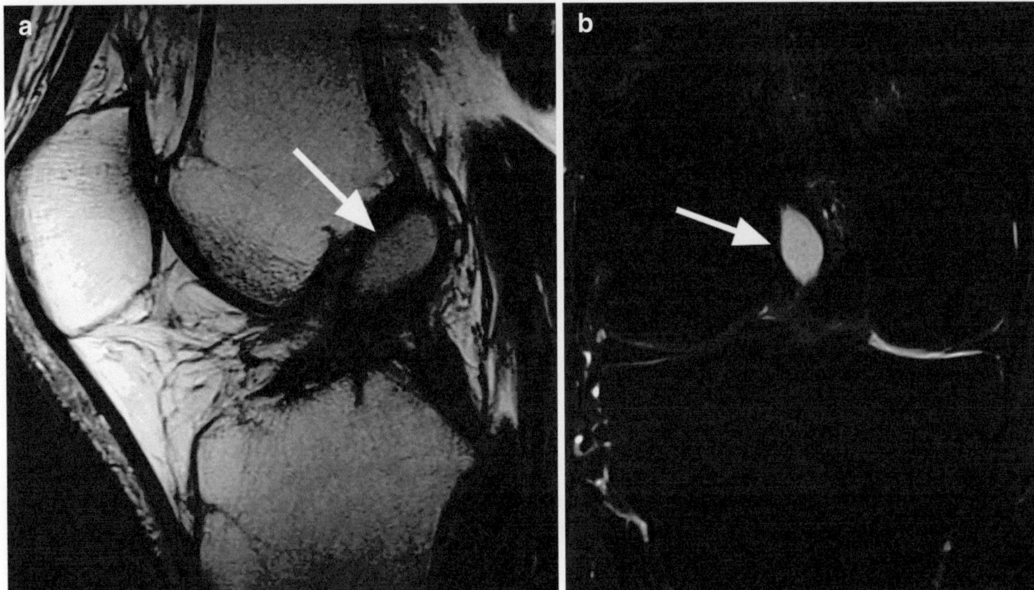

Fig. 1.21 Ganglion cyst of anterior cruciate ligament (ACL) in a 51 year old male with posterior knee pain. *S*agittal proton-density (PD) FSE image (**a**) and coronal proton-density (PD) FSE fat-suppressed image (**b**) show a well-delineated cystic lesion within the proximal anterior cruciate ligament (*arrow*). The lesion appears as homogeneous fluid-filled lesion

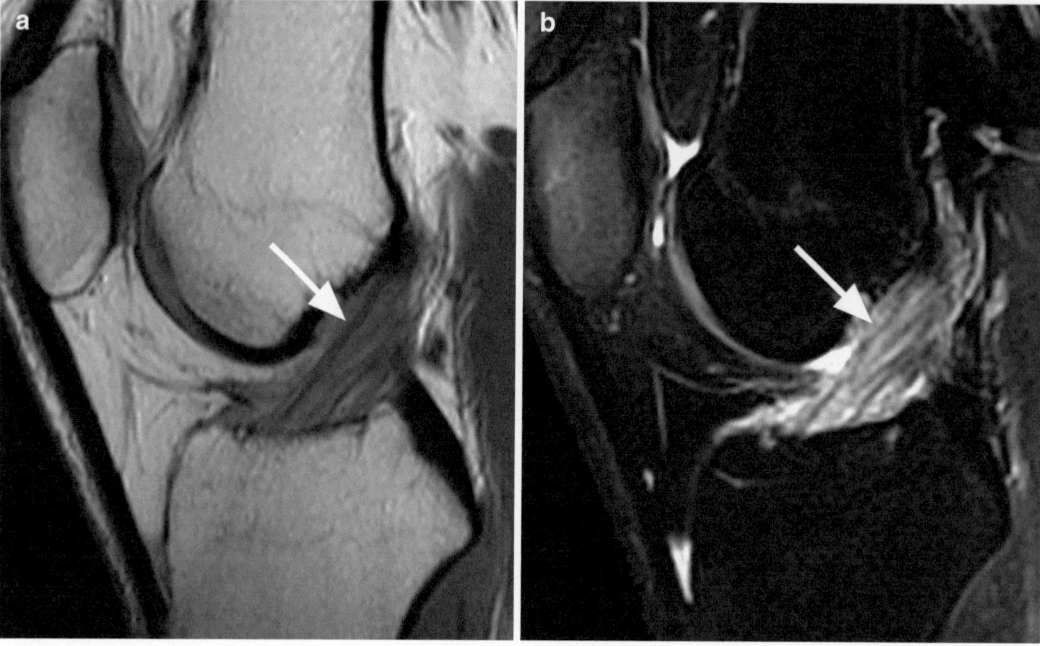

Fig. 1.22 Mucoid degeneration of anterior cruciate ligament (ACL) in a 24 year old female. *Sagittal proton-density (PD) FSE image (**a**) and sagittal T2-weighted FSE* fat-suppressed image (**b**) show typical linear signal changes on both intermediate- and T2-weighted images (*arrow*) known as the "celery stalk" sign

The ACL Graft's Signal Intensity

In the case of bone-patellar tendon-bone, the ACL graft shows low signal intensity during the first 3 months after surgery due to the avascular nature of the graft [14]. When hamstring autografts (distal semitendinosus or gracilis tendon) are used, the ACL graft does not necessarily exhibit low signal intensity on T1- and T2-weighted images.

During the next 12–18 months, the ACL graft usually shows a mildly increased signal intensity on T1- and T2-weighted images as a result of remodeling and vascularization (Fig. 1.24) [15]. After this period, approximately 2 years after ACL reconstruction, the signal intensity often becomes similar to a native ACL [16].

The hamstring tendon graft demonstrates layered appearance, and small fluid between the bundles of hamstring graft and fluid collections within the femoral and tibial tunnels during the first year are normal postoperative findings [17].

1.3.2 MRI Pathological Postoperative Findings

Tunnel Misplacement

If the femoral tunnel is too anteriorly, excessive strain occurs during knee flexion. If the femoral tunnel is positioned too posteriorly, the ACL graft is too tight in extension, and the graft may fail as a result of posterior wall breaking (Fig. 1.25). In the case of a slope higher than 75°, the graft tension will be affected.

When the tibial tunnel is too far anteriorly positioned, there are difficulties of knee extension due to roof impingement (Fig. 1.26). The MR images might show posterior bowing of the graft, spurring of the anterior margin of the intercondylar roof, and signal-intensity alteration of the anterior two thirds of the graft [18]. A tibial tunnel positioned too posteriorly leads to graft laxity and knee instability (Fig. 1.27).

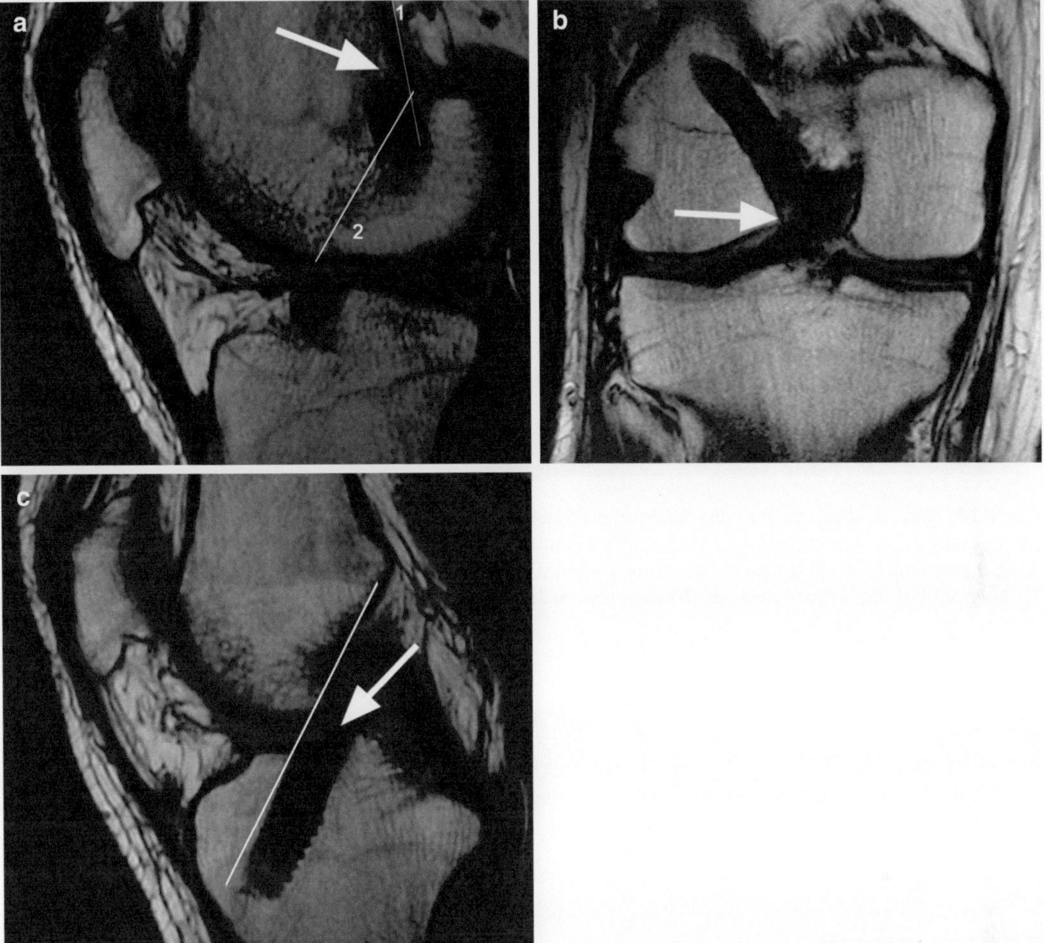

Fig. 1.23 Correct location of the tunnels in a 22 year old male after right knee anterior cruciate ligament (ACL) reconstruction. *S*agittal proton-density (PD) FSE image (**a**) shows the correct location of the femoral tunnel (*arrow*) posterior to the intersection a line parallel to the posterior femoral cortex (*line 1*) and the Blumensaat's line (*line 2*). On coronal proton-density (PD) FSE MR image (**b**), the correct position of the femoral tunnel for the right knee is at 11 o'clock (*arrow*). *S*agittal proton-density (PD) FSE image (**c**) shows the correct location of the tibial tunnel on sagittal plane (*arrow*) with the anterior border of the tibial tunnel located posterior to the Blumensaat's line (*line*)

Tear of the ACL Graft

A partial graft tear appears as focal areas of increased signal intensity at T2-weighted images with intact fibers still present. A complete acute tear of the ACL graft is seen as a complete disruption of the fibers and a fluid-filled defect (Fig. 1.26). Bone marrow edema in the lateral tibial plateau is a finding of recurrent trauma which has and a great positive predictive value for complete ACL graft tear. In chronic graft tears, the ACL lies horizontally, and the MR images may show a resorption of graft fibers (Fig. 1.26).

Tunnel Cysts and Tunnel Enlargement

The tunnel cyst is the result of the extrusion of joint fluid into the tunnel and can cause postoperative pain. Femoral tunnel cysts are rare

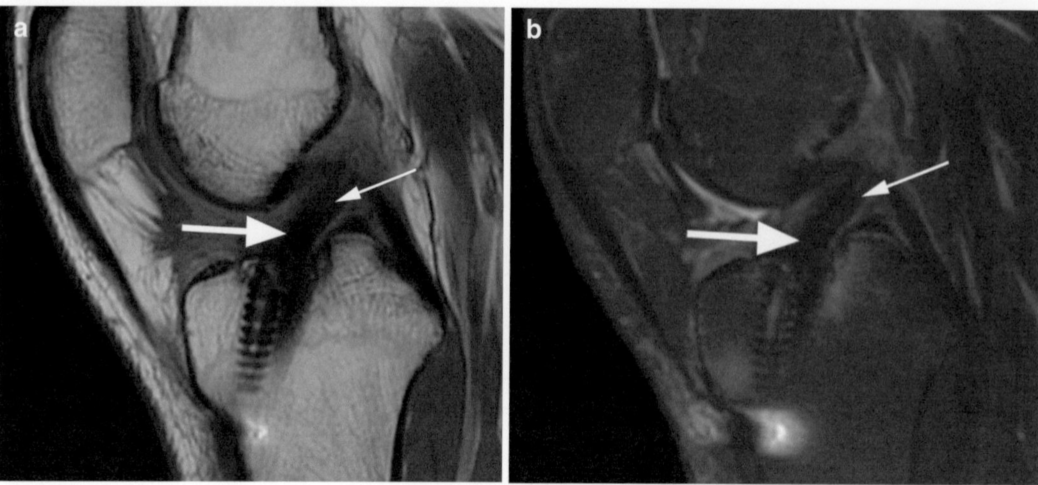

Fig. 1.24 Normal appearance of the anterior cruciate (ACL) graft 1 year after surgery in a 37 year old patient. *Sagittal proton-density (PD) FSE image (a) and sagittal T2-weighted FSE fat-suppressed image (b) show a normal course of the graft with predominantly low signal intensity (*large arrow*). Note a mild increased signal intensity within the graft (*small arrow*) which is normal at 1 year after reconstruction

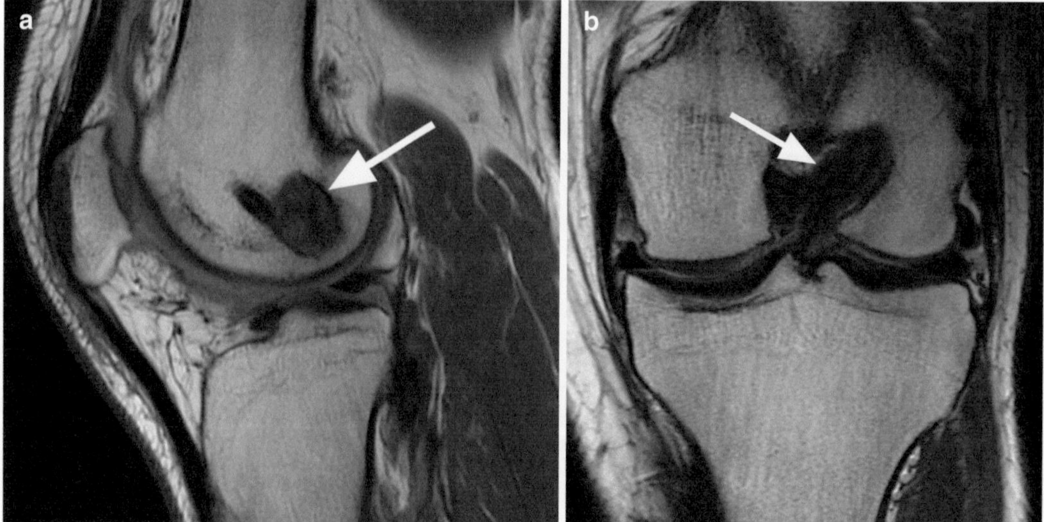

Fig. 1.25 Misplacement of the femoral tunnel of the anterior cruciate (ACL) graft of the left knee in a 23 year old male. *Sagittal proton-density (PD) FSE image (a) shows the femoral tunnel too posteriorly and too distally (*arrow*) from the ideal location of the tunnel. In this case, the ACL graft is too tight in extension, and the graft may fail as a result of posterior wall breaking. Coronal proton-density (PD) FSE MR image (b) in the same patient shows a femoral tunnel (*arrow*) misplaced at 2 o'clock (normal position at 1 o'clock for the left knee)

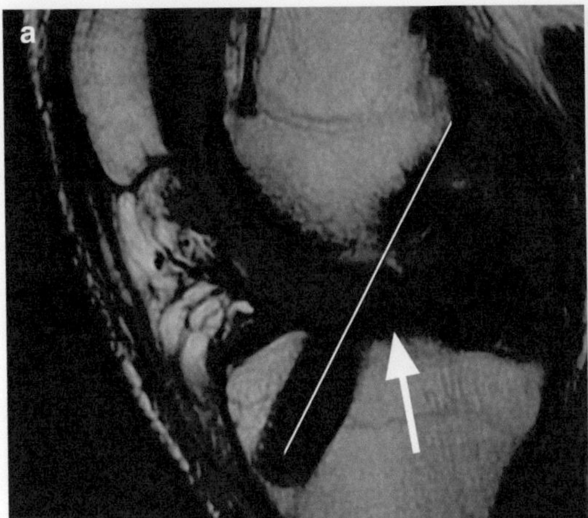 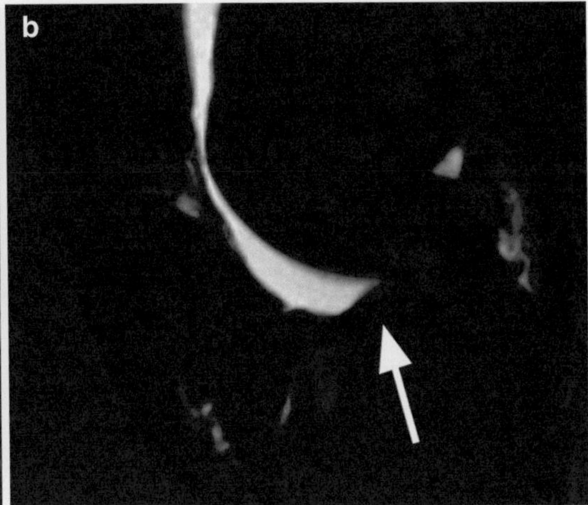

Fig. 1.26 Too anteriorly positioned tibial tunnel in a 31 year old male with nontraumatic clinical instability after anterior cruciate ligament (ACL) reconstruction. *S*agittal proton-density (PD) FSE image (**a**) and sagittal T2-weighted FSE fat-suppressed image (**b**) show tibial tunnel misplaced anteriorly to the Blumensaat's line (*line* in **a**). There is complete tear of ACL graft probably due to the roof impingement during extension. The ACL graft (*arrow*) lies horizontally, and the MR images show a resorption of graft fibers

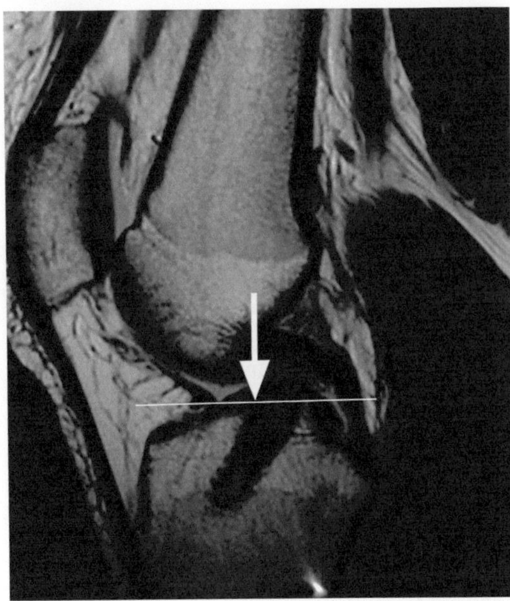

Fig. 1.27 Tibial tunnel too posteriorly positioned in a 17 year old female with knee instability after anterior cruciate ligament (ACL) reconstruction. *S*agittal proton-density (PD) FSE image shows that the anterior margin of the tunnel is situated just posterior to the midpoint of tibial plateau (*arrow*). The misplaced tunnel may lead to graft laxity and knee instability

compared to tibial tunnel cysts but are frequently associated with complete disruption of the graft (Fig. 1.28).

Tibial tunnel cysts may be incidentally found at MR imaging. Large cysts may manifest as palpable pretibial soft tissue mass, i.e., when they extend distally beyond the osseous border of the tunnel [19].

Arthrofibrosis

The second common cause of impaired knee extension after the graft impingement is the presence of localized arthrofibrosis, also known as cyclops lesion. It represents a focal fibrosis situated anterior to the distal portion of the ACL graft, often in the midline of the joint space. The pathogenesis is uncertain, but one of the causes is considered the impingement and debris raised by drilling the tibial tunnel [20].

Arthrofibrosis appears in 1–10 % of patients with ACL reconstruction and can be classified in two histological types: true cyclops lesions and soft cyclopoid scars (Figs. 1.29 and 1.30) [21].

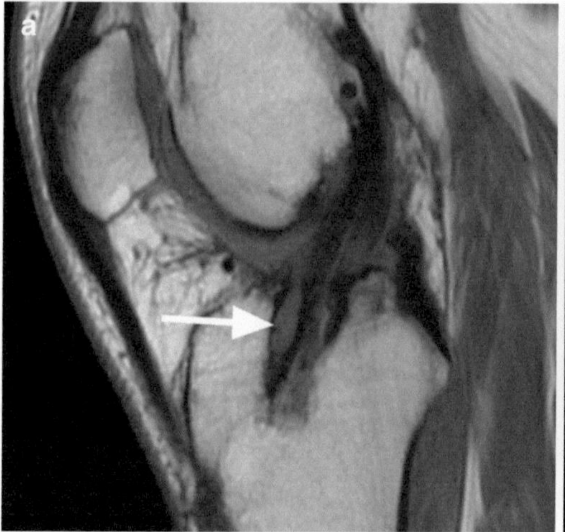 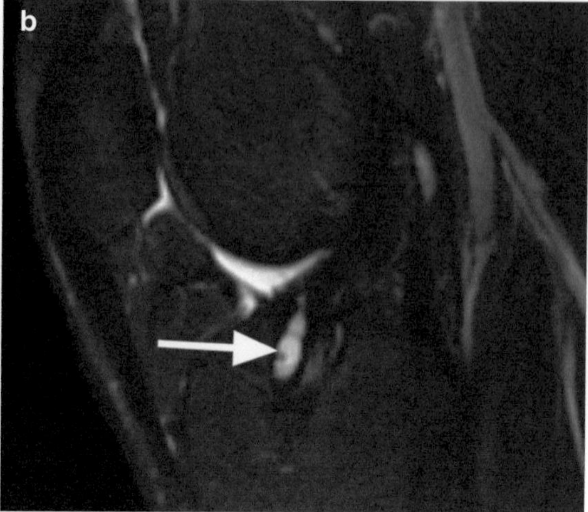

Fig. 1.28 Ganglion cyst and enlargement of the tibia tunnel in a 31 year old female after anterior cruciate ligament (ACL) reconstruction. *S*agittal proton-density (PD) FSE image (**a**) and sagittal T2-weighted FSE fat-suppressed image (**b**) show a cystic lesion within the tunnel (*arrow*). The lesion is well delineated, is septate, and has similar signal intensity with the joint fluid

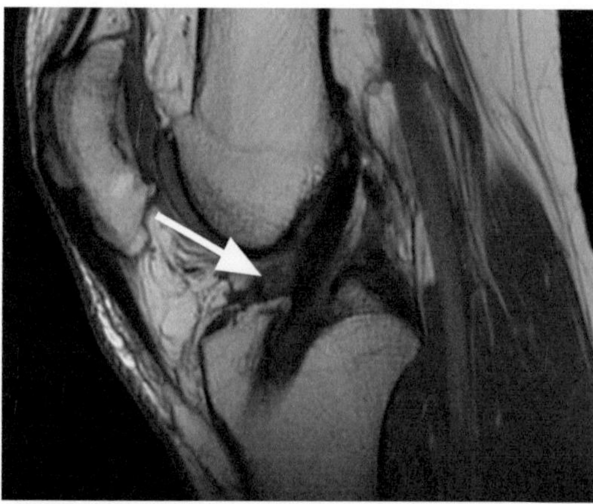

Fig. 1.29 Small cyclops lesion in a 30 year old male after anterior cruciate ligament (ACL) reconstruction. *S*agittal proton-density (PD) FSE image shows a focal round lesion of intermediate signal intensity anterior to the ACL graft representing fibrosis (*arrow*)

Infections

Septic arthritis after ACL reconstruction has a cumulative incidence of 0.1–0.9 %. MR imaging validates the clinical diagnosis and determines the extent of infection [19]. MR images show soft tissue edema, soft tissue abscesses, sinus tracts, synovitis, bone erosions, and bone marrow edema (Fig. 1.31).

Hardware-Related Complications and Iliotibial Band Friction Syndrome

Fixation devices such as bioabsorbable screws, metallic screws, and pins may be loosen or displaced requiring revision surgery. Iliotibial band friction syndrome typically occurs at the lateral aspect of the distal femur where the femoral transfixion devices for reconstructed ACL grafts are located [22]. The iliotibial band courses over the device which causes inflammation, pain, and structural changes to the iliotibial band. This friction syndrome affects, in the majority of cases, patients with hamstring grafts since the fixation device for it might be larger and more superficial to the femoral cortex than in patients with bone-patellar-bone grafts. Incorrect positioning and rupture of the femoral bioabsorbable cross-pin might also be a cause for the friction syndrome [22]. There is usually no sign for knee instability. MR images show edema and contrast enhancement of the surrounding soft tissue and allow direct visualization of the fixation device failure [22]. Often, surgery is needed for removal of offending fragment.

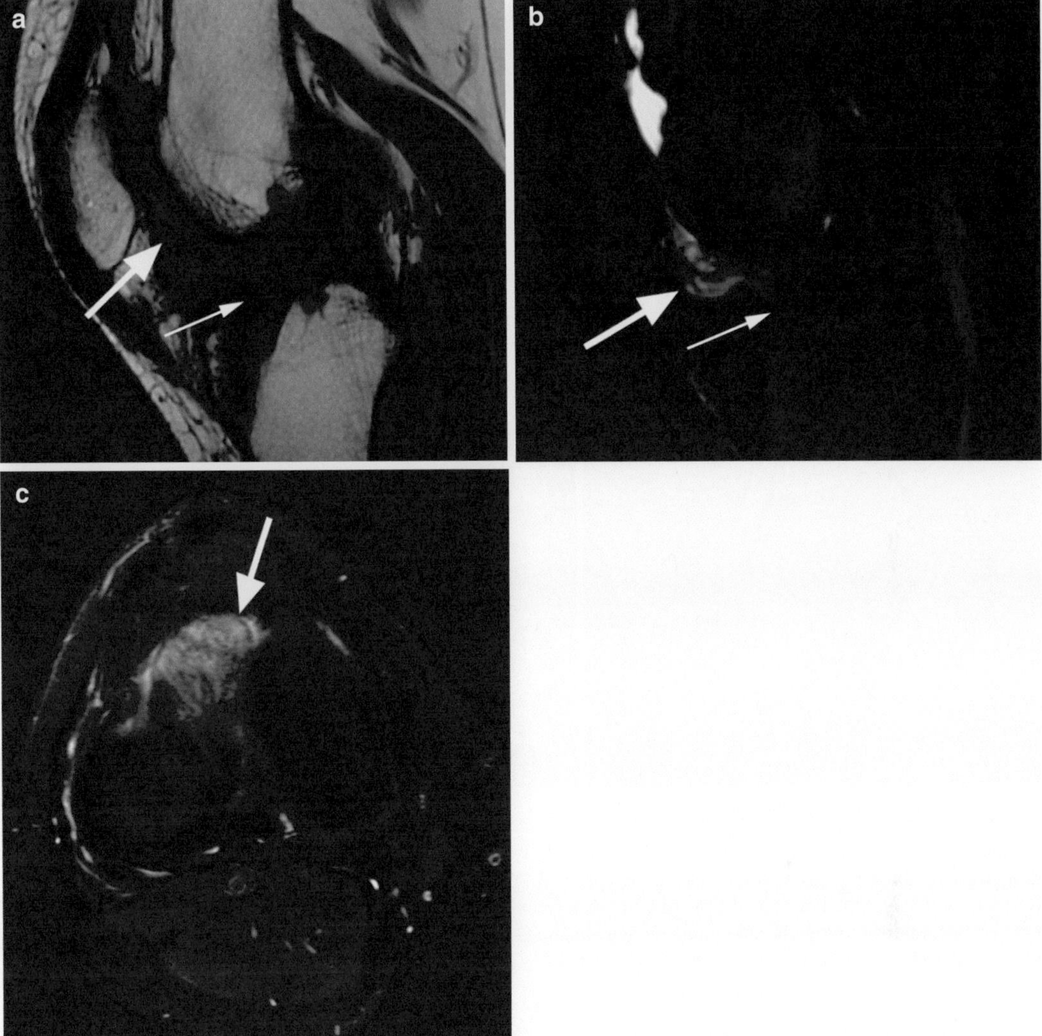

Fig. 1.30 Large cyclops lesion in a 30 year old female after anterior cruciate ligament (ACL) reconstruction. Sagittal proton-density (PD) FSE image (**a**), sagittal T2-weighted FSE fat-suppressed image (**b**), and axial proton-density (PD) FSE fat-suppressed image (**c**) show a large postoperative cyclops lesion (*large arrow*). Note that the tibial tunnel is misplaced being too anteriorly (*small arrow*)

1.4 MRI Impression

1.4.1 Nonsurgical ACL

1. Acute complete tear of ACL (femoral insertion tear, midsubstance tear, or tibial insertion tear)
2. Partial tear of ACL (anteromedial or posterolateral bundle, percentage of the injured ACL substance)
3. Chronic tear of ACL
4. Ganglion cyst of ACL
5. Mucoid degeneration of ACL
6. Tibial avulsion fractures (type I, II, or III) with normal/injured ACL

1.4.2 Postoperative ACL

1. Normal postoperative appearance – normal positioning of the tunnels and normal ACL graft without any signs of postoperative complications

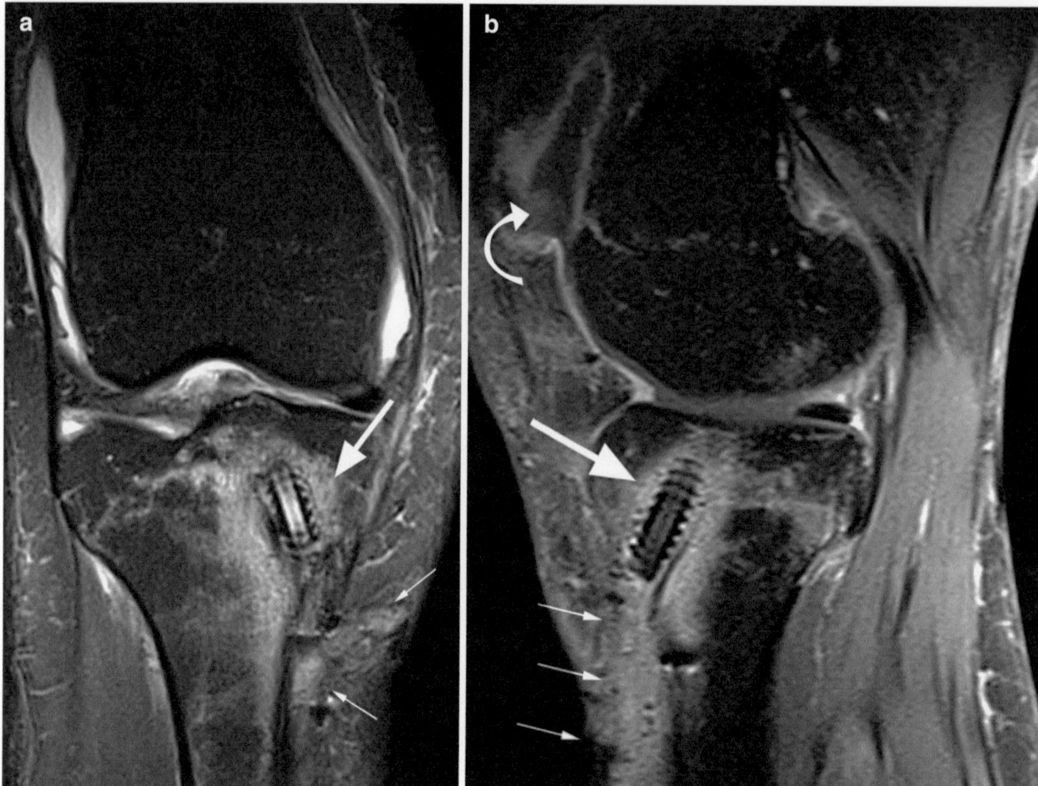

Fig. 1.31 Septic arthritis in a 32 year old female 4 months after anterior cruciate ligament (ACL) reconstruction. Coronal proton-density (PD) FSE fat-suppressed image (**a**) and sagittal T1-weighted FSE MR image after i.v. contrast administration (**b**) show enlargement of the tibial tunnel with diffuse bone marrow edema hyperintense on T2-weighted image with enhancement after contrast administration (*large arrow*). The inflammatory changes extend into the anterior soft tissue with formation of sinus tract (*small arrows*). Note the thickening and enhancement of the synovium as a result of the arthritis (*curved arrow*)

2. Partial or complete tear of the ACL graft
3. The femoral/tibial tunnels misplaced with normal or abnormal ACL graft
4. Postoperative complications (e.g., tunnel cysts, arthrofibrosis, possible infectious arthritis, displaced screws, iliotibial friction syndrome)

References

1. Gentili A, et al. Anterior cruciate ligament tear: indirect signs at MR imaging. Radiology. 1994;193(3):835–40.
2. Kim HK, et al. Anterior and posterior cruciate ligaments at different patient ages: MR imaging findings. Radiology. 2008;247(3):826–35.
3. Cohen SB, et al. MRI measurement of the 2 bundles of the normal anterior cruciate ligament. Orthopedics. 2009;32(9). Doi:10.3928/01477447-20090728-35.
4. Umans H, et al. Diagnosis of partial tears of the anterior cruciate ligament of the knee: value of MR imaging. AJR Am J Roentgenol. 1995;165(4):893–7.
5. Thomas NP, Jackson AM, Aichroth PM. Congenital absence of the anterior cruciate ligament. A common component of knee dysplasia. J Bone Joint Surg Br. 1985;67(4):572–5.
6. Huang GS, et al. Acute anterior cruciate ligament stump entrapment in anterior cruciate ligament tears: MR imaging appearance. Radiology. 2002;225(2):537–40.
7. Murphy BJ, et al. Bone signal abnormalities in the posterolateral tibia and lateral femoral condyle in complete tears of the anterior cruciate ligament: a specific sign? Radiology. 1992;182(1):221–4.
8. Meyers MH, Mc KF. Fracture of the intercondylar eminence of the tibia. J Bone Joint Surg Am. 1959;41-A(2):209–20; discussion 220–2.
9. Bui-Mansfield LT, Youngberg RA. Intraarticular ganglia of the knee: prevalence, presentation, etiology, and management. AJR Am J Roentgenol. 1997;168(1):123–7.

10. Kaatee R, Kjartansson O, Brekkan A. Intraarticular ganglion between the cruciate ligaments of the knee. A case report. Acta Radiol. 1994;35(5):434–6.
11. Bergin D, et al. Anterior cruciate ligament ganglia and mucoid degeneration: coexistence and clinical correlation. AJR Am J Roentgenol. 2004;182(5):1283–7.
12. Papadopoulou P. The celery stalk sign. Radiology. 2007;245(3):916–7.
13. Gnannt R, et al. MR imaging of the postoperative knee. J Magn Reson Imaging. 2011;34(5):1007–21.
14. Saupe N, et al. Anterior cruciate ligament reconstruction grafts: MR imaging features at long-term follow-up–correlation with functional and clinical evaluation. Radiology. 2008;249(2):581–90.
15. Jansson KA, et al. MRI of anterior cruciate ligament repair with patellar and hamstring tendon autografts. Skeletal Radiol. 2001;30(1):8–14.
16. Trattnig S, et al. Magnetic resonance imaging of the postoperative knee. Top Magn Reson Imaging. 1999;10(4):221–36.
17. Sanders TG, et al. Fluid collections in the osseous tunnel during the first year after anterior cruciate ligament repair using an autologous hamstring graft: natural history and clinical correlation. J Comput Assist Tomogr. 2002;26(4):617–21.
18. Papakonstantinou O, et al. Complications of anterior cruciate ligament reconstruction: MR imaging. Eur Radiol. 2003;13(5):1106–17.
19. Bencardino JT, et al. MR imaging of complications of anterior cruciate ligament graft reconstruction. Radiographics. 2009;29(7):2115–26.
20. Recht MP, Kramer J. MR imaging of the postoperative knee: a pictorial essay. Radiographics. 2002;22(4):765–74.
21. Muellner T, et al. Cyclops and cyclopoid formation after anterior cruciate ligament reconstruction: clinical and histomorphological differences. Knee Surg Sports Traumatol Arthrosc. 1999;7(5):284–9.
22. Pelfort X, et al. Iliotibial band friction syndrome after anterior cruciate ligament reconstruction using the transfix device: report of two cases and review of the literature. Knee Surg Sports Traumatol Arthrosc. 2006;14(6):586–9.

Posterior Cruciate Ligament (PCL) and Meniscofemoral Ligaments

Nicolae Bolog, Gustav Andreisek, Erika Ulbrich, and René Roth

2.1 Anatomy and Normal MRI Appearance

2.1.1 Posterior Cruciate Ligament (PCL)

The posterior cruciate ligament (PCL) is the strongest ligament of the knee. It is intra-articular and extrasynovial. The PCL arises from the anterolateral surface of the medial femoral condyle and reaches the posterior intercondylar area of the tibia. The femoral origin is more anterior than that of anterior cruciate ligament (ACL), and in contrast to the ACL, the PCL is larger at its femoral origin than at its tibial insertion [1]. The tibial attachment is extra-articular, and it is approximately 1 cm distal to the plane of the articular surface [2]. The PCL is the primary restraint to posterior tibial translation relative to the femur and becomes more important in preventing distraction of the joint as the knee reaches higher degrees of flexion [3, 4].

The PCL consists of two functional bundles: the anterolateral and the posteromedial bundle [5]. The anterolateral bundle (65 %) is usually thicker and stronger than the posteromedial bundle (35 %) [6]. Most PCL fibers are not isometric and the bundles have different functions that enable the PCL to resist posterior translation [5]. The length of the ligament is similar to that of the ACL (mean length, 38 mm) [7].

The PCL is seen as a band of low signal intensity in all MR sequences and is usually visualized in its entire length on one or two consecutive sagittal images (Fig. 2.1). The two-bundle anatomy is often well visualized on axial planes, and all axial planes should thoroughly be evaluated for partial (uni-bundle) rupture. To assess the intact attachments of the PCL, axial, sagittal, and coronal images should be evaluated (Fig. 2.1). The axial images are especially helpful for the femoral attachment, whereas the sagittal images are especially helpful for assessing the tibial attachment.

Since the PCL appears as an angulated structure on sagittal MR images, several indirect signs have been described to detect other ligament abnormalities, one of which is the PCL angle. The mean PCL angle is 123° and is smaller in patients with acute anterior cruciate ligament (ACL) tear but also in younger patients without ACL abnormalities [8]. Due to this overlap, indirect signs for ACL tears, i.e., quantitative and semiquantitative signs, should be used with care, especially in the skeletally immature patient [8].

2.1.2 Meniscofemoral Ligaments

The posterior meniscofemoral ligament (Wrisberg ligament) attaches proximally separately from the posteromedial bundle of the PCL [9]. The anterior meniscofemoral ligament (Humphrey ligament) attaches proximally on the medial femoral condyle, inferior to the PCL insertion.

N.V. Bolog et al., *MRI of the Knee: A Guide to Evaluation and Reporting*,
DOI 10.1007/978-3-319-08165-6_2, © Springer International Publishing Switzerland 2015

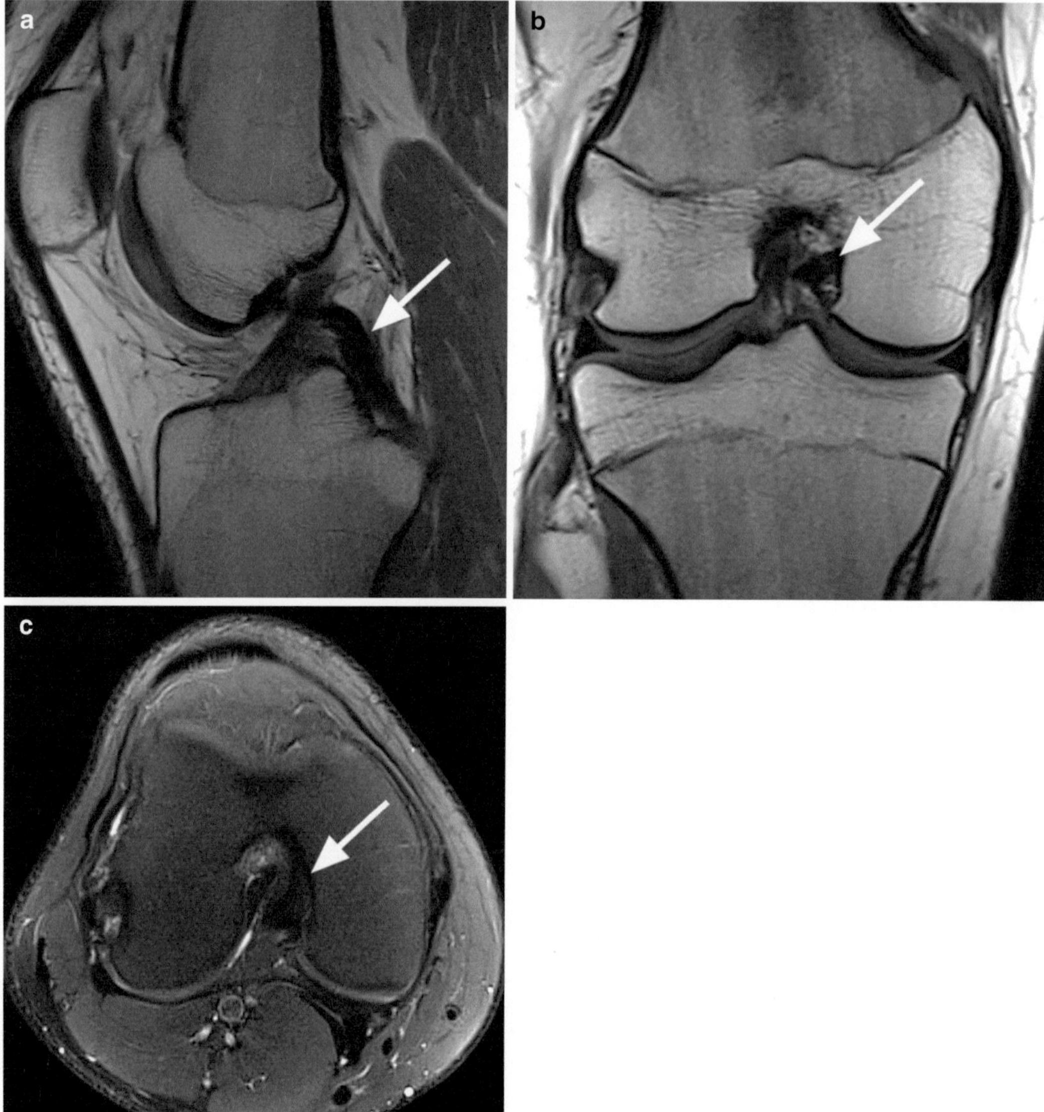

Fig. 2.1 Normal posterior cruciate ligament (PCL) in a 17 year old male. Sagittal proton-density (PD) FSE image (**a**) shows the PCL as a band of low signal intensity (*arrow*). Coronal (**b**) and axial images (**c**) should always be assessed especially for the femoral (*arrow* in **b**) and tibial attachments (*arrow* in **c**)

Both ligaments attach distally to the posterior horn of the lateral meniscus and contribute to posterior drawer stability [10]. At least one meniscofemoral ligament is present in 70–93 % of knees [4, 7, 11].

The meniscofemoral ligaments are best seen on sagittal and coronal images as low-signal-intensity bands anterior and posterior to the PCL (Figs. 2.2 and 2.3).

The orientation and characteristic localization of meniscofemoral ligaments should be taken into account in order to differentiate intra-articular lesions such as cartilage displaced and meniscal fragments or pseudotears of the lateral meniscus.

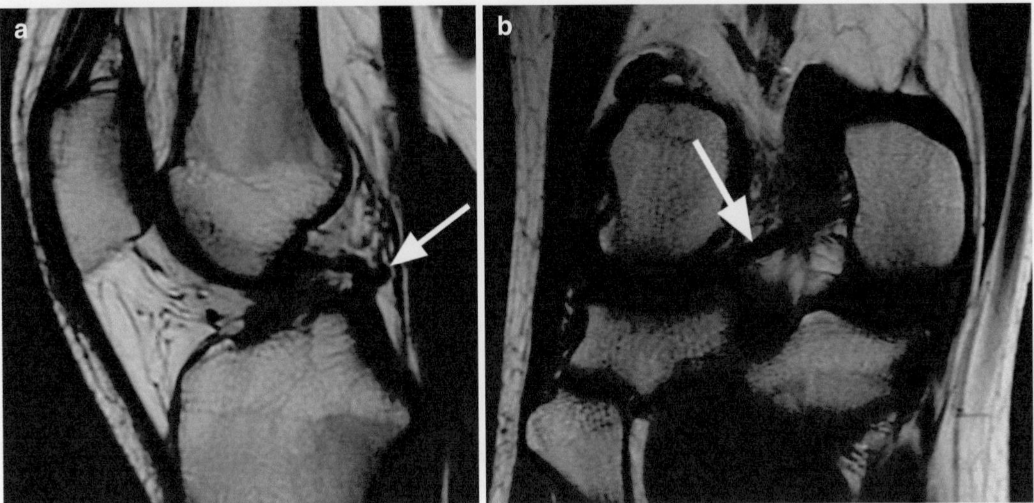

Fig. 2.2 Posterior meniscofemoral ligament (Wrisberg ligament) in a 19 year old female. Sagittal proton-density (PD) FSE image (**a**) and coronal proton-density (PD) FSE image (**b**) show the posterior meniscofemoral ligament (*arrow*) posterior to the posterior cruciate ligament (**a**) with the distal insertion on the posterior horn of the lateral meniscus and the proximal insertion on the medial femoral condyle (**b**)

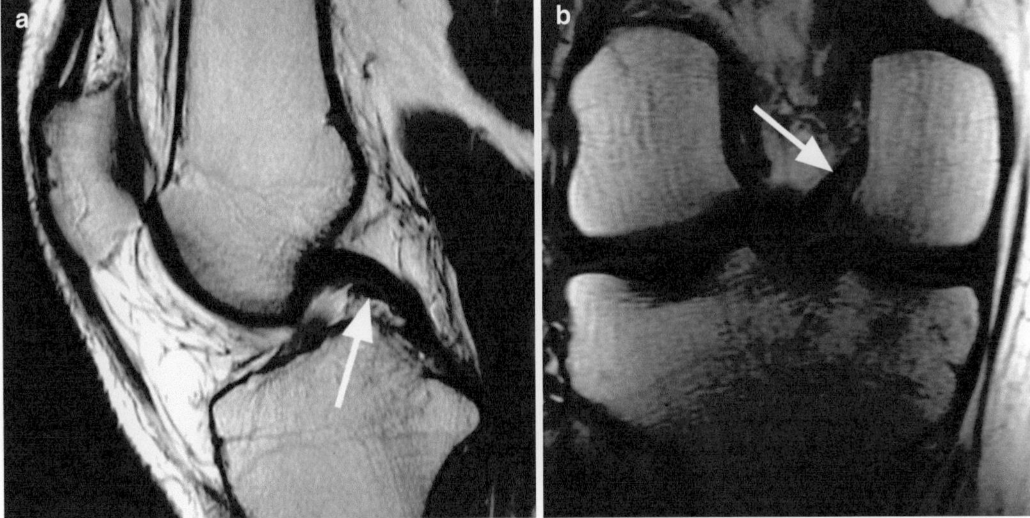

Fig. 2.3 Anterior meniscofemoral ligament (Humphrey ligament) in a 40 year old male. Sagittal proton-density (PD) FSE image (**a**) and coronal proton-density (PD) FSE image (**b**) show the anterior meniscofemoral ligament (*arrow*) anterior to the posterior cruciate ligament (**a**) with the proximal insertion on the medial femoral condyle (**b**)

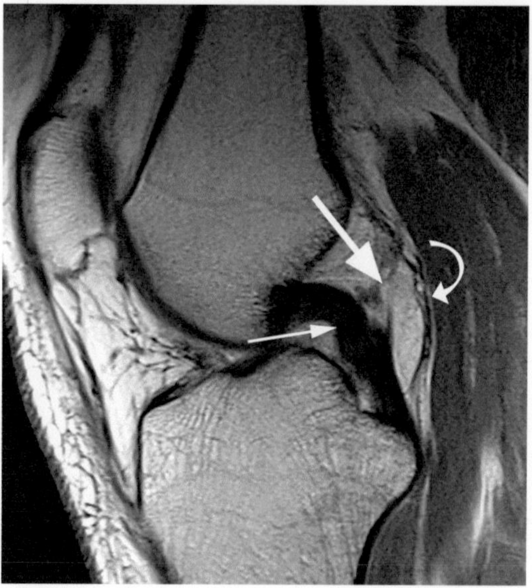

Fig. 2.4 Normal retrocruciate fat pad in a 27 year old male. Sagittal proton-density (PD) FSE image shows the retrocruciate fat pad (*arrow*) situated between the posterior cruciate ligament (*small arrow*) and the posterior joint capsule (*curved arrow*). The signal is similar to the subcutaneous fat in all sequences

2.1.3 Retrocruciate Fat Pad

Retrocruciate fat pad is situated between the PCL and the posterior joint capsule (Fig. 2.4) [12]. The fat pad may be involved in several pathological intra-articular changes (e.g., fluid collections, inflammation).

2.2 MRI Pathological Findings

2.2.1 Acute Tear

Complete Tear

Focal discontinuity and an amorphous high signal intensity due to hemorrhage and edema without visualization of the ligamentous fibers are signs of PCL tear (Figs. 2.5 and 2.6). Isolated PCL tears are found in 24 % of patients [13], and they can be localized at the femoral insertion, in the midsubstance, or at the tibial insertion. The associated findings of other coexisting knee injuries may be present in 76 % of cases and include involvement

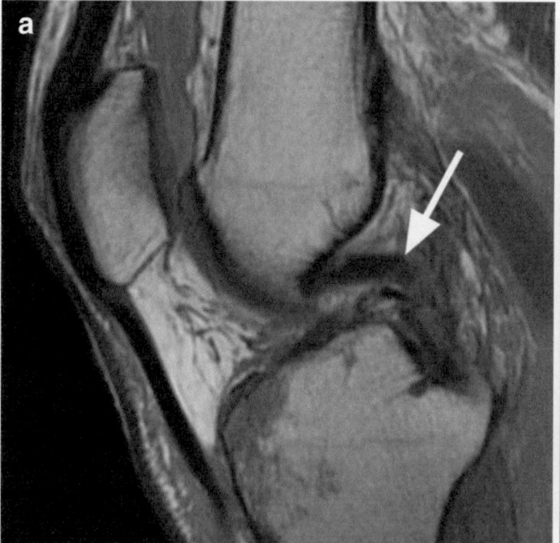

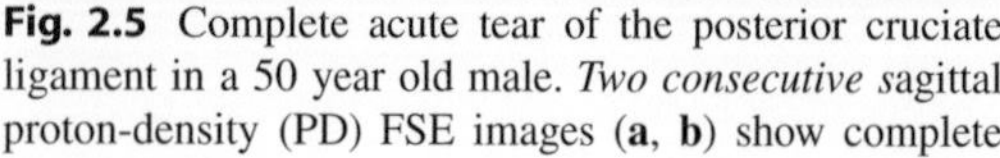

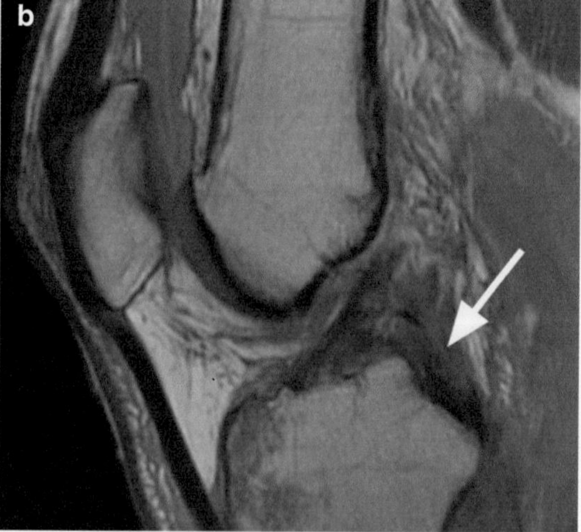

Fig. 2.5 Complete acute tear of the posterior cruciate ligament in a 50 year old male. *Two consecutive* sagittal proton-density (PD) FSE images (**a**, **b**) show complete discontinuity of the fibers (*arrow*) (**a**) with hemorrhage and edema in the midsubstance and at the femoral insertion of the ligament (**b**)

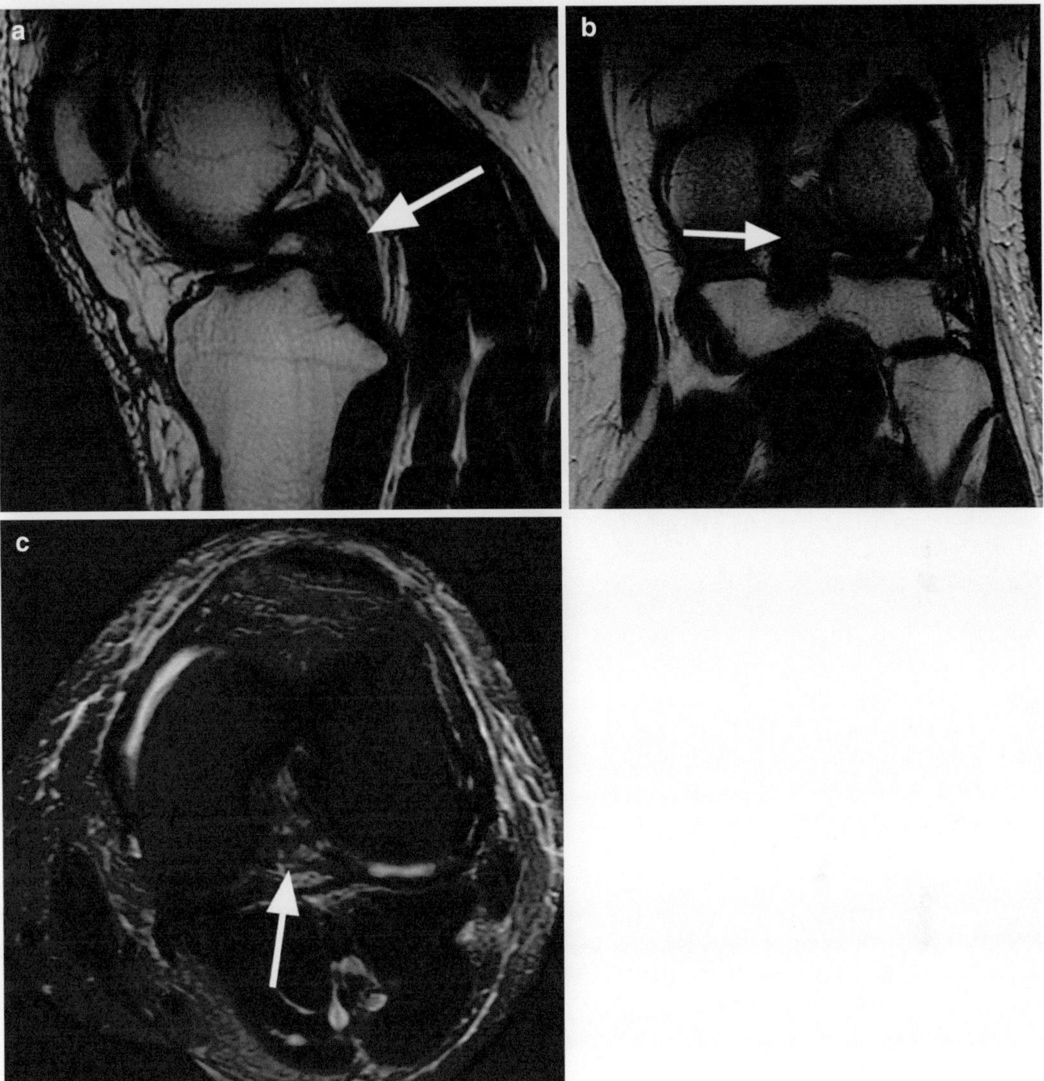

Fig. 2.6 Complete acute tear of the posterior cruciate ligament in a 44 year old female. *S*agittal proton-density (PD) FSE images (**a**) and coronal proton-density (PD) FSE image (**b**) show diffuse-signal-intensity changes within the ligament (*arrow*). Although there is the impres-sion of fiber continuity on both sagittal and coronal images (**a, b**) on axial proton-density (PD) FSE fat-sup-pressed image (**c**), there is a complete absence of the fibers with hemorrhage within the distal portion (*arrow*)

of medial collateral ligament more often than the lateral collateral ligament and medial meniscus more commonly than the lateral meniscus [13].

Partial Tear

Partial tears represent 55 % of all PCL tears [13]. Criteria of diagnosis include the presence of increased signal intensity with discernible fibers along the course of the ligament. The partial tear can be interstitial or can involve one of the above described PCL bundles. In partial interstitial tears, there is an increased longitudinal ligamentous sig-nal intensity without disruption of the fibers (Fig. 2.7). In these cases, the PCL bundles can be separated by the signal-intensity changes. The findings of interstitial tear of the PCL must be

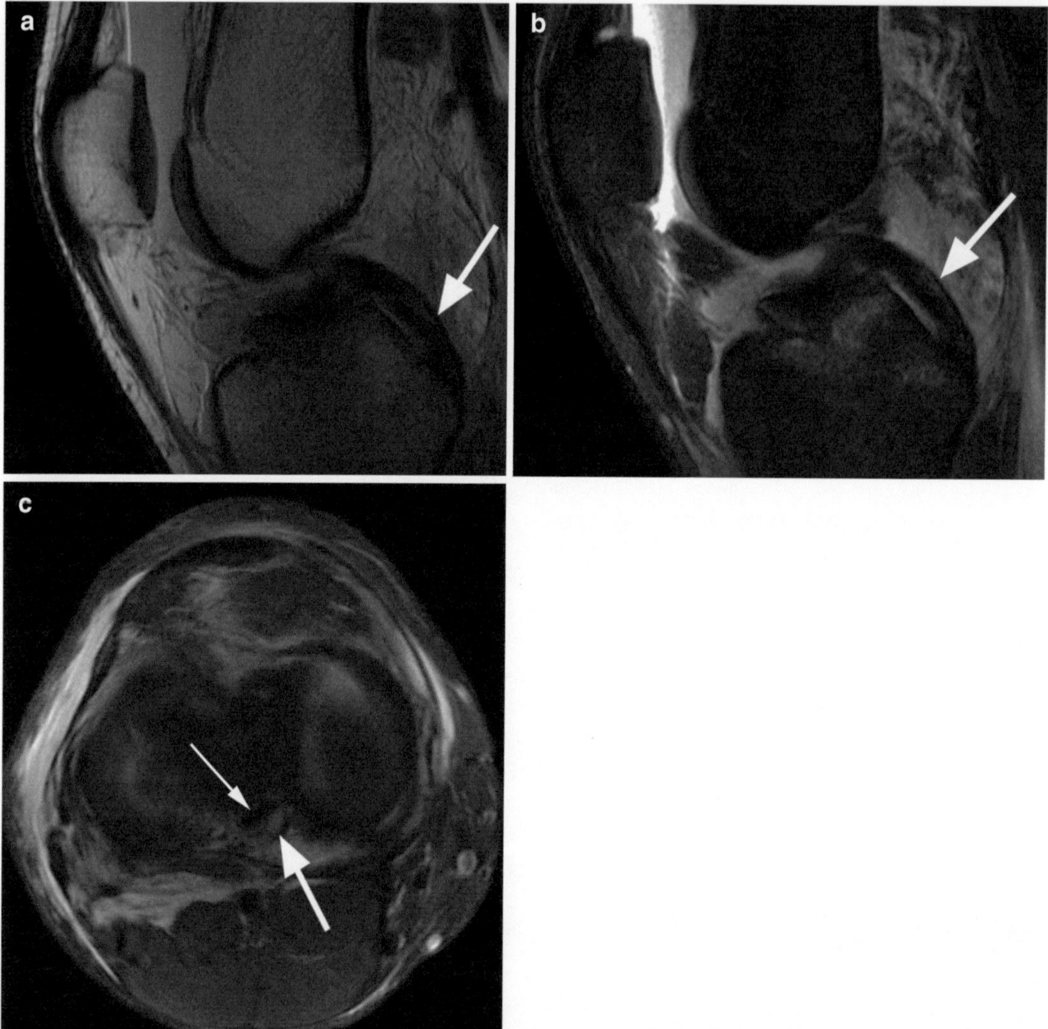

Fig. 2.7 Partial interstitial acute tear of the posterior cruciate ligament involving the posteromedial bundle in an 18 year old male with recent knee trauma. *Sagittal proton-density (PD) FSE image (**a**), sagittal T2-weighted FSE fat-suppressed image (**b**), and axial proton-density (PD) FSE fat-suppressed image (**c**) show increased longitudinal signal-intensity changes within the ligament (*arrow*) without complete discontinuity of the fibers (*small arrow* in **c**)

correlated with an appropriate history of trauma in order to differentiate from a mucoid degeneration of PCL, i.e., in middle-aged patients.

2.2.2   Posterior Cruciate Ligament Avulsion Fracture

The PCL avulsion fracture involves the detachment of the tibial plateau that results from the pulling of PCL from its attachment point. The mechanisms include a severe hyperextension or a direct blow to the anterior tibia with the knee flexed [14]. An early diagnosis is usually possible on standard radiographs where a bony fragment may be visible. At MR imaging, bone marrow edema and a small bone fragment attached to PCL is seen in acute trauma (Fig. 2.8). In chronic cases, the bone marrow edema is usually absent (Fig. 2.9).

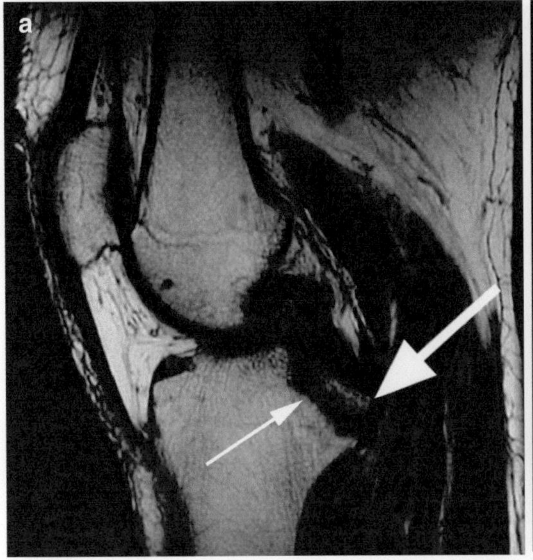
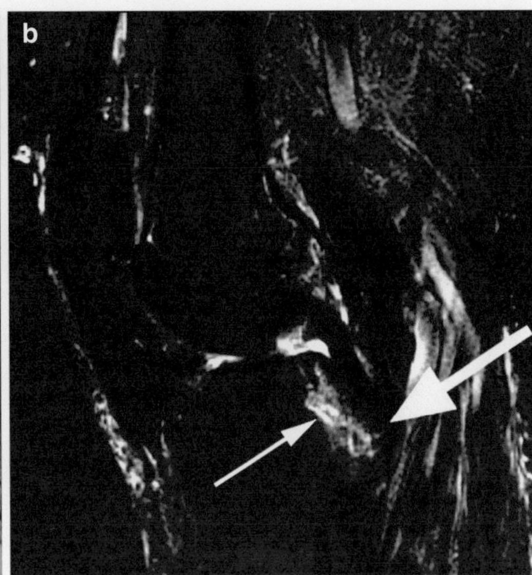

Fig. 2.8 Acute posterior cruciate ligament (PCL) avulsion fracture from pulling from its tibial attachment in a 35 year old female with acute knee trauma. *S*agittal proton-density (PD) FSE image (**a**) and sagittal T2-weighted FSE fat-suppressed image (**b**) show a bone fragment attached (*arrow*) to a normal PCL. Bone marrow edema is present at the site of the tibial avulsion (*small arrow*)

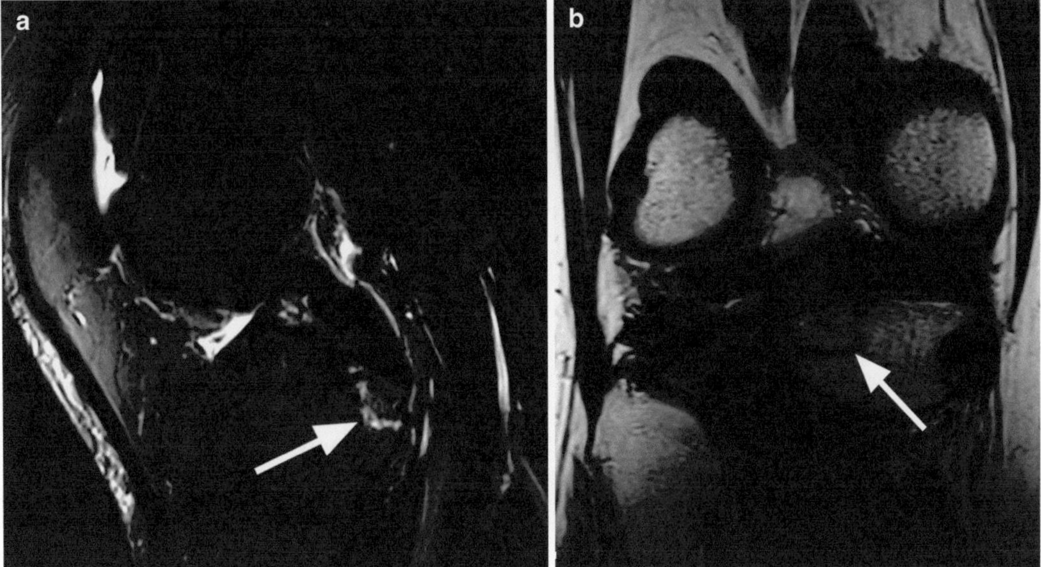

Fig. 2.9 Chronic posterior cruciate ligament (PCL) avulsion fracture in a 68 year old female. *S*agittal T2-weighted FSE fat-suppressed image (**a**) and coronal T1-weighted image (**b**) show a small bone fragment detached from the tibial attachment (*arrow*) without adjacent bone marrow edema

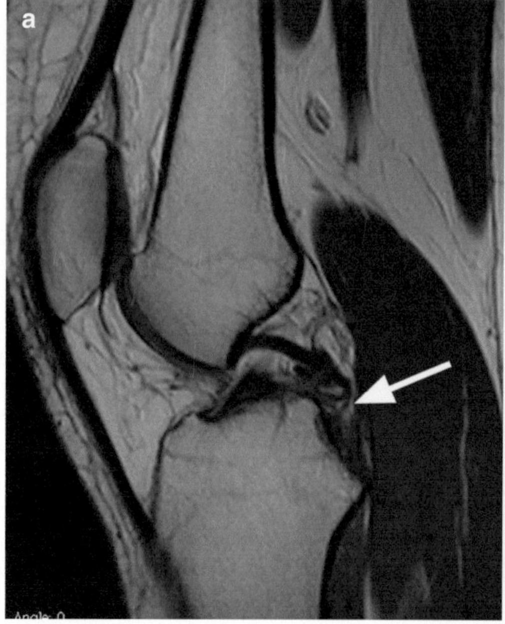
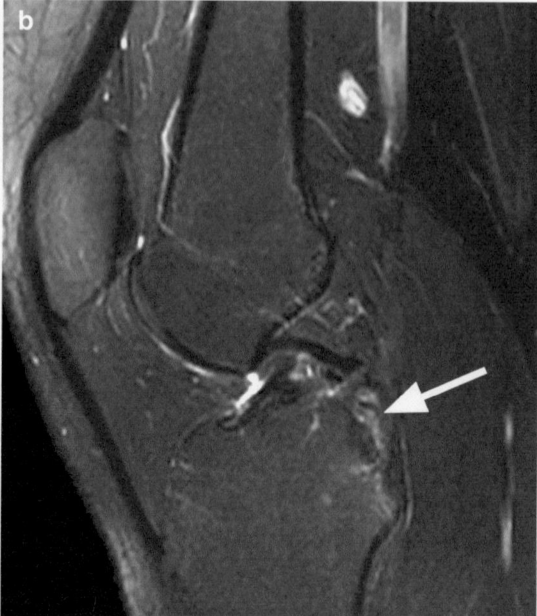

Fig. 2.10 Chronic tear of the posterior cruciate ligament (PCL) in a 17 year old female. *S*agittal proton-density (PD) FSE image (**a**) and sagittal T2-weighted fat-suppressed image (**b**) show discontinuity of the ligament with focal fibrotic changes without hemorrhage and edema (*arrow*)

2.2.3 Chronic Tear and Mucoid Degeneration

Diffuse thickening (more than 7 mm on sagittal plane) with low or intermediate signal, often seen as focal changes of the PCL, is suggestive for chronic PCL tear [15]. MR imaging shows focal or diffuse changes of low signal intensity on T1-weighted images and intermediate-high signal intensity on T2-weighted images (Fig. 2.10).

Mucoid degeneration is a rare cause of pain in the middle-aged patients without knee instability [16]. The signal intensity on T2-weighted images is different from that of a joint effusion and enables the differentiation from a ganglion cyst (Fig. 2.11) [16].

2.2.4 Ganglion Cyst

The ganglion cyst of the PCL is uncommon, and the clinical manifestations are variable and nonspecific and the most consistent symptom is knee pain [17]. PCL ganglion cysts are less common than anterior cruciate ganglion cysts. MR imaging is the most sensitive, specific, and accurate method for diagnosis and is superior to arthroscopy. Ganglion cyst demonstrates fluid characteristic signal intensity on T2-weighted images and intermediate signal intensity on T1-weighted images (Fig. 2.12). The cysts may be inhomogeneous due to fibrous or myxoid changes [18].

2.2.5 Retrocruciate Fat Pad Impingement

Posteriorly, the joint capsule is not in contact with the joint cavity on one or more sagittal MR images [12]. The retrocruciate fat pad which is situated at this level, behind the PCL, may be distorted by distension of the posterior synovial recess resulting from large intra-articular fluid collections [12]. In cases of inflammation of the retrocruciate fat pad, the MR imaging shows a diffuse increased signal intensity of the fat with or without edema of the soft tissue superficial to the joint capsule (Fig. 2.13) [19]. Clinically, the patients may complain of posterior pain during deep flexion as a result of the fat pad impingement [19].

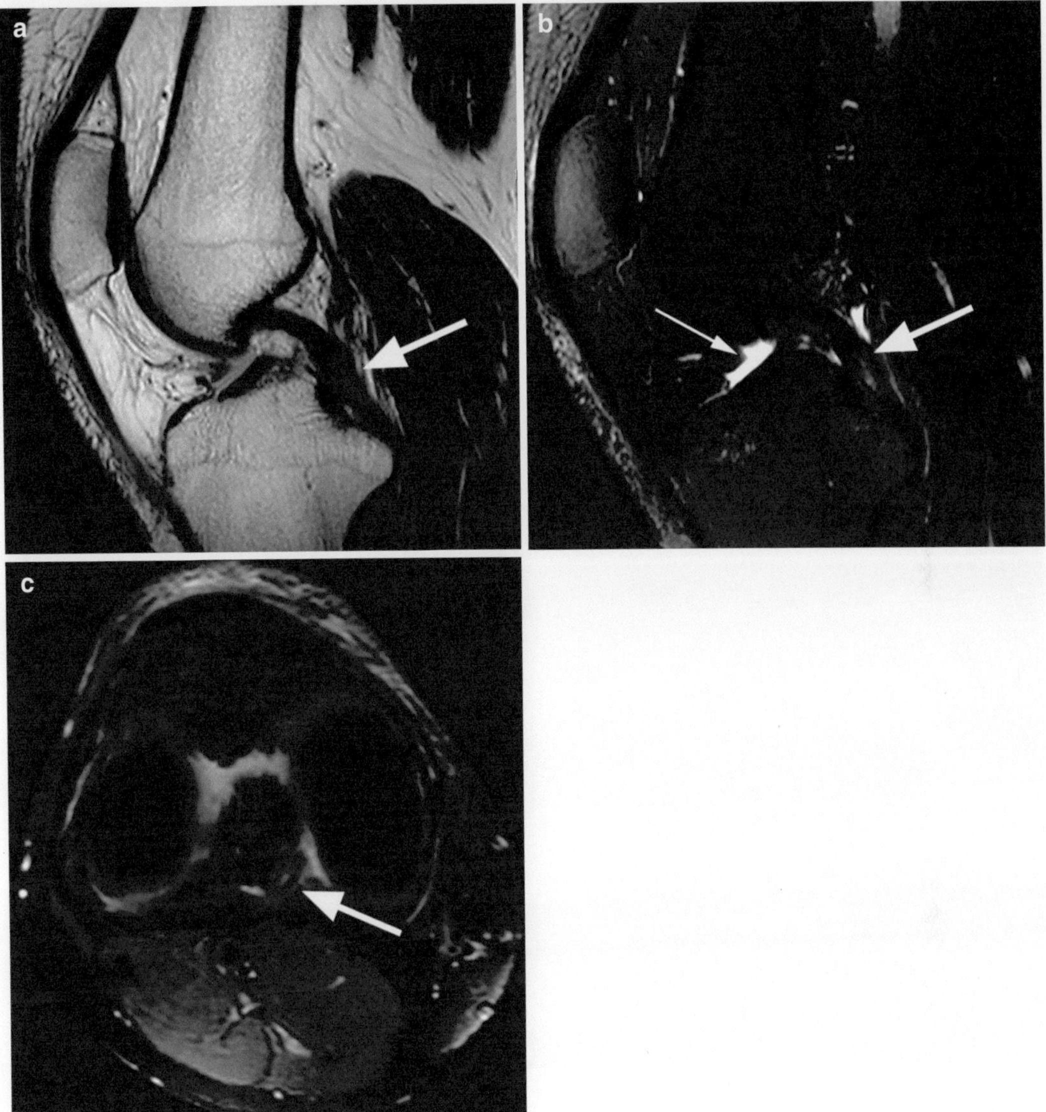

Fig. 2.11 Mucoid degeneration of the posterior cruciate ligament (PCL) in a 29 year old male without history of knee trauma and without knee instability. *S*agittal proton-density (PD) FSE image (**a**), sagittal T2-weighted fat-suppressed image (**b**), and axial proton-density (PD) FSE fat-suppressed image (**c**) show a diffuse thickening of the ligament with intermediate signal changes (*large arrow* in **a**, **b**, and **c**) that are different from that of a joint effusion (*small arrow* in **b**)

2.3   Postoperative Posterior Cruciate Ligament (PCL)

Repair of the PCL is performed less often than that of the ACL. Nonoperative treatment is recommended for acute isolated injuries. However, it has been shown that complete PCL tears with greater than 12 mm of posterior subluxation are less likely to heal completely and the nonsurgical management of PCL tears leads to early degenerative changes [20, 21]. Surgical treatment is indicated for symptomatic chronic PCL injury, acute bony avulsion, and combined ligament injuries. The surgical techniques vary according to the tibial fixation technique, to the single or two-bundle technique, to the type of the graft, and to the fixation material.

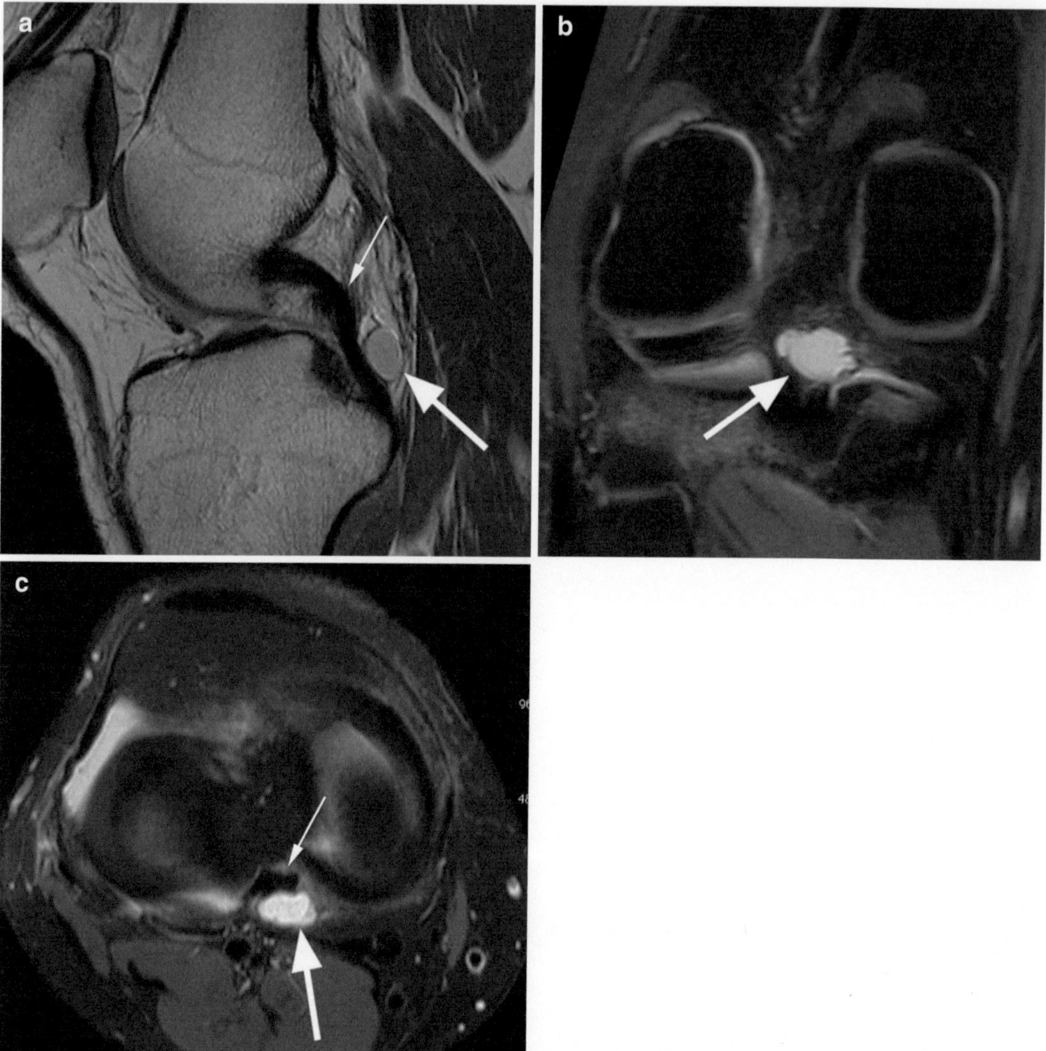

Fig. 2.12 Ganglion cyst of the posterior cruciate ligament (PCL) in a 25 year old male. *S*agittal proton-density (PD) FSE image (**a**) and coronal (**b**) and axial proton-density (PD) FSE fat-suppressed images (**c**) show a well-delineated lobulated cystic lesion (*arrow*) with signal intensity similar to the joint effusion. The lesion is in contact with the normal PCL (*small arrow* in **a**, **c**)

2.3.1 Normal Postoperative PCL Graft and MRI Appearance

Femoral and Tibial Tunnels

The ideal femoral graft origin is the most anterior zone of the normal PCL insertion on the medial femoral condyle. The femoral tunnel should be located on the anterior third of the medial condyle on axial images and 5–10 mm from the articular edge of the medial femoral condyle on sagittal images (Fig. 2.14) [22]. In the case in which two-bundle Y-type bone-patellar tendon-bone technique is used, there are two tunnels at the femoral insertion, and in the case of two-bundle reconstruction using double-double tunnel, there are two tunnels at the femoral

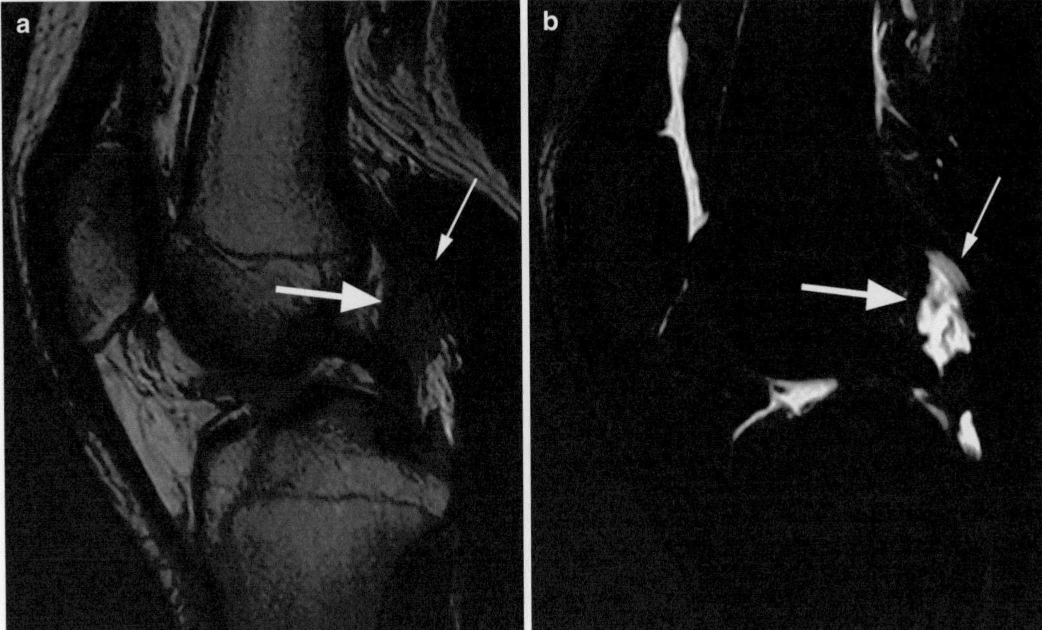

Fig. 2.13 Retrocruciate fat pad impingement in a 22 year old female with pain during flexion. *S*agittal proton-density (PD) FSE image (**a**) and sagittal T2-weighted fat-suppressed image (**b**) show changes of the normal signal intensity of the retrocruciate fat pad suggestive for fluid collection at this level (*large arrow*). Note the distended capsule (*small arrow*) due to fat pad inflammation

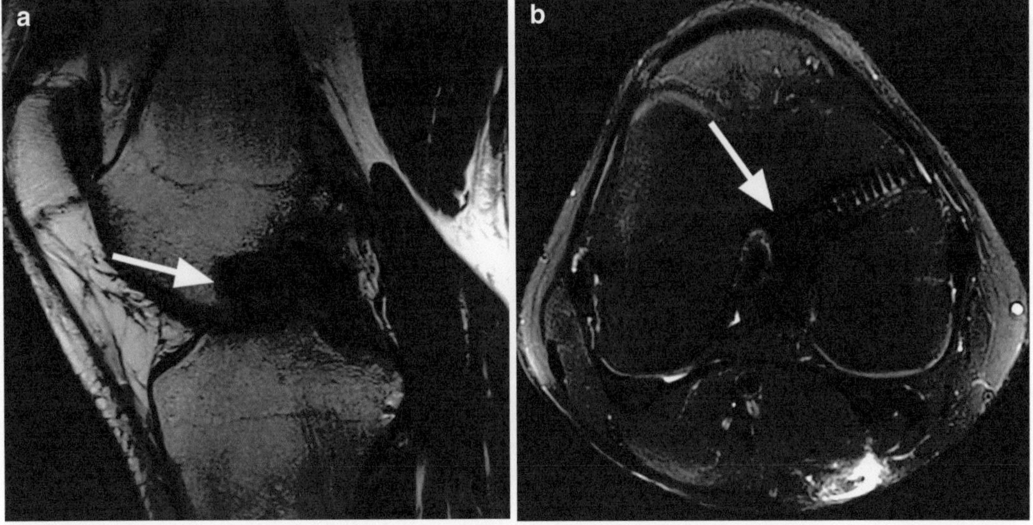

Fig. 2.14 Normal femoral tunnel position in posterior cruciate ligament (PCL) one-bundle reconstruction in a 25 year old male. On sagittal proton-density (PD) FSE image (**a**), the femoral tunnel is positioned 5 mm from the articular edge of the medial femoral (*arrow*) which is within the normal range (5–10 mm). On axial proton-density (PD) FSE fat-suppressed image (**b**), the tunnel is located on the anterior third of the medial condyle (*arrow*)

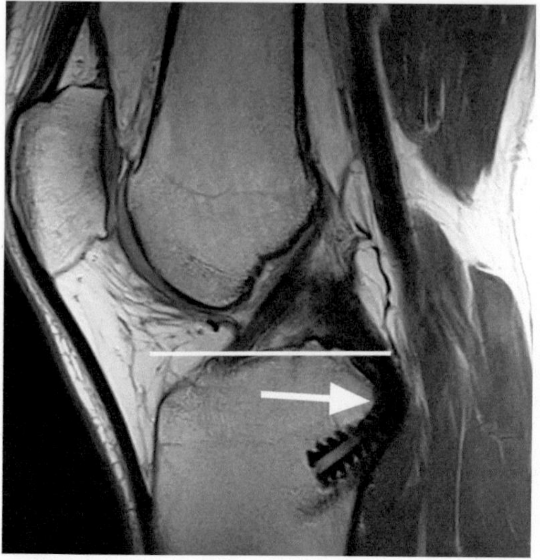

Fig. 2.15 Normal femoral tunnel position in posterior cruciate ligament (PCL) one-bundle reconstruction in a 25 year old male. Sagittal proton-density (PD) FSE image shows the tibial tunnel (*arrow*) at 10 mm distally to the articular surface of the tibial plateau (*line*)

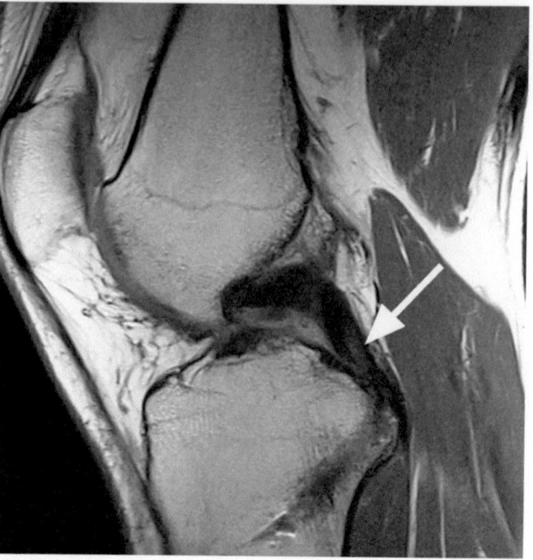

Fig. 2.16 Normal posterior cruciate ligament (PCL) autograft appearance in posterior cruciate ligament (PCL) one-bundle reconstruction in 25 year old male 9 months after intervention. Sagittal proton-density (PD) FSE image shows a normal thickness of the graft with diffuse intrasubstance signal-intensity changes (*arrow*) which are normal during the first postoperative year

insertion and two tunnels at the tibial insertion [23]. There are two techniques for tibial fixation. In the inlay technique, the graft is directly fixated to the tibia. In the transtibial technique, a tunnel is drilled through the tibia. The tibial fixation and the tibial tunnel should be located at the site of the PCL insertion, 10 mm distal to the articular surface of the tibial plateau on sagittal images (Fig. 2.15) [24].

The PCL Graft's Signal Intensity

The appearance of PCL grafts depends on the graft material used. Currently, autograft and allograft tissues are most frequently used for PCL reconstruction, whereas synthetic graft materials are avoided by most surgeons due to their high complication rate. Bone-patellar tendon-bone grafts and hamstring and quadriceps tendon grafts are used with various fixation techniques [25].

If bone-patellar tendon-bone grafts are used, the initial signal at postoperative MR images is similar to the normal patellar tendon, namely, homogeneous low signal intensity. Within a year, there might be neovascularization which usually causes an increase in signal intensity with

however a preserved structure. PCL graft from hamstrings or quadriceps tendon however may have during the first postoperative year an initial increased intrasubstance signal intensity and a thickened graft (Fig. 2.16) [26].

2.3.2 MRI Pathological Postoperative Findings

Tunnels Misplacement and Tear of PCL Graft

The femoral attachment of the PCL graft covers a broad area, and therefore, a tunnel with a diameter of 10 mm can be placed in a multitude of sites and still be considered within the anatomic position [27]. However, a proximal alteration of the femoral tunnel position correlates with a decrease in graft tension. In these cases, graft impingement may appear with tears in the graft bundles and fibrosis. The misplacement of the femoral tunnel in the anterior-posterior direction has little effect on the graft tension [27]. A tibial tunnel placed in a wrong position is very rarely seen, and variations in the tibial attachment site produce only minor changes in the posterior motion limits. Assessment of tunnel misplacement in patients with two-bundle reconstructions is quite difficult in the clinical routine in the authors experience as these cases are relatively seldom seen. There is also a lack of evidence in the literature about the appropriate assessment parameters and criteria. In such cases, discussion with the referring surgeon is strongly recommended.

The tear of the PCL graft is seen on MR images as an area of high signal intensity similar to that of fluid traversing the graft or as an area of absence of visualization of the fibers on sagittal and coronal images [26].

Tunnel Cysts and Tunnel Enlargement

Ganglion cyst formation after PCL reconstruction is rare and appears more common with hamstring tendon grafts and allografts [28]. Presence of a ganglion cyst may cause widening of the tunnel, which is considered significant when more than 50 % of the area of the tunnel is increased [29]. The cysts are formed in the tibial tunnel, and in some cases, they can communicate with the subcutaneous tissue anterior and posterior to the tibia as a result of the failed osteointegration of the graft [30, 31]. In these particular cases, the cysts are seen as fluid-containing masses located anterior and posterior to the tibia. The complication is usually asymptomatic.

Arthrofibrosis, Loose Bodies, and Infection

In PCL reconstruction, a mild grade of arthrofibrosis around the PCL graft may be a normal finding and is even considered to improve knee joint stability [32]. Similar to the ACL reconstruction, there might be a localized fibrosis anterior in the midline of the joint space ("cyclops lesion") or a diffuse ill-defined lesion within the Hoffa's fat space.

Other pathological MR image findings after PCL reconstruction include the presence of intra-articular loose bodies (cartilage or meniscal fragments) and septic arthritis.

2.4 MRI Impression

2.4.1 Nonsurgical PCL

1. Acute tear
   (a) Complete tear of PCL (femoral insertion tear, midsubstance tear, or tibial insertion tear)
   (b) Partial tear (interstitial, tear of anterolateral/posteromedial bundle)
2. Chronic tear
3. Mucoid degeneration of PCL
4. Ganglion cyst of PCL
5. Retrocruciate fat pad inflammation

2.4.2 Postoperative PCL

1. Normal postoperative appearance – normal positioning of the tunnels and normal PCL graft without any signs of postoperative complications
2. Partial or complete tear of the PCL graft
3. The femoral/tibial tunnels misplaced with normal or abnormal PCL graft
4. Postoperative complications (e.g., tunnel cysts, arthrofibrosis, loose bodies, septic arthritis)

References

1. Harner CD, et al. The human posterior cruciate ligament complex: an interdisciplinary study. Ligament morphology and biomechanical evaluation. Am J Sports Med. 1995;23(6):736–45.
2. Tajima G, et al. Morphology of the tibial insertion of the posterior cruciate ligament. J Bone Joint Surg Am. 2009;91(4):859–66.
3. Andriacchi TP. Knee joint, anatomy and biomechanics. In: Pellicci PM, Tria AJ, Garvin KL, editors. Orthopaedic knowledge update. Hip and Knee reconstruction 2. Rosemont, IL: American Academy of Orthopaedic Surgeons; 2000. p. 239–49.
4. Amis AA, et al. Anatomy of the posterior cruciate ligament and the meniscofemoral ligaments. Knee Surg Sports Traumatol Arthrosc. 2006;14(3):257–63.
5. Fanelli GC, Beck JD, Edson CJ. Current concepts review: the posterior cruciate ligament. J Knee Surg. 2010;23(2):61–72.
6. Race A, Amis AA. The mechanical properties of the two bundles of the human posterior cruciate ligament. J Biomech. 1994;27(1):13–24.
7. Girgis FG, Marshall JL, Monajem A. The cruciate ligaments of the knee joint. Anatomical, functional

and experimental analysis. Clin Orthop Relat Res. 1975;106:216–31.

8. Kim HK, et al. Anterior and posterior cruciate ligaments at different patient ages: MR imaging findings. Radiology. 2008;247(3):826–35.

9. Edwards A, Bull AM, Amis AA. The attachments of the fiber bundles of the posterior cruciate ligament: an anatomic study. Arthroscopy. 2007;23(3):284–90.

10. Gupte CM, et al. The meniscofemoral ligaments: secondary restraints to the posterior drawer. Analysis of anteroposterior and rotary laxity in the intact and posterior-cruciate-deficient knee. J Bone Joint Surg Br. 2003;85(5):765–73.

11. Heller L, Langman J. The menisco-femoral ligaments of the human knee. J Bone Joint Surg Br. 1964;46:307–13.

12. de Abreu MR, et al. Posterior cruciate ligament recess and normal posterior capsular insertional anatomy: MR imaging of cadaveric knees. Radiology. 2005;236(3):968–73.

13. Sonin AH, et al. MR imaging of the posterior cruciate ligament: normal, abnormal, and associated injury patterns. Radiographics. 1995;15(3):551–61.

14. Gottsegen CJ, et al. Avulsion fractures of the knee: imaging findings and clinical significance. Radiographics. 2008;28(6):1755–70.

15. Rodriguez Jr W, et al. MRI appearance of posterior cruciate ligament tears. AJR Am J Roentgenol. 2008;191(4):1031.

16. Shoji T, Fujimoto E, Sasashige Y. Mucoid degeneration of the posterior cruciate ligament. Knee Surg Sports Traumatol Arthrosc. 2010;18(7):1001–2.

17. Durante JA. Ganglion cyst on the posterior cruciate ligament: a case report. J Can Chiropr Assoc. 2009;53(4):334–8.

18. Friedman L, Finlay K, Jurriaans E. Ultrasound of the knee. Skeletal Radiol. 2001;30(7):361–77.

19. Resnick D, Kand HS, Pretterklieber ML. Knee. Internal derangements of joints, vol. 2. Philadelphia: Elsevier Inc.; 2007.

20. Keller PM, et al. Nonoperatively treated isolated posterior cruciate ligament injuries. Am J Sports Med. 1993;21(1):132–6.

21. Mariani PP, et al. Evaluation of posterior cruciate ligament healing: a study using magnetic resonance imaging and stress radiography. Arthroscopy. 2005;21(11):1354–61.

22. Trus P, Petermann J, Gotzen L. Posterior cruciate ligament (PCL) reconstruction–an in vitro study of isometry. Part I. Tests using a string linkage model. Knee Surg Sports Traumatol Arthrosc. 1994;2(2):100–3.

23. Makino A, et al. Anatomic double-bundle posterior cruciate ligament reconstruction using double-double tunnel with tibial anterior and posterior fresh-frozen allograft. Arthroscopy. 2006;22(6):684.e1–5.

24. Berg EE. Posterior cruciate ligament tibial inlay reconstruction. Arthroscopy. 1995;11(1):69–76.

25. Hoher J, Scheffler S, Weiler A. Graft choice and graft fixation in PCL reconstruction. Knee Surg Sports Traumatol Arthrosc. 2003;11(5):297–306.

26. Sherman PM, et al. MR imaging of the posterior cruciate ligament graft: initial experience in 15 patients with clinical correlation. Radiology. 2001;221(1):191–8.

27. Burns 2nd WC, et al. The effect of femoral tunnel position and graft tensioning technique on posterior laxity of the posterior cruciate ligament-reconstructed knee. Am J Sports Med. 1995;23(4):424–30.

28. Sanders TG. MR imaging of postoperative ligaments of the knee. Semin Musculoskelet Radiol. 2002;6(1):19–33.

29. Noyes FR, Barber-Westin SD. Posterior cruciate ligament revision reconstruction, part 2: results of revision using a 2-strand quadriceps tendon-patellar bone autograft. Am J Sports Med. 2005;33(5):655–65.

30. Thaunat M, Chambat P. Pretibial ganglion-like cyst formation after anterior cruciate ligament reconstruction: a consequence of the incomplete bony integration of the graft? Knee Surg Sports Traumatol Arthrosc. 2007;15(5):522–4.

31. Ahn JH, Lee YS, Chang MJ. Post-tibial cyst formation over 2 years after posterior cruciate ligament reconstruction. Knee Surg Sports Traumatol Arthrosc. 2008;16(11):996–8.

32. Buess E, Imhoff AB, Hodler J. Knee evaluation in two systems and magnetic resonance imaging after operative treatment of posterior cruciate ligament injuries. Arch Orthop Trauma Surg. 1996;115(6):307–12.

Medial Collateral Ligament (MCL) and Medial Supporting Structures

Nicolae Bolog, Gustav Andreisek, and Erika Ulbrich

3.1 Anatomy and Normal MRI Appearance

The medial supporting structures of the knee can be divided into three layers [1]. Layer 1 consists of the deep crural fascia that is seen on MR images as a thin low-intensity structure on all MR sequences (Fig. 3.1). Anteriorly, the deep crural fascia joins the superficial layer of MCL into the medial patellar retinaculum that appears on MR images as a low-signal-intensity structure that extends from the vastus medialis muscle to the tibia inferiorly (Fig. 3.2) [2]. In some cases, two band-like structures may be seen [2].

The MCL is beneath the deep crural fascia (layer 1), from which it is separated by a variable amount of fat (Fig. 3.1). The MCL is composed of the superficial layer (layer 2 of the medial supporting structures) and the deep layer (layer 3 of the medial supporting structures).

The superficial layer of MCL (layer 2), also known as the vertical component of MCL, is about 12 cm long, 1–2 cm wide, and 2–4 mm thick and extends from its medial femoral epicondyle origin to its attachment at the tibial plateau, just posterior to the pes anserinus insertion (Fig. 3.1) [2]. It is the strongest part of MCL. Anteriorly, the superficial layer of MCL joins the deep crural fascia to form the medial patellar retinaculum which is part of the anterior third of the medial joint capsule (Fig. 3.2) [3]. Posteriorly, the superficial layer (layer 2) and the deep layer of MCL (layer 3) merge forming

the posterior oblique portion, also known as the posterior oblique ligament (POL), that is closely attached to the posteromedial meniscus (Fig. 3.3) [4]. The posterior oblique ligament (POL) is part of the posterior third of the joint capsule and is formed by the superficial, the tibial, and the capsular arms [4]. The POL maintains medial stability and resists anteromedial tibial subluxation.

All the above-described structures are structures of the so-called posteromedial corner. The posteromedial corner of the knee is reinforced by the semimembranosus tendon and the medial head of the gastrocnemius muscle (Fig. 3.4) [5].

Layer 2 or the superficial layer of MCL appears on MR images as a homogeneous low-signal band and is separated from layer 3 or the deep layer of MCL by a variable amount of fat and the MCL bursa (Fig. 3.5). The MCL bursa is not apparent on normal MR images but may be outlined on MR images in the cases of bursitis [6].

The deep layer of the MCL (layer 3 of the medial supporting structures) is located close to the meniscus and represents the middle third of the deepest capsular layer of the knee. The medial meniscus is closely related to this layer. The deep layer of MCL includes the meniscofemoral ligament, meniscotibial ligament, and patellomeniscal ligament (Fig. 3.6). The meniscofemoral ligament originates from the superior margin of the meniscus and inserts on the femoral condyle or the superficial layer of MCL 1–2 cm above the joint line (Fig. 3.6) [2]. The meniscotibial ligament

N.V. Bolog et al., *MRI of the Knee: A Guide to Evaluation and Reporting*,
DOI 10.1007/978-3-319-08165-6_3, © Springer International Publishing Switzerland 2015

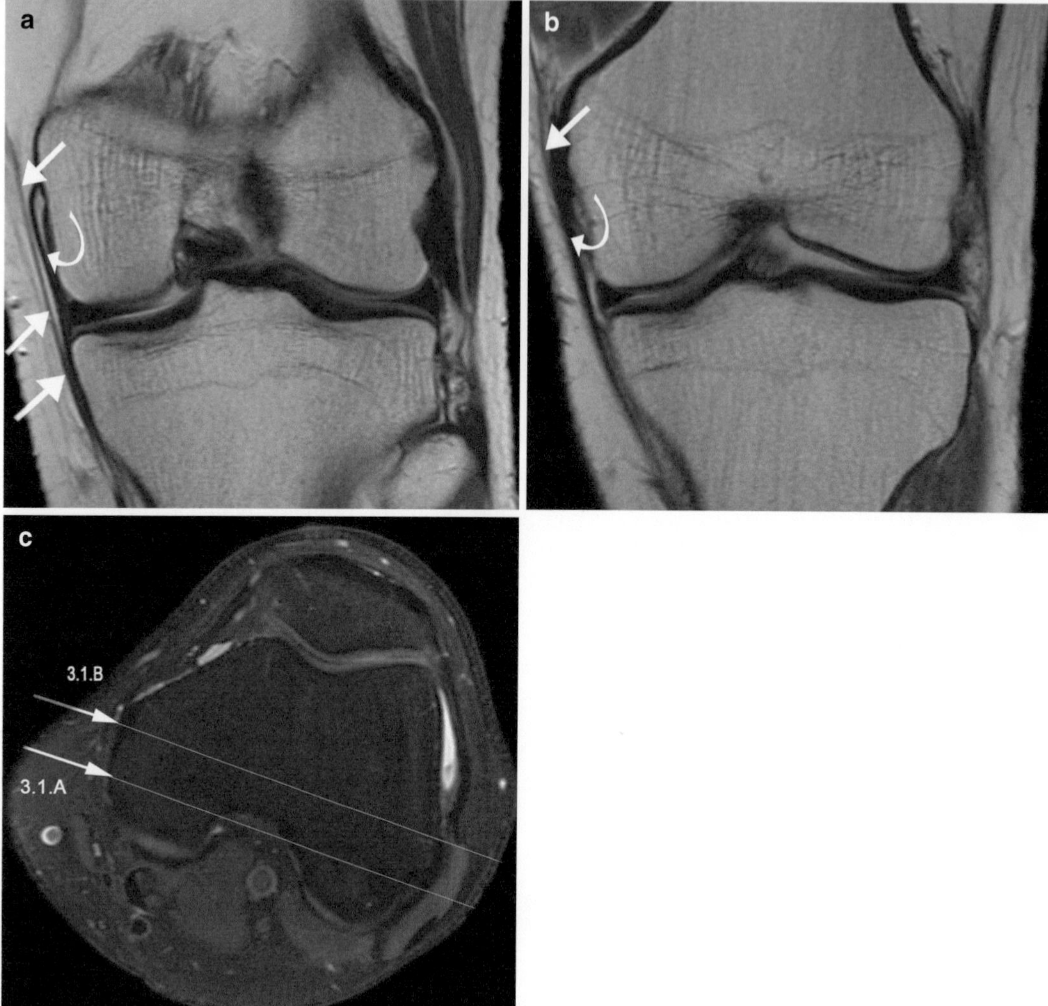

Fig. 3.1 Normal superficial layer of the medial supporting structures or layer 1 represented by deep crural fascia in a 36 year old male. Coronal proton-density (PD) FSE image (**a**) obtained posteriorly through the joint – the plane is drawn in **c** as *line 3.1.A*. At this level, the deep crural fascia that is seen on MR images as a thin low-intensity structure (*arrows*) separated by a variable amount of fat from the superficial layer of medial collateral ligament known also as the vertical part of the ligament (*curved arrow*). Anteriorly, mid-coronal proton-density (PD) FSE image (**b**) – the plane is drawn in **c** as *line 3.1.B* – the deep crural fascia (*arrow*) joins the medial collateral ligament (*curved arrow in* **b**)

is shorter, and it extends from the inferior margin of the meniscus to tibial cortex inferior to the joint line (Fig. 3.6) [2]. The patellomeniscal ligament is seen anteriorly and extends from the medial meniscus to the patellar margin (Fig. 3.7) [7]. Anteriorly, the deep layer is continuous with the capsule of the suprapatellar recess [2]. The meniscofemoral, the meniscotibial, and the patellomeniscal ligaments are seen as thin low-signal-intensity bands on all MRI sequences (Figs. 3.6 and 3.7). The outer mar-gin of the medial meniscus can typically not be distinguished from the deep layer of the MCL on MR images (Fig. 3.8).

The MCL provides primary valgus stability. A secondary function of the MCL is resistance to anterior and posterior stress, supplementing the primary function of the cruciate ligaments, and therefore, in cases with ACL tears, the MCL and the medial supporting structures function as secondary restraints to anterior tibial translation [8–10].

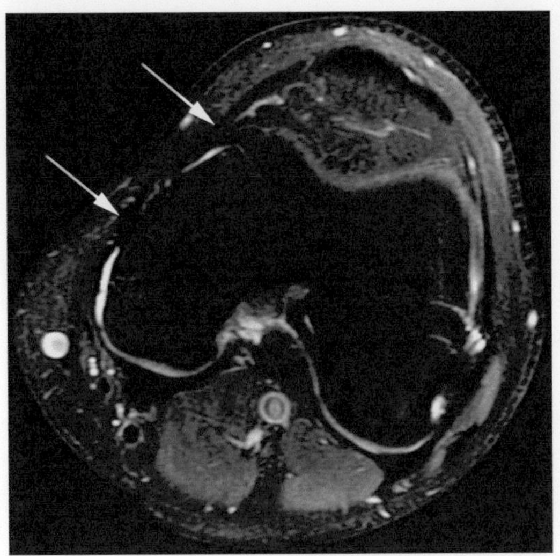

Fig. 3.2 Normal medial retinaculum. Axial proton-density (PD) FSE fat-suppressed image shows the medial retinaculum as a thin low-signal-intensity structure (*arrows*) which results from the crural fascia and the superficial layer of the MCL. The medial patellar retinaculum is part of the anterior third of the medial joint capsule

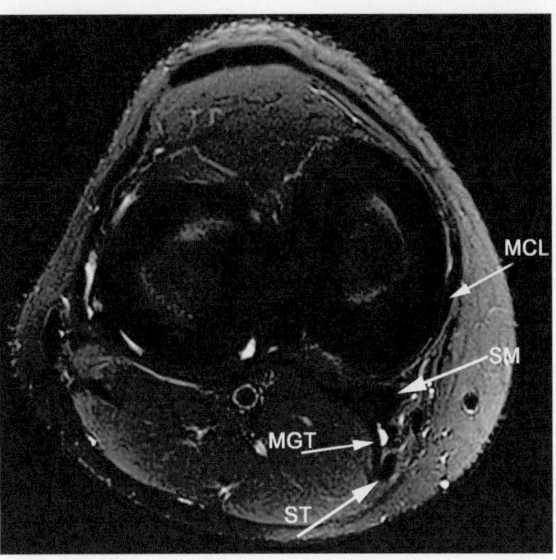

Fig. 3.4 The main structures of the posteromedial corner of the knee. Axial proton-density (PD) FSE fat-suppressed image through the meniscus shows the MCL and the semimembranosus tendon (*SM*). The posteromedial corner is reinforced by the medial gastrocnemius tendon (*MGT*). The semitendinosus tendon (*ST*) is identified posteriorly

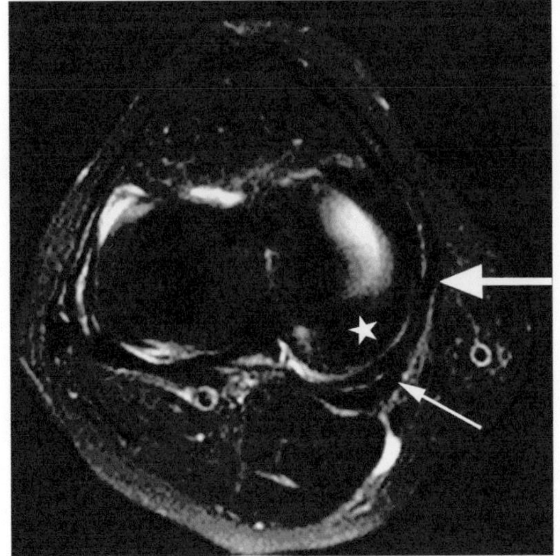

Fig. 3.3 The posterior oblique ligament (POL). Axial proton-density (PD) FSE fat-suppressed image through the meniscus shows the POL (*large arrow*) which results from the join of the superficial layer (layer 2) and the deep layer of medial collateral ligament (layer 3). Proximally, POL inserts at the semimembranosus tendon (*small arrow*). The POL is part of the posterior joint capsule and is closely attached to the medial meniscus (*star*)

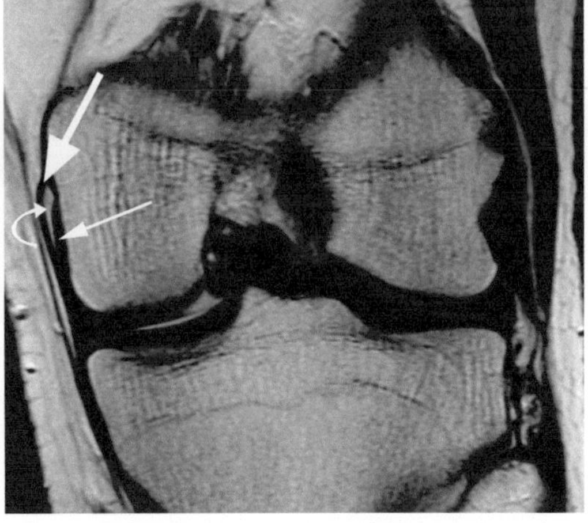

Fig. 3.5 The two layers of the MCL. Coronal proton-density (PD) FSE image shows the superficial layer of MCL or layer 2 (*large arrow*) separated from layer 3 or the deep layer of MCL (*small arrow*) by a variable amount of fat (*curved arrow*)

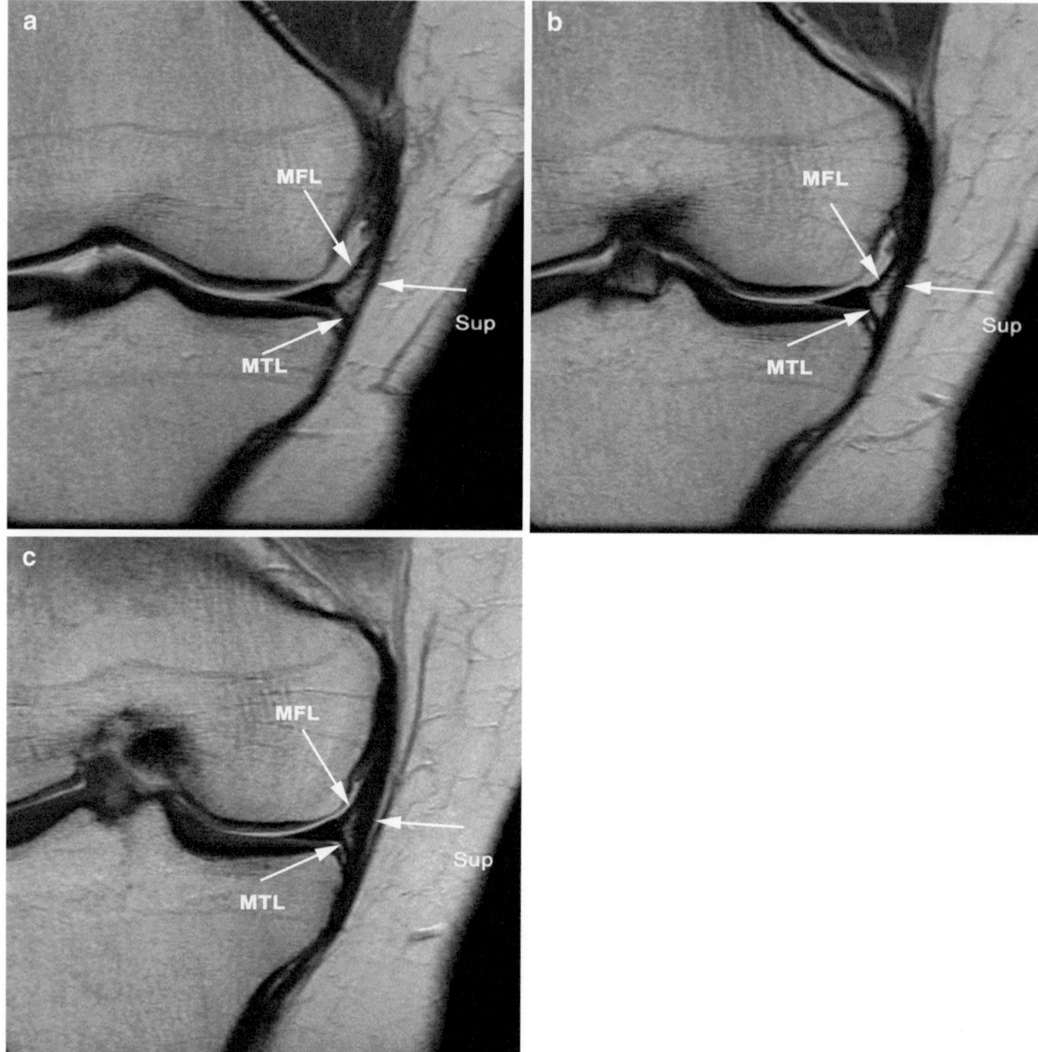

Fig. 3.6 The meniscofemoral and the meniscotibial ligaments. Coronal proton-density (PD) FSE images through the anterior (**a**), mid-coronal (**b**), and posterior (**c**) joints. The superficial layer of the medial collateral ligament (*Sup*) is clearly separated by the meniscofemoral ligament which originates from the femoral condyle (*MFL*) and the meniscotibial ligament (*MTL*) which is shorter, and it extends from the inferior margin of the meniscus to tibial cortex inferior to the joint line

3.2 MRI Pathological Findings

3.2.1 Acute Tear

The MCL is the most frequently injured knee ligament. Although, the treatment of the injuries is mostly nonoperatively, MR imaging is unavoidable in managing the patients. The interest in classifying the MCL injuries has declined since the treatment moves toward conservative approach for all grades of isolated injuries [11]. The MCL injuries may be classified into isolated or combined injuries. The most frequently associated lesions are ACL tears, medial meniscal lesions, meniscocapsular separations, medial retinaculum teas, disruption

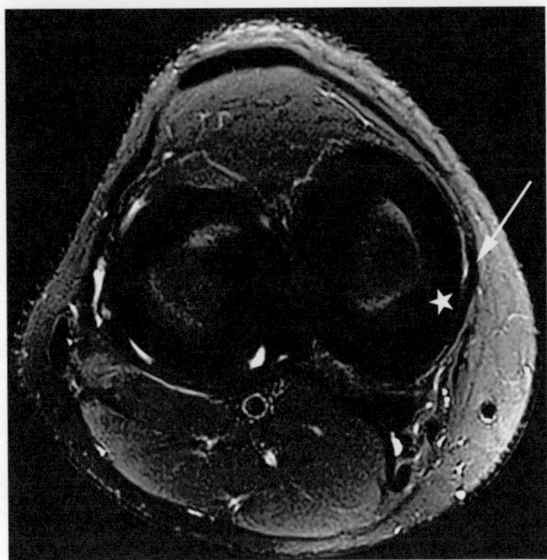

Fig. 3.7 The patellomeniscal ligament. Axial proton-density (PD) FSE fat-suppressed image through the meniscus shows the origin of the patellomeniscal ligament (*arrow*) extending anteriorly from the medial meniscus (*star*)

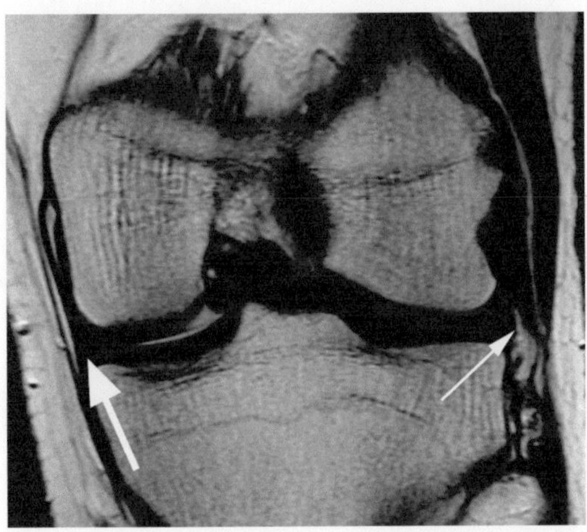

Fig. 3.8 Coronal proton-density (PD) FSE image demonstrates that the outer margin of the medial meniscus cannot be typically distinguished from the deep layer of MCL (*large arrow*) in comparison with the lateral side where is a clear demarcation between the lateral meniscus and the lateral collateral ligament (*small arrow*)

of the posteromedial joint capsule, and tears of pes anserinus [12].

Commonly, the MCL injuries are classified into the following three types or grades: sprain, partial tear, and complete tear.

Sprain with Intact Fibers

A MCL sprain with intact fibers is referred to as grade I MCL tear. It corresponds to ligamentous fibers that are stretched but still in continuity [12]. A MCL sprain is typically associated with pain but not with medial laxity on physical examination. The treatment is nonoperative. On MR images, the ligament is of almost normal thickness, and a diffuse edema or hemorrhage of high signal intensity on T2-weighted images parallel to superficial layer of MCL is seen (Fig. 3.9). There is a loss of clear demarcation between the MCL and the subcutaneous fat, but the ligament is still closely attached to the femoral and tibial bone at its origin and insertion, respectively (Fig. 3.9).

Partial (or Incomplete) Tear

A partial tear of the MCL is referred to as grade II MCL tear. It implies an incomplete disruption of the fibers and some form of laxity on physical examination. An incomplete tear of the MCL is usually treated conservatively. MR images show a poorly defined internal signal intensity and morphologic disruption with focal abnormalities of hyperintensity of some but not all fibers [13]. The fibers are displaced from the adjacent bone at the ligaments origin or insertion, and diffuse edema and hemorrhage of high signal intensity is seen superficially and deeply to the MCL (Fig. 3.10). When the inner fibers are involved, the MCL bursa may be separated from the joint with fluid in the bursa [13]. Partial MCL tears may involve both, the superficial and the deep layer of MCL, with tear of the meniscofemoral and/or meniscotibial ligaments (Fig. 3.11). The latter two can also be affected in rare cases in isolation with an otherwise intact superficial portion of the MCL (Figs. 3.10 and 3.11). Contusion edema of the medial femoral condyle may be seen as an associated finding in partial tears of MCL. It might be noted that some authors use the expression "low-grade" and "high-grade" partial tears to address cases where partial tearing involves only few fibers or many fibers of the MCL. This is however of little consequence for patient management.

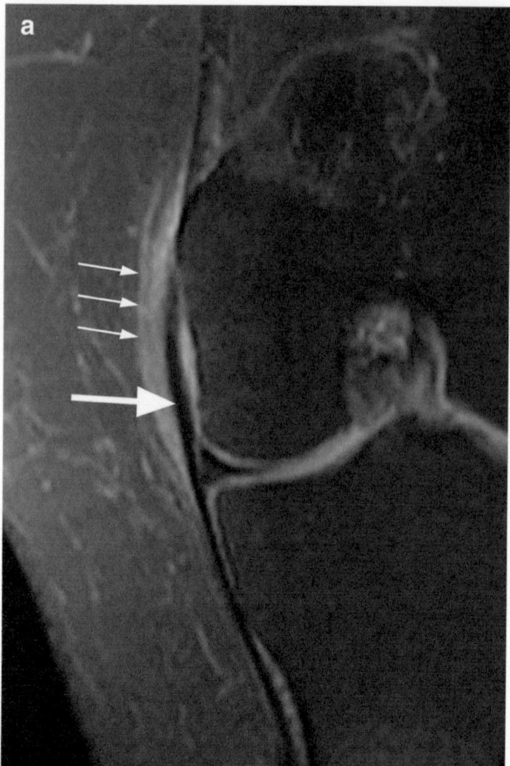

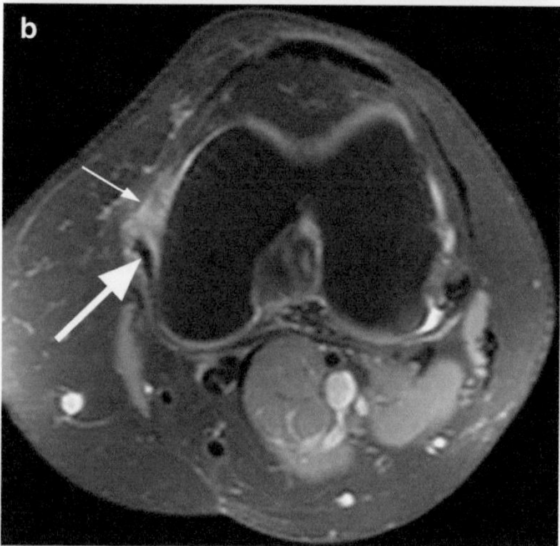

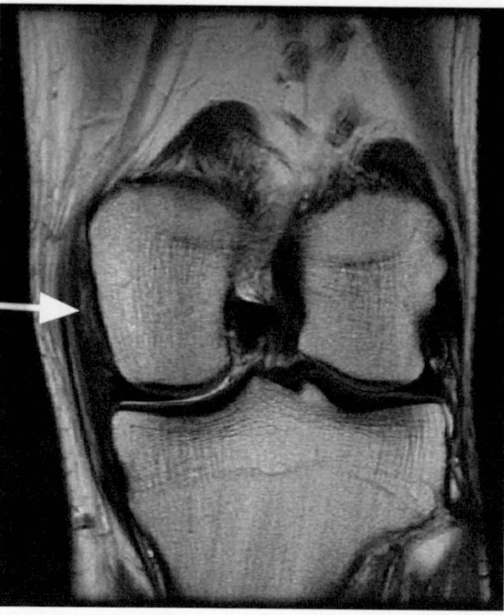

Fig. 3.10 Partial tear of the medial collateral ligament (MCL) or grade II tear in a 22 year old female. Coronal proton-density (PD) FSE image shows focal signal abnormalities of the ligament involving the deep layer (*arrow*). There is a poorly defined internal structure of the ligament, and the fibers are displaced from the adjacent bone at the femoral insertion. However, the superficial layer is still in continuity

Fig. 3.9 Sprain of the medial collateral ligament (MCL) or grade I tear in a 36 year old female. Coronal proton-density (PD) fat-suppressed image (**a**) and axial proton-density (PD) FSE fat-suppressed image (**b**) show diffuse edema and hemorrhage of high signal intensity parallel to the medial collateral ligament (*small arrows* in **a** and **b**). The ligament fibers are intact (*large arrow*), and the ligament is still closely attached to the femoral and tibial bone as well as to the medial meniscus

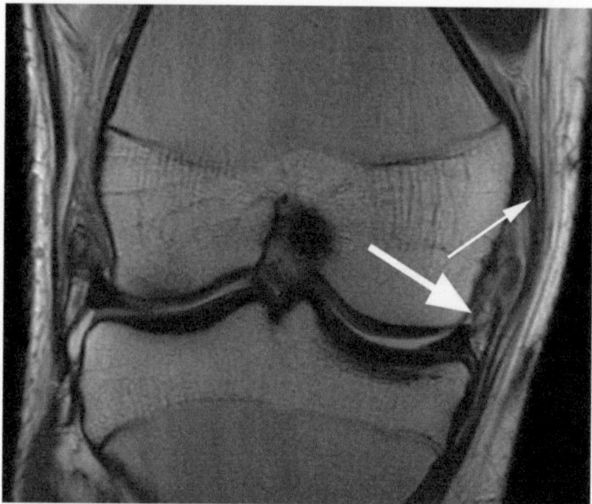

Fig. 3.11 Partial tear of the medial collateral ligament (MCL) or grade II tear in a 16 year old male. Coronal proton-density (PD) FSE image shows an incomplete tear of MCL involving the meniscofemoral ligament (*large arrow*) with displacement from the adjacent bone. Note that the superficial layer (*small arrow*) is intact

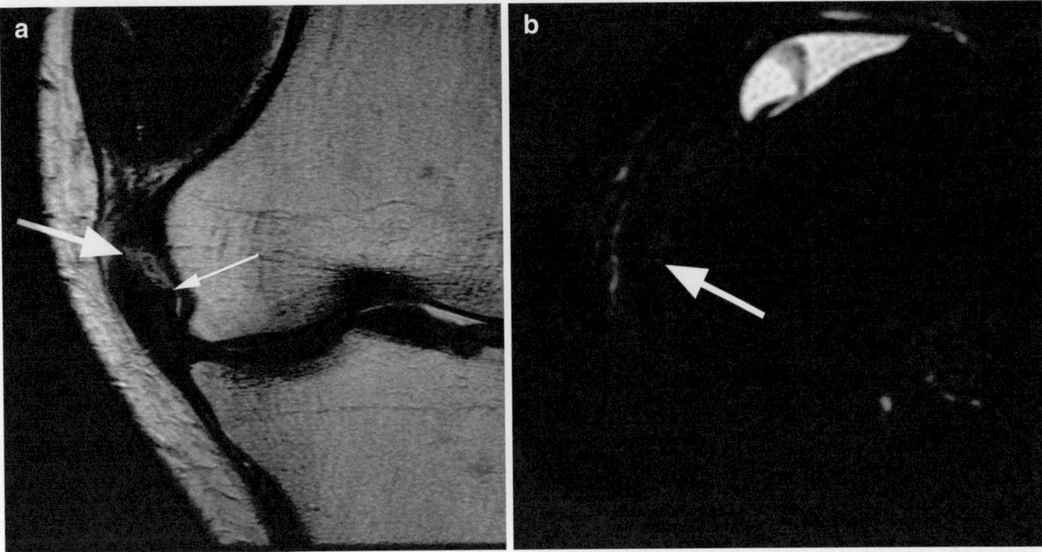

Fig. 3.12 Complete tear of the medial collateral ligament (MCL) or grade III tear in a 16 year old male. Coronal proton-density (PD) FSE image (**a**) and axial proton-density (PD) FSE fat-suppressed image (**b**) show complete disruption of both superficial and deep layers of the femoral portion of the ligament (*large arrow* in **a** and **b**). Note the wavy contour of the deep meniscofemoral ligament (*small arrow* in **a**)

Complete Tear

Complete tears are referred to as grade III MCL tears with complete loss of continuity of the fibers and medial knee instability on physical examination. Ligament discontinuity and the presence of edema and/or hemorrhage of high signal intensity are signs of complete tear of MCL on MR images (Fig. 3.12) [13]. The torn MCL has a wavy contour, and sometimes the torn end of the MCL can be entrapped between the femoral condyle and the tibia.

Since the surgical treatment of MCL tears depends on the exact site of the lesion as well as the distance between the torn ends of the fibers, the role of MRI is to accurately assess these features in order to support the clinicians in their therapeutic decision making. Tears located at the femoral origin are thereby the most common type of tears and are often associated with a small bony avulsion fragment [12]. On MR images, an avulsed bone fragment from the femoral epicondyle may be seen together with subchondral edema (Fig. 3.13). However, in many cases it is pretty difficult to detect the avulsed fragment on MR images. Thus, we still recommend to perform plain radiographs of the acutely injured knee for small bone fragment detection.

When an anteromedial rotatory instability is present at the physical examination, there is almost always an injury of the posterior oblique ligament (POL) concomitant with the MCL lesion. The posterior oblique ligament lesions can be classified similar to the MCL lesion as strain (grade I), partial tear (grade II), and complete tear (grade III) (Figs. 3.14 and 3.15) [14].

Other MCL-associated lesions that are often displayed on MR images are the capsular disruption with or without associated medial meniscal tear, meniscocapsular separation (Fig. 3.16), and bony avulsion at the level of the meniscotibial insertion (the so-called reverse Segond fracture) (Fig. 3.17) [15].

3.2.2 Chronic Injury of MCL

In some cases, the injury may be more gradual in onset, resulting from repetitive use injuries and microtears [16], and the MCL may appear thickened on MR images. Ossification of the proximal attachment of the MCL is also caused by chronic trauma. The presence of bone formation at the femoral attachment is known as Pellegrini-Stieda

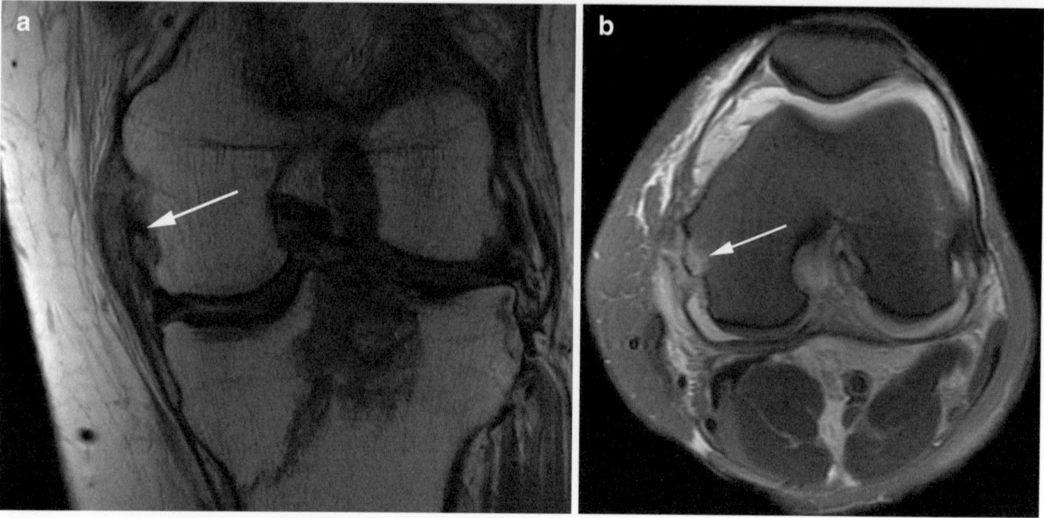

Fig. 3.13 Complete tear of the medial collateral ligament (MCL) with bone avulsion in a 40 year old female. Coronal proton-density (PD) FSE image (**a**) and axial proton-density (PD) FSE fat-suppressed image (**b**) show a small cortical bone fragment avulsed from the femoral insertion of MCL. The fragment is difficult to be identified on proton-density (PD) FSE image (*arrow* in **a**) but is confirmed on axial proton-density (PD) FSE fat-suppressed image (*arrow* in **b**) due to the presence of bone marrow edema

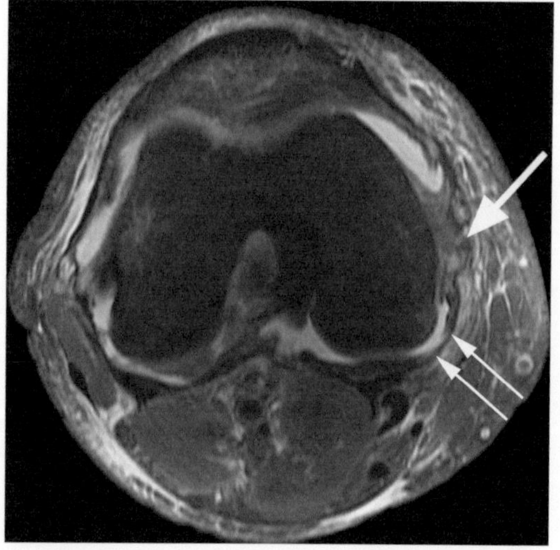

Fig. 3.14 Partial tear of the posterior oblique ligament (POL) concomitant with medial collateral ligament (MCL) tear in a 45 year old male. Axial proton-density (PD) FSE fat-suppressed image shows a complete tear of the MCL (*large arrow*) and high-signal-intensity changes within the posterior oblique ligament (POL) (*small arrows*) suggestive for partial tear or grade II tear of POL

sign (Fig. 3.18) [17]. Although most are asymptomatic, a few patients will develop pain and restricted movements that are characteristic of Pellegrini-Stieda disease, which can be severely limiting [18]. However, the ossification in Pellegrini-Stieda disease is not only confined to the MCL but may also involve the adductor magnus tendon [19]. Appearance on MR images depends on the size of the lesion. Smaller calcifications are seen as hypointensities on T1- and T2-weighted images. In the cases of more significant bone formation, marrow fat signal intensity may be detected on MR images. Although in mild cases conservative treatment is often successful, patients with persistent symptoms require surgical excision.

3.2.3 Healing Stages of MCL

All three types or grades of MCL injury can be treated conservatively after careful exclusion of any associated injuries that may require surgical treatment. Treatment options include bracing, activity modification, and rehabilitation. Although there is time variation of the healing time during individuals, the torn MCL undergoes three stages of healing [20]. Initially, there is a short phase of hemorrhage and inflammation within the first days of injury. Then, after 2 weeks there is an intermediate phase which is characterized by

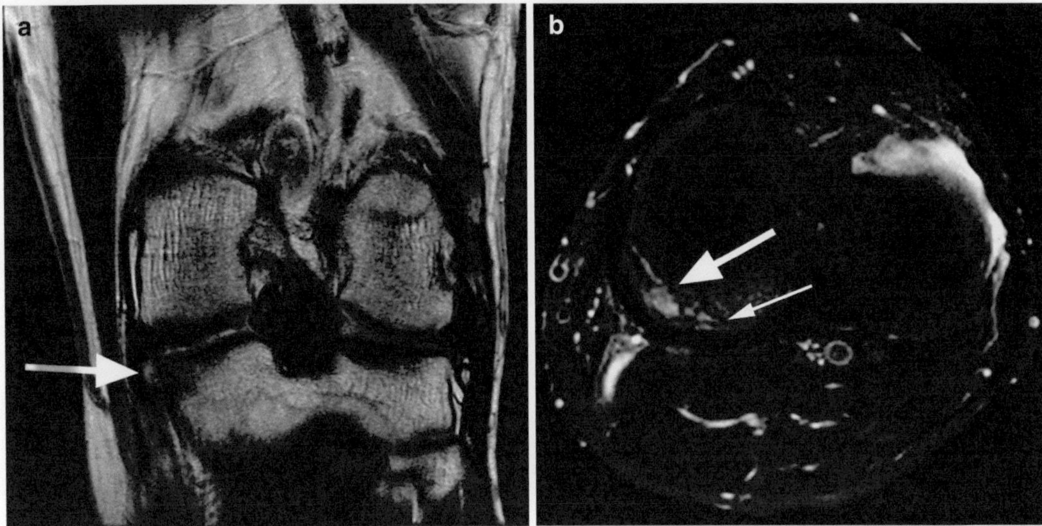

Fig. 3.15 Posterior oblique ligament (POL) injury in a 35 year old male. Coronal proton-density (PD) FSE image (**a**) and axial proton-density (PD) FSE fat-suppressed image (**b**) show posterior oblique ligament (POL) injury with fracture of the medial and posterior tibial plateau (*arrow*)

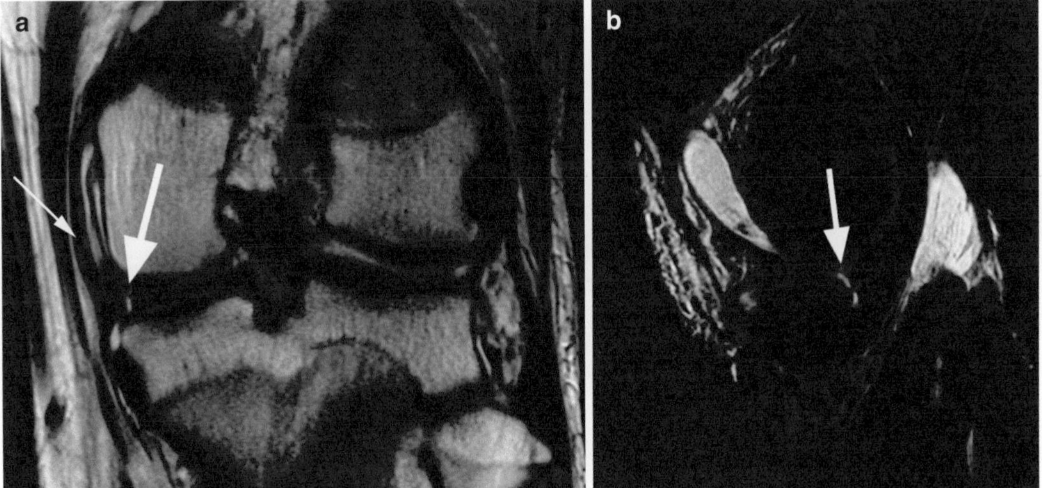

Fig. 3.16 Meniscocapsular separation in an 18 year old male. Coronal proton-density FSE image (**a**) and sagittal T2-weighted FSE fat-suppressed image (**b**) show a complete plane of fluid (*large arrow*) separating the medial meniscus and medial and posterior capsule. Note the strain of the medial collateral ligament without discontinuity of the fibbers (*small arrow* in **a**)

proliferation and replacement of type III with type I collagen fibers (Fig. 3.19) [21]. The last stage is a prolonged phase of remodeling that results in bridging scar formation (Fig. 3.19) [20]. Similar to tendons, the healing process does not imply a true ligament regeneration but a fibrous scar tissue formation. Therefore, the healed MCL is biomechanically inferior to the native MCL which means it is weaker and more prone to reinjuries (Fig. 3.20) [21]. Appearance of the healing MCL on MR images depends on the stage, but there might be thickening and persistent or prolonged intermediate signal intensity compared to the ligaments' normal hypointensity after the first short stage of inflammation (Fig. 3.19).

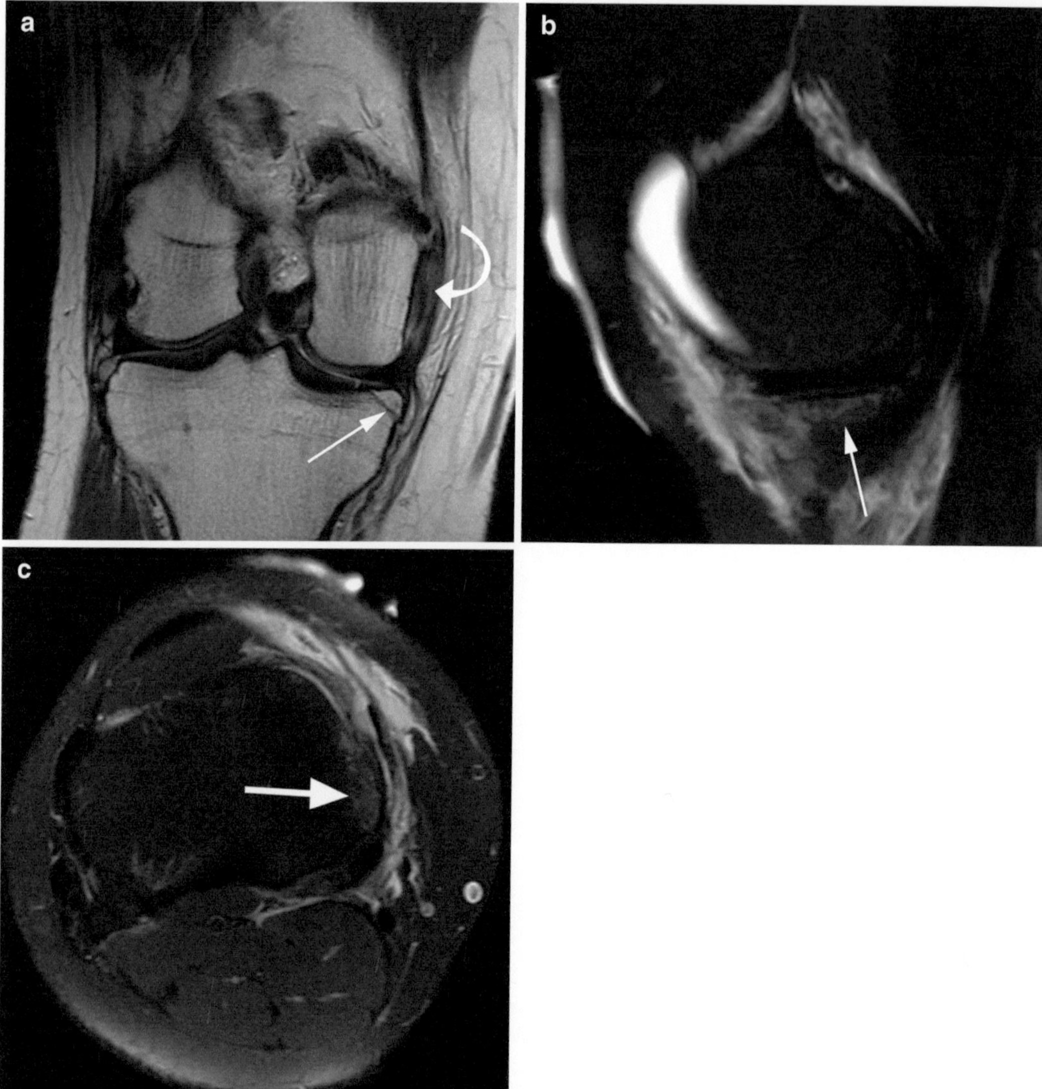

Fig. 3.17 Reverse Segond fracture in a 30 year old female. Coronal proton-density (PD) FSE image (**a**), sagittal T2-weighted FSE fat-suppressed image (**b**), and axial proton-density (PD) FSE fat-suppressed image (**c**) show a fracture of the medial articular proximal tibia (*arrow*) resulting from avulsion of the deep layer of the medial collateral ligament. Note the tear of the medial collateral ligament (*curved arrow* in **a**)

3.3   MRI Postoperative Findings

The surgical treatment depends on the location of the tear and the associated lesions. Tears from the femoral origin are the most common type of tears and are often associated with a bony avulsion fragment and may be treated with reattachment to the femur (Fig. 3.21) [12]. Ligament disruption in the midportion of the ligament is typically repaired with end-to-end suturing [12]. Tears of the distal portion of MCL may be associated with pes anserinus tendon tears, and the treatment consists of reattaching the ligament to the bone.

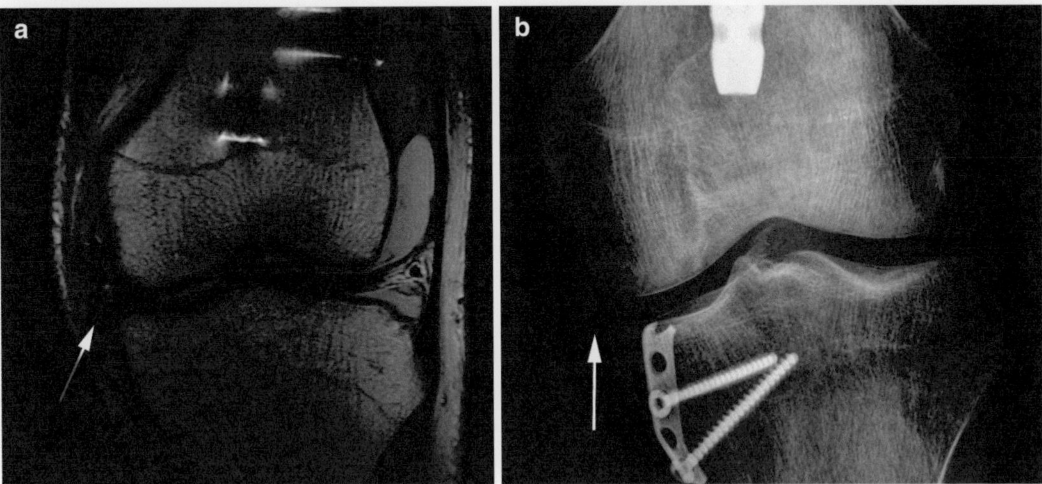

Fig. 3.18 Pellegrini-Stieda disease in a 39 year old female with medial knee pain. Coronal proton-density (PD) FSE image (**a**) and plain radiography (**b**) show calcification in the medial collateral ligament (*arrow*)

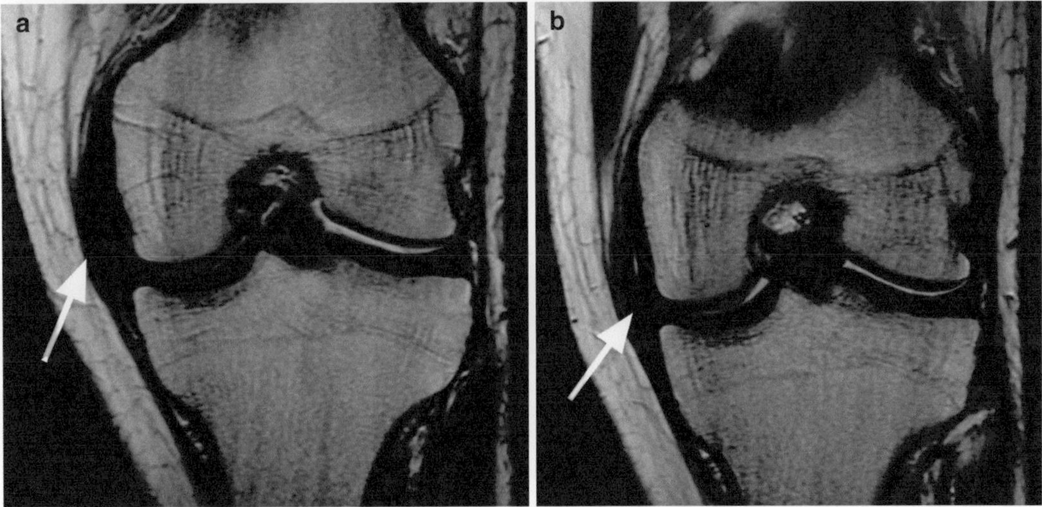

Fig. 3.19 Healing stages of the medial collateral ligament in a 40 year old male after complete tear. Coronal proton-density (PD) FSE image (**a**) 4 weeks after injury shows thickening of the ligament and diffuse intrasubstance signal-intensity changes due to the inflammatory changes (*arrow*). One year after injury, coronal proton-density (PD) FSE image (**b**) shows a decrease of the inflammatory process with a remaining thickening suggestive for bridging scar formation (*arrow*)

For reconstruction of the superficial MCL, multiple reconstruction techniques have been described with quadriceps tendon autograft, hamstring autograft, hamstring allograft, or Achilles allograft [22]. The presence of metallic hardware may cause degradation of image quality on MR imaging resulting from susceptibility artifacts (Fig. 3.21). However, as with native MCL, the presence of increased signal intensity (equal to that of fluid) interrupting the ligament should be taken as evidence of recurrent disruption [23].

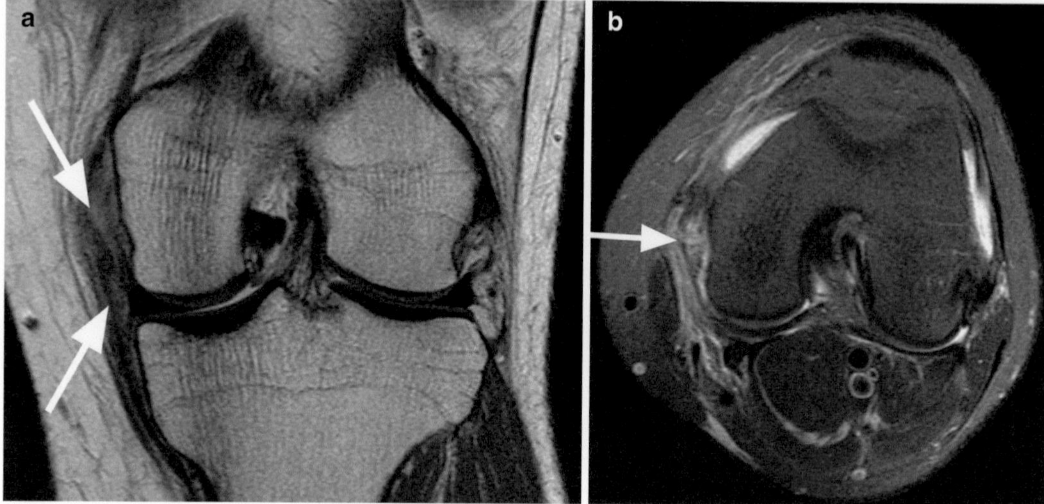

Fig. 3.20 Re-tear of the medial collateral ligament (MCL) in 34 year old male. Coronal proton-density (PD) FSE image (**a**) and axial proton-density (PD) FSE fat-suppressed image (**b**) show complete disruption of the ligament continuity with hemorrhage between the ligament and bone. The entire ligament is thickened with inhomogeneous signal intensity (*arrows* in **a, b**)

3.4   MRI Impression

3.4.1   Nonoperative MCL

1. Acute tear
   - (a) Sprain with intact fibers
   - (b) Partial tear (superficial or deep layer) with or without MCL bursitis
   - (c) Complete tear (femoral insertion, in the midsubstance, or at the tibial insertion) with or without capsular disruption
2. Chronic tear
3. Calcifications at the femoral insertion – Pellegrini-Stieda sign
4. Healed MCL – normal/abnormal appearance regarding the time from the injury; scar formation

3.4.2   Post-Injury Nonoperative MCL

1. Normal healed MCL regarding the time from the injury (scar formation)
2. Recurrence of the tear

3.4.3   Postoperative MCL

1. Normal postoperative appearance
2. Tear of the MCL graft

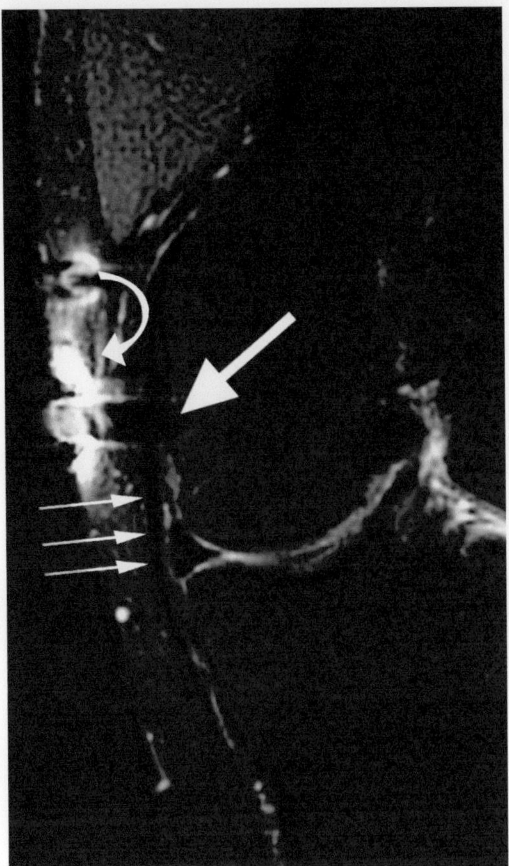

Fig. 3.21 Medial collateral ligament (MCL) reattachment in a 39 year old male. Coronal proton-density (PD) fat-suppressed image shows the femoral reattachment of MCL (*large arrow*) and the normal continuity of the ligament (*small arrows*). The presence of metallic hardware and the susceptibility artifacts (*curved arrow*) does not influence in this case the ligament assessment

References

1. Warren LA, Marshall JL, Girgis F. The prime static stabilizer of the medical side of the knee. J Bone Joint Surg Am. 1974;56(4):665–74.
2. De Maeseneer M, et al. Three layers of the medial capsular and supporting structures of the knee: MR imaging-anatomic correlation. Radiographics. 2000;20(Spec No):S83–9.
3. Ruiz ME, Erickson SJ. Medial and lateral supporting structures of the knee. Normal MR imaging anatomy and pathologic findings. Magn Reson Imaging Clin N Am. 1994;2(3):381–99.
4. LaPrade RF, et al. The anatomy of the medial part of the knee. J Bone Joint Surg Am. 2007;89(9):2000–10.
5. Robinson JR, et al. The posteromedial corner revisited. An anatomical description of the passive restraining structures of the medial aspect of the human knee. J Bone Joint Surg Br. 2004;86(5):674–81.
6. De Maeseneer M, et al. MR imaging of the medial collateral ligament bursa: findings in patients and anatomic data derived from cadavers. AJR Am J Roentgenol. 2001;177(4):911–7.
7. Starok M, et al. Normal patellar retinaculum: MR and sonographic imaging with cadaveric correlation. AJR Am J Roentgenol. 1997;168(6):1493–9.
8. Haimes JL, et al. Role of the medial structures in the intact and anterior cruciate ligament-deficient knee. Limits of motion in the human knee. Am J Sports Med. 1994;22(3):402–9.
9. Ritchie JR, et al. Isolated sectioning of the medial and posteromedial capsular ligaments in the posterior cruciate ligament-deficient knee. Influence on posterior tibial translation. Am J Sports Med. 1998;26(3):389–94.
10. Bauer KL, Stannard JP. Surgical approach to the posteromedial corner: indications, technique, outcomes. Curr Rev Musculoskelet Med. 2013;6(2):124–31.
11. Sims WF, Jacobson KE. The posteromedial corner of the knee: medial-sided injury patterns revisited. Am J Sports Med. 2004;32(2):337–45.
12. Beall DP, et al. Magnetic resonance imaging of the collateral ligaments and the anatomic quadrants of the knee. Radiol Clin North Am. 2007;45(6):983–1002, vi.
13. Schweitzer ME, et al. Medial collateral ligament injuries: evaluation of multiple signs, prevalence and location of associated bone bruises, and assessment with MR imaging. Radiology. 1995;194(3):825–9.
14. House CV, Connell DA, Saifuddin A. Posteromedial corner injuries of the knee. Clin Radiol. 2007;62(6):539–46.
15. Geiger D, et al. Posterolateral and posteromedial corner injuries of the knee. Radiol Clin North Am. 2013;51(3):413–32.
16. Duffy PS, Miyamoto RG. Management of medial collateral ligament injuries in the knee: an update and review. Phys Sportsmed. 2010;38(2):48–54.
17. Wang JC, Shapiro MS. Pellegrini-Stieda syndrome. Am J Orthop (Belle Mead NJ). 1995;24(6):493–7.
18. Theivendran K, Lever CJ, Hart WJ. Good result after surgical treatment of Pellegrini-Stieda syndrome. Knee Surg Sports Traumatol Arthrosc. 2009;17(10):1231–3.
19. Mendes LF, et al. Pellegrini-Stieda disease: a heterogeneous disorder not synonymous with ossification/calcification of the tibial collateral ligament-anatomic and imaging investigation. Skeletal Radiol. 2006;35(12):916–22.
20. Frank C, Schachar N, Dittrich D. Natural history of healing in the repaired medial collateral ligament. J Orthop Res. 1983;1(2):179–88.
21. Stoller DW, Anderson LJ, Cannon WD. The knee. In: Stoller DW, editor. Magnetic resonance imaging in orthopaedics and sports medicine, vol. 1. 3rd ed. Philadepllphia: Lippincott Williams & Wilkins; 2007.
22. Phisitkul P, et al. MCL injuries of the knee: current concepts review. Iowa Orthop J. 2006;26:77–90.
23. Frick MA, Collins MS, Adkins MC. Postoperative imaging of the knee. Radiol Clin North Am. 2006;44(3):367–89.

Lateral Collateral Ligament (LCL) and Posterolateral Corner (PLC)

Nicolae Bolog, Gustav Andreisek, Erika Ulbrich, and Brian M. Devitt

4.1 Anatomy and Normal MRI Appearance

The posterolateral corner (PLC) of the knee is a complex functional unit consisting of several important ligaments and is responsible for posterolateral stabilization of the joint [1]. There is some variability in the definition of the posterolateral corner (PLC) in the literature, but most descriptions include *the lateral collateral ligament* (LCL), *the anterior oblique band* (AOB), *the popliteal tendon* (PT) with *the anterolateral ligament* (ALL), *the popliteomeniscal fascicles*, and *the popliteofibular ligament* (PFL), as well as the posterolateral capsule including *the arcuate ligament* (AL) and *the fabellofibular ligament* (FFL) [1]. These structures are reinforced by the biceps femoris tendon and the iliotibial tract.

The posterolateral corner limits posterior translation, varus angulation, and excessive external rotation. The popliteal tendon (PT) is considered to be a dynamic stabilizer, and the lateral collateral ligament (LCL), the fabellofibular ligament (FFL), the popliteofibular ligament (PFL), and the arcuate ligament (AL) represent static posterolateral stabilizers [1].

4.1.1 Lateral Collateral Ligament (LCL) and the Anterior Oblique Band (AOB)

With the knee in extension, *the lateral collateral ligament* (LCL) is approximately 6 cm long and 3–5 mm thick [2–7]. The ligament is superficially located and is a static stabilizer during varus angulation. Lateral collateral ligament extends from the lateral femoral condyle, posterior to the lateral epicondyle and 2 cm above the joint line to the fibular head (Fig. 4.1) [8, 9]. At the fibular insertion, the lateral collateral ligament and the biceps tendon form a conjoined tendon (Fig. 4.1) [10]. Between the two structures, the lateral collateral ligament-biceps femoris bursa is constantly described [8].

The anterior oblique band (AOB) is a band of fibrous tissue that extends from the lateral collateral ligament to the lateral portion of tibia [11]. Some fibers of the anterior oblique band (AOB) blend with posterior fibers of the iliotibial tract [11].

On MR images, the lateral collateral ligament appears as a straight homogeneous hypointense structure on all sequences (Fig. 4.2). The anterior oblique band (AOB) is seen on axial MR images as a thin hypointense band extending from the lateral collateral ligament to the lateral tibia and the iliotibial tract (Fig. 4.3).

4.1.2 Popliteal Tendon (PT), Anterolateral Ligament (ALL), Popliteomeniscal Fascicles (PMF), and Popliteofibular Ligament (PFL)

The popliteal tendon (PT) has its proximal attachment on the lateral femoral condyle, anteroinferiorly to the lateral collateral ligament. Two separate bundles are described at the proximal attachment:

N.V. Bolog et al., *MRI of the Knee: A Guide to Evaluation and Reporting*,
DOI 10.1007/978-3-319-08165-6_4, © Springer International Publishing Switzerland 2015

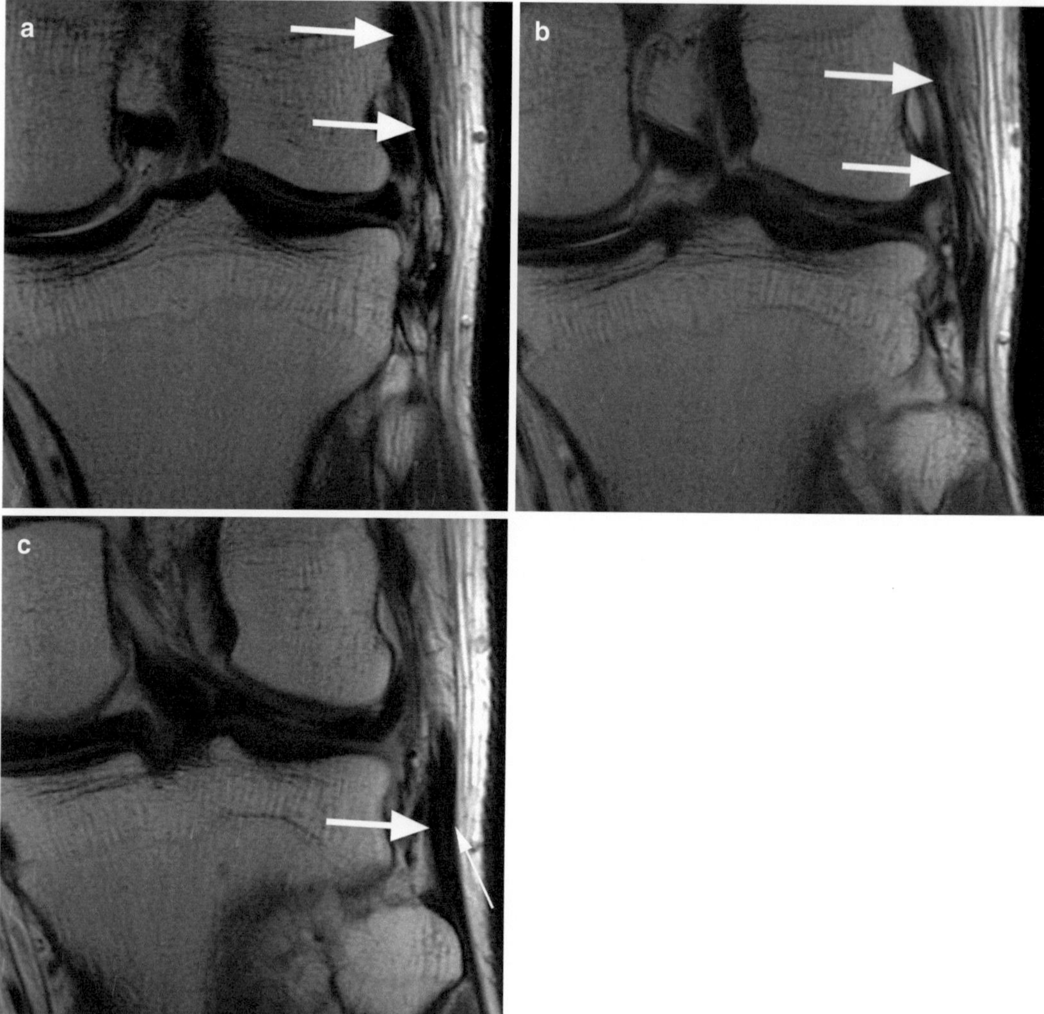

Fig. 4.1 Normal lateral collateral ligament (LCL) in a 21 year old male. Three consecutive coronal proton-density (PD) FSE images from anterior to posterior (**a–c**) show the normal LCL extending from the lateral femoral condyle to the fibular head (*large arrows* in **a** and **b**). At the fibular insertion LCL (*large arrow* in **c**) forms a conjoined tendon with the biceps tendon (*small arrow* in **c**)

the posterior superficial bundle and the anterior deep bundle [12]. The popliteal tendon (PT) is intra-articular and extrasynovial at the level of the femorotibial joint and is surrounded by the popliteal bursa [13]. Distally, the tendon is extra-artic-ular, deep to the fabellofibular ligament and the arcuate ligament [14]. It extends to the popliteal muscle. An extension of the synovial membrane between the posterior horn of the lateral meniscus and the popliteus tendon, known as popliteus or subpopliteus bursa, surrounds the tendon and may communicate with the superior tibiofibular joint

(Fig. 4.4) [13]. On MR images, the tendon is hypointense on all sequences (Fig. 4.4). However, magic angle artifacts may occur due to its curved and oblique course especially at the proximal part. Thus, signal intensity irregularities should not be mistaken as tendinopathy or rupture per se but need to be verified on other sequences.

The anterolateral ligament (ALL) is a relatively consistent structure that is found during knee arthroplasty [15]. It was first described as a reinforcement of the lateral capsule. The antero-lateral ligament (ALL) takes origin from the

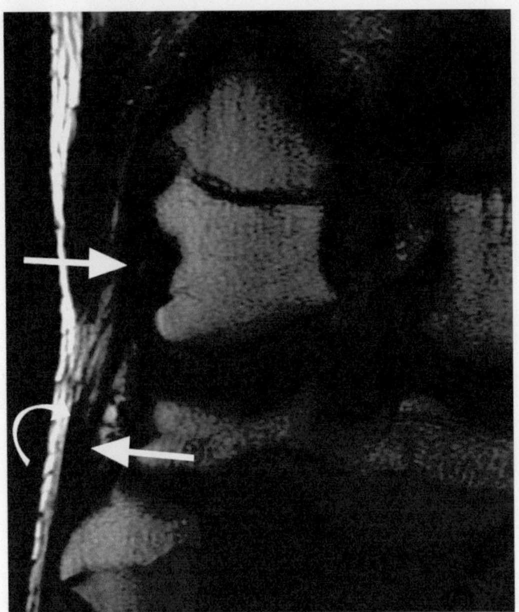

Fig. 4.2 Normal lateral collateral ligament (LCL) in a 22 year old male. In this case, the LCL is visualized on a single coronal proton-density (PD) FSE image as a continuous hypointense band (*large arrows*). At the distal insertion, the LCL and the biceps tendon (*curved arrow*) form a conjoined tendon

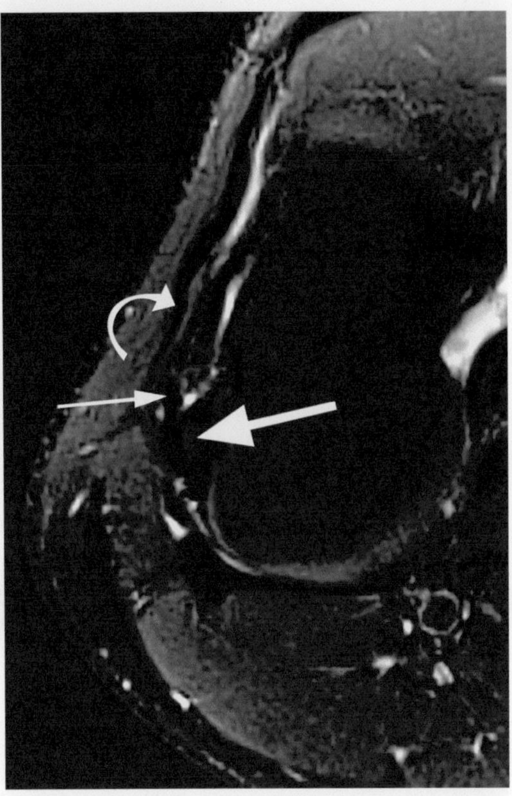

Fig. 4.3 Normal anterior oblique band (AOB) in a 17 year old male. Axial proton-density (PD) FSE fat-suppressed image shows the anterior oblique band (AOB) (*small arrow*) extending from the lateral collateral ligament (LCL) (*large arrow*) to the iliotibial tract (*curved arrow*)

lateral femoral condyle just anterior to and blending with the popliteus tendon, and it inserts distally to the lateral meniscus and lateral tibial plateau, typically about 5 mm distal to the joint line [15]. It can be seen on coronal MR images as a thin hypointense linear structure anterior to the popliteal tendon (PT) (Fig. 4.5).

The popliteal tendon (PT) is strongly attached to the lateral meniscus through the two *popliteomeniscal fascicles* (PMF). The posterosuperior popliteomeniscal fascicle extends from the popliteal tendon to the posterolateral aspect of the lateral meniscus. The anteroinferior popliteomeniscal fascicle is stronger and shorter and extends from the popliteal tendon to the middle third of the lateral meniscus [12, 16]. On MR images, the popliteomeniscal fascicles are inconsistently seen as hypointense structures on sagittal planes (Fig. 4.6).

The popliteofibular ligament (PFL) attaches the popliteal tendon (PT) to the fibular head. It originates proximal to the myotendinous junction of the popliteus muscle and attaches to the medial

fibular styloid [17]. The popliteofibular ligament (PFL) is approximately 10 mm long having a thickness similar to the lateral collateral ligament [12, 18]. The ligament is inconsistently identified on coronal MR images as a hypointense band (Fig. 4.7).

4.1.3   Arcuate Ligament (AL) and Fabellofibular Ligament (FFL)

The arcuate ligament (AL) is a Y-shaped thickening of the capsule with a medial and a lateral limb. The body of the arcuate ligament (AL) originates from the lateral edge of the styloid process of the fibula [19]. The lateral limb blends

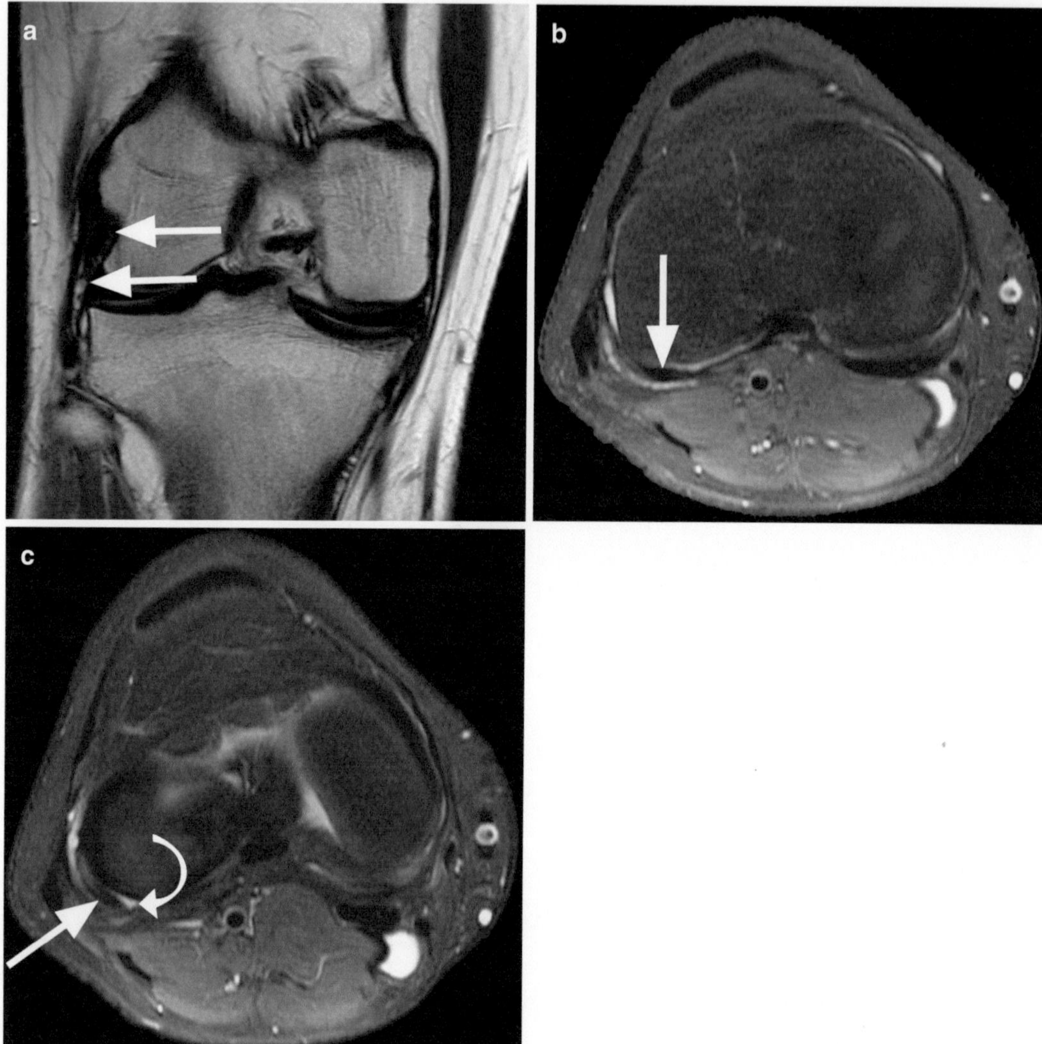

Fig. 4.4 Normal popliteal tendon (PT) and popliteus or subpopliteus bursa in a 19 year old female. Coronal proton-density (PD) FSE image (**a**) shows the hypointense PT at its femoral insertion (*large arrows*). On axial proton-density (PD) FSE fat-suppressed images (**b, c**), the PT is seen in contact with the lateral femoral condyle (*large arrows* in **b**, **c**). A small subpopliteus bursa (*curved arrow* in **c**) is seen between PT and posterior horn of lateral meniscus

with the capsule and inserts to the lateral femoral condyle near the lateral gastrocnemius muscle (Fig. 4.8). The medial limb attaches to the posterior capsule.

The fabellofibular ligament (FFL) attaches proximally to the fabella and extends inferiorly and vertically to the fibular styloid process (Fig. 4.9). However, the fabellofibular ligament (FFL) may be present even in the absence of fabella [8, 20].

The arcuate ligament (AL) and the fabellofibular ligament (FFL) are not always present in anatomical studies. When present, the normal arcuate ligament (AL) and fabellofibular ligament (FFL) are depicted on MR images on coronal (arcuate ligament and fabellofibular ligament) and sagittal planes (fabellofibular ligament) as hypointense homogeneous bands (Figs. 4.8 and 4.9). However, in the authors' experience, it remains

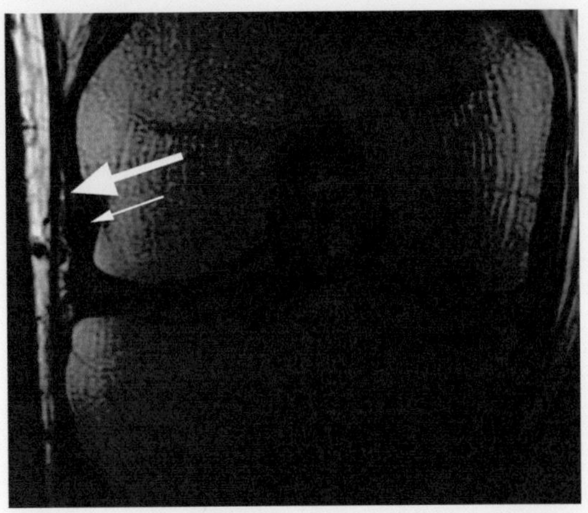

Fig. 4.5 The anterolateral ligament (ALL) in a 22 year old male. Coronal proton-density (PD) FSE image shows the ALL (*large arrow*) with its insertion on the lateral femoral condyle. The ligament blends with the popliteus tendon (*small arrow*)

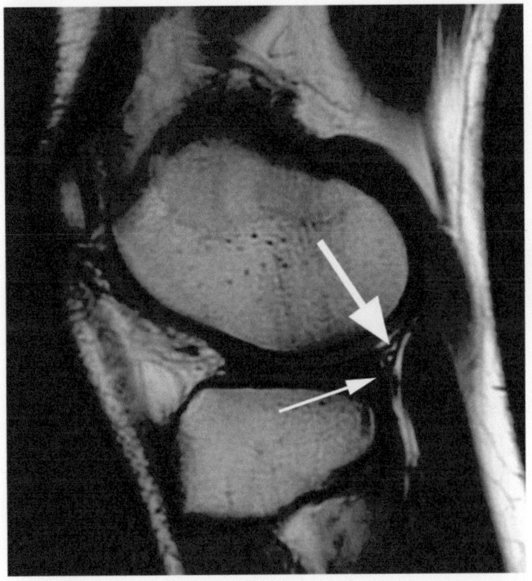

Fig. 4.6 The popliteomeniscal fascicles in a 19 year old female. Sagittal proton-density (PD) FSE image shows the posterosuperior popliteomeniscal fascicle (*large arrow*) and the anteroinferior popliteomeniscal fascicle (*small arrow*) strongly attached to the lateral meniscus

difficult to identify both structures in the clinical routine imaging. One has to look specifically for these structures, and high-resolution images are mandatory for that.

4.2 MRI Pathological Findings

Although posterolateral corner injuries are not as common as injuries to the medial collateral ligament, they are more complex and more difficult to diagnose on physical examination. The most typical injury mechanism is a direct varus force to the anteromedial aspect of the hyperextended knee.

Almost all posterolateral corner lesions are associated with other injuries. The more common associated lesions are anterior and posterior cruciate ligament tears, medial collateral and medial meniscus injuries, anteromedial tibial plateau contusion or fracture, and the Segond fracture [1]. Untreated posterolateral injuries may be associated with chronic instability of the knee, failure of cruciate ligament reconstructions, and osteoarthritis [21, 22].

Appearance on MR images depends upon what structures are injured and the degree of injury. Lesions involving well-defined and well-delineated structures such as the lateral collateral ligament (LCL) and popliteal tendon (PT) can be classified on MR images into partial or complete tear. In the case of all the small structures mentioned above which, in addition, are inconsistently present and part of the capsule, the MR description should only refer to as "probably torn" based mainly on indirect signs.

4.2.1 Sprain and Partial Tears

The sprain with intact fibers of the lateral collateral ligament (LCL) implies the presence of edema around the ligament with intact fibers (Fig. 4.10). A partial tear of the lateral collateral ligament (LCL) is seen on MR images as inhomogeneous signal intensity within the ligament. The ligament may be thinned or thickened without complete interruption of the fibers, and high-signal-intensity edema around the ligament is typically present (Figs. 4.11 and 4.12).

Most lesions of the popliteal tendon (PT) are extra-articular at the myotendinous junction. In the case of a partial tear of the popliteal tendon

Fig. 4.7 The popliteofibular ligament (PFL) in a 19 year old female. Sagittal proton-density (PD) FSE image (**a**) shows the thick hypointense PFL (*large arrow*) inserting on the fibular head. On coronal proton-density (PD) FSE image (**b**) through the same level (*line* in **a**), the PFL (*large arrow*) is identified and connects the fibular head with the popliteal tendon (*small arrow*)

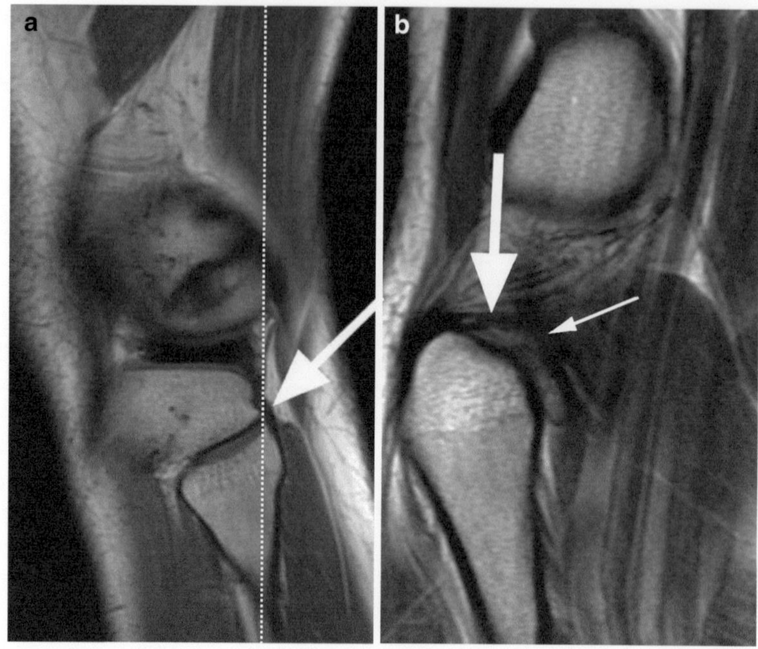

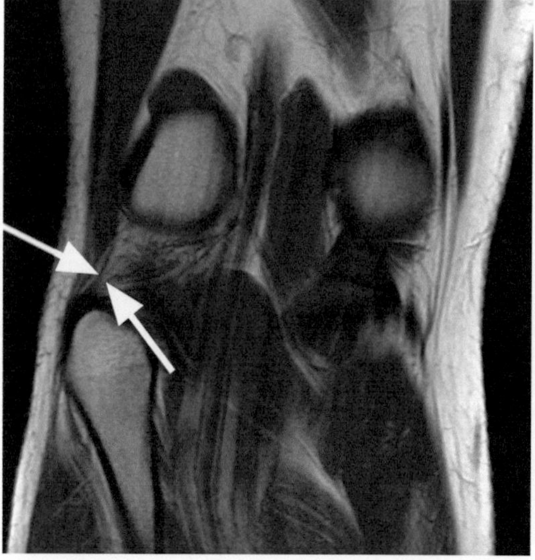

Fig. 4.8 The arcuate ligament (AL) in a 19 year old female. Coronal proton-density (PD) FSE image shows a thin hypointense band representing the lateral limb of AL (*arrows*) which originates from the lateral edge of the styloid process of the fibula and inserts to the lateral femoral condyle

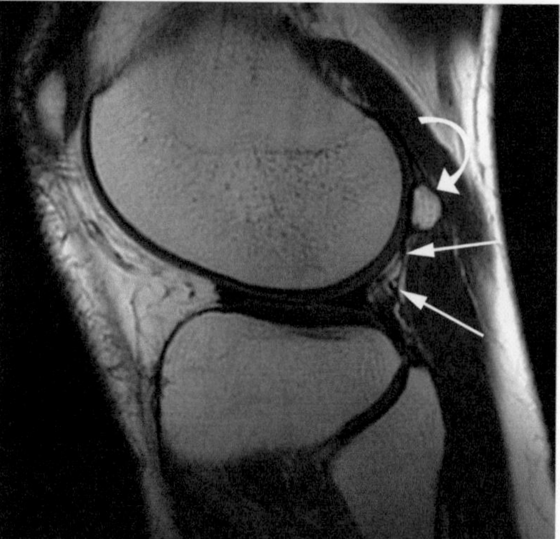

Fig. 4.9 The fabellofibular ligament (FFL) in a 35 year old male. Sagittal proton-density (PD) FSE image shows the FFL (*arrows*) which extends from the fabella (*curved arrow*) to the fibular styloid process on the fibular head. The fabellofibular ligament (FFL) may be present even in the absence of fabella

(PT), the injury is associated with edema and hemorrhage within the tendon and the musculotendinous junction. On MR images, the partial tear is seen as an amorphous or feathery signal intensity changes that may extend also into the muscle belly (Fig. 4.13).

4.2.2   Complete Tears

In complete tears, there is a discontinuity of the involved anatomical structures that can be associated with waviness of the remaining ligament. In complete LCL tears, there is a discontinuity of the fibers, and edema or hemorrhage of high

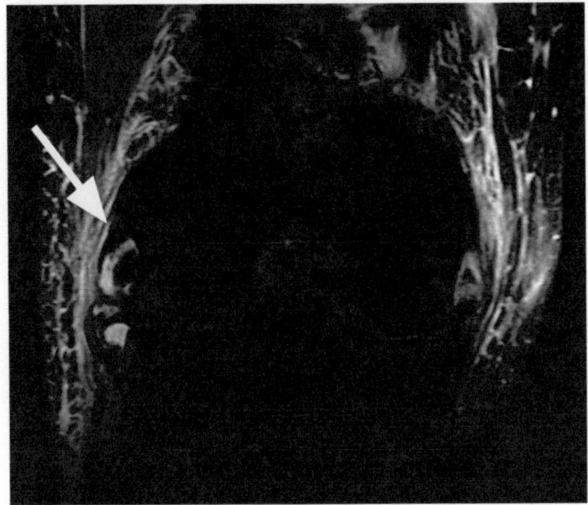

Fig. 4.10 Lateral collateral ligament (LCL) sprain in a 21 year old male. Coronal proton-density (PD) FSE fat-suppressed image shows extensive edema (*arrow*) around the proximal portion of LCL with intact fibers

signal intensity on fluid-sensitive MR images is detected at the tendon defect (Figs. 4.14 and 4.15). A complete discontinuity of the popliteus musculotendinous junction with tendon retraction indicates a complete tear. When a hematoma is present, enlarged muscle volume and perifascial fluid collections are frequently seen [1]. In some cases, avulsion of the femoral insertion of popliteal tendon (PT) may be present.

Individual assessment of the integrity of the anterolateral ligament (ALL), arcuate ligament (AL), popliteofibular ligament (PFL), and fabellofibular ligament (FFL) may not be possible [17]. MR signal abnormalities around the capsule, surrounding soft tissue edema or hemorrhage, and the lack of visualization of these structures are suggestive for popliteomeniscal fascicles (PMF) (Fig. 4.16), anterolateral ligament (ALL), arcuate ligament (AL), and fabellofibular ligament (FFL) tears. Normally, there should be fat tissue in this region which presents as homogeneous low signal intensity on fat-suppressed T2-weighted images (Fig. 4.17). Hyperintense signal on fat-suppressed T2-weighted MR images located posterior to the popliteal tendon (PT) suggests capsular tearing.

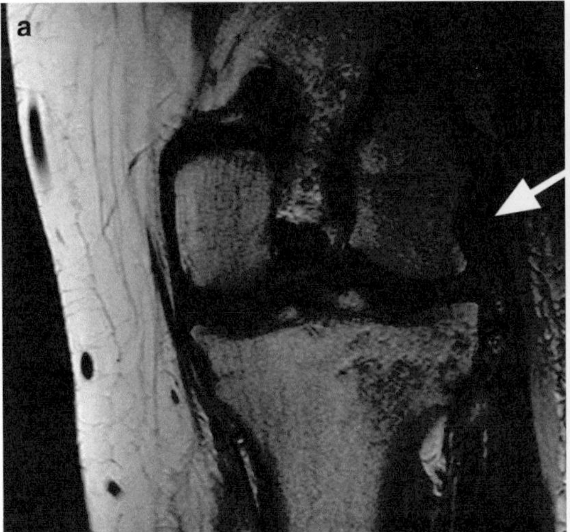
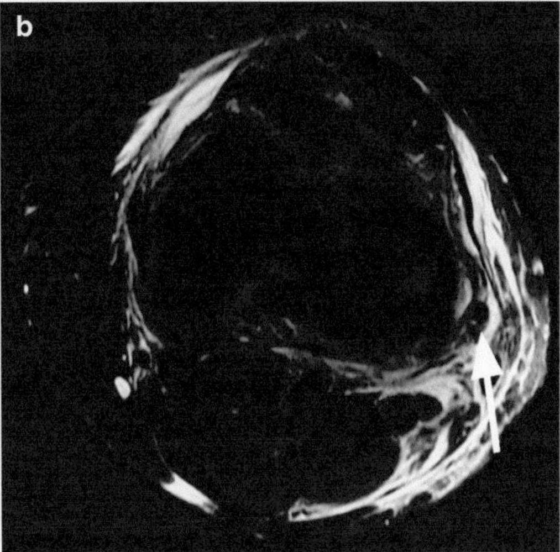

Fig. 4.11 Lateral collateral ligament (LCL) partial tear in a 29 year old female. Coronal proton-density (PD) FSE fat-suppressed image (**a**) shows intrasubstance signal changes (*arrow*) at the proximal insertion of LCL without complete discontinuity of the ligament. The lesion is confirmed on axial proton-density (PD) FSE fat-suppressed image (**b**) where the tear is seen as a hyperintense linear signal lesion within the ligament (*arrow*)

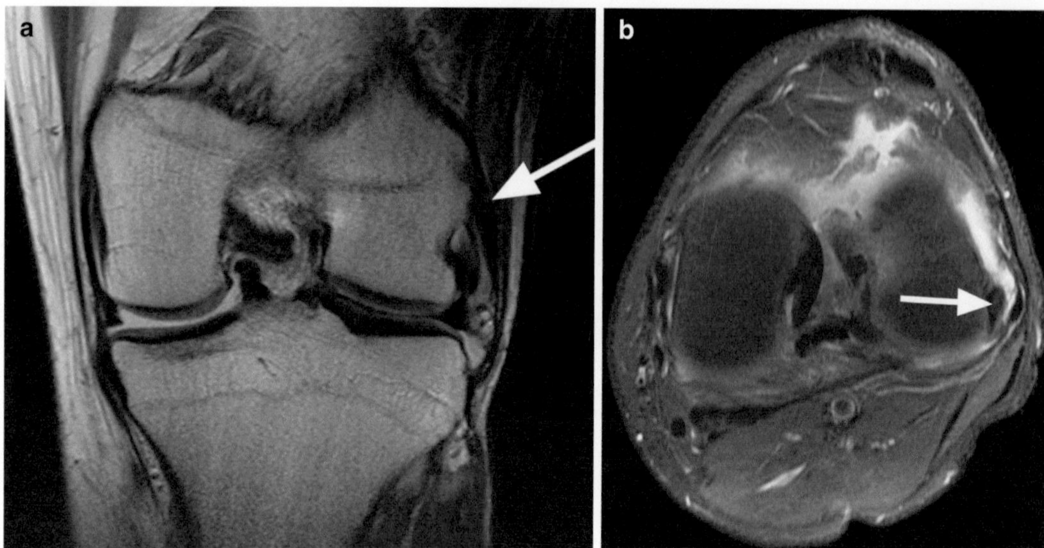

Fig. 4.12 Lateral collateral ligament (LCL) partial tear in a 17 year old male. Coronal proton-density (PD) FSE fat-suppressed image (**a**) and axial proton-density (PD) FSE fat-suppressed image (**b**) show intrasubstance signal changes (*arrow* in **a**, **b**) at the proximal insertion of LCL without complete interruption of the fibers and high-signal-intensity edema around the ligament

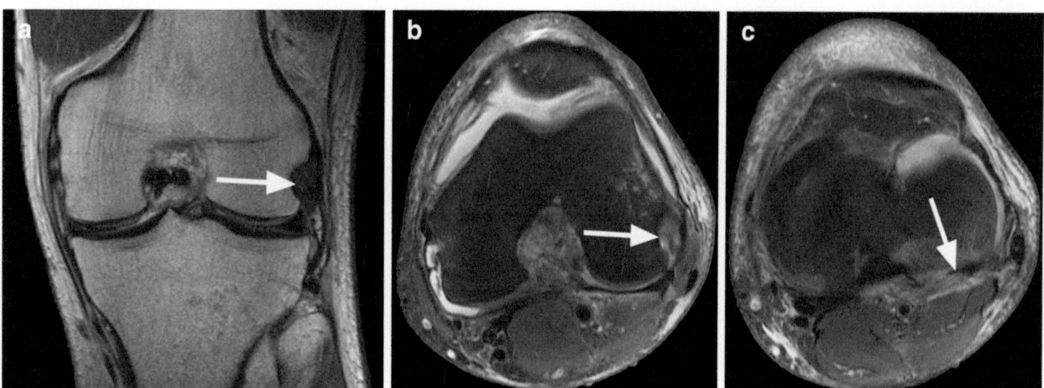

Fig. 4.13 Partial tear of the popliteal tendon (PT) in a 45 year old male. Coronal proton-density (PD) FSE fat-suppressed image (**a**) and axial proton-density (PD) FSE fat-suppressed image at the level of the femoral insertion (**b**) show intrasubstance signal changes (*arrow* in **a**, **b**). The lesion extension is usually better evaluated on serial axial images as in this case in which a more caudally axial (PD) FSE fat-suppressed image (**c**) shows the intrasubstance partial tear (*arrow*)

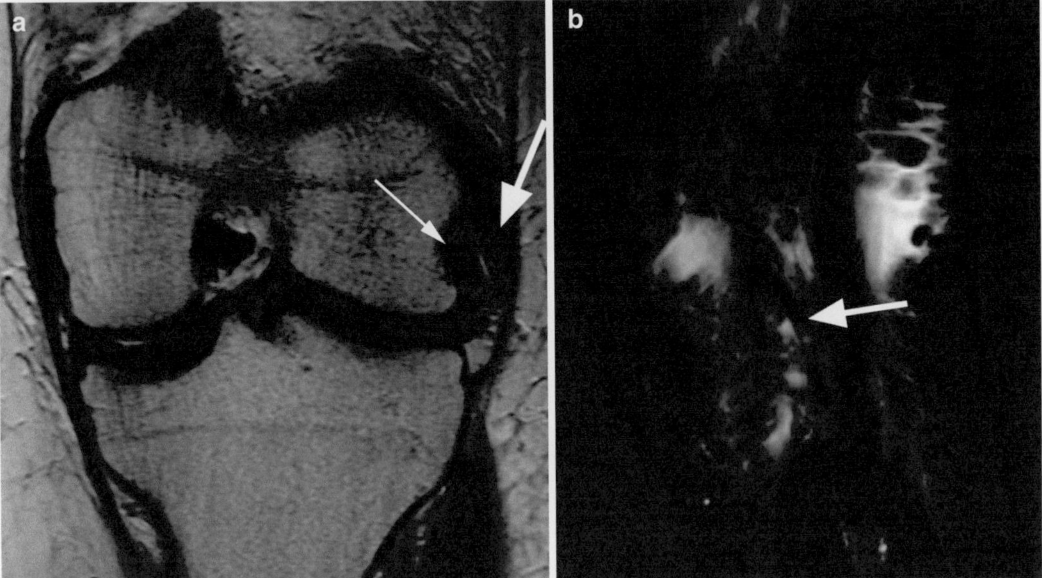

Fig. 4.14 Complete tear of the lateral collateral ligament (LCL) in a 25 year old soccer player. Coronal proton-density (PD) FSE image (**a**) shows discontinuity of the ligament (*large arrow*). Note the normal popliteal tendon (*small arrow*). Sagittal T2-weighted fat-suppressed image (**b**) demonstrates the interruption of the fibers (*arrow*) without a wavy contour of the ligament

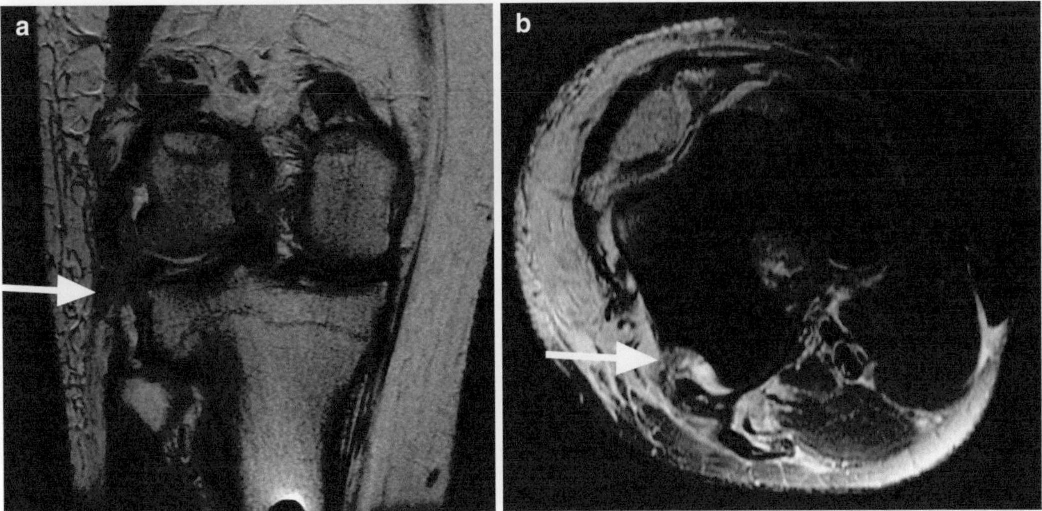

Fig. 4.15 Complete tear of the lateral collateral ligament (LCL) in a 22 year old male. Coronal proton-density (PD) FSE fat-suppressed image (**a**) and axial proton-density (PD) FSE fat-suppressed image (**b**) show a complete tear of LCL with edema or hemorrhage at the site of the lesion (*arrow* in **a, b**)

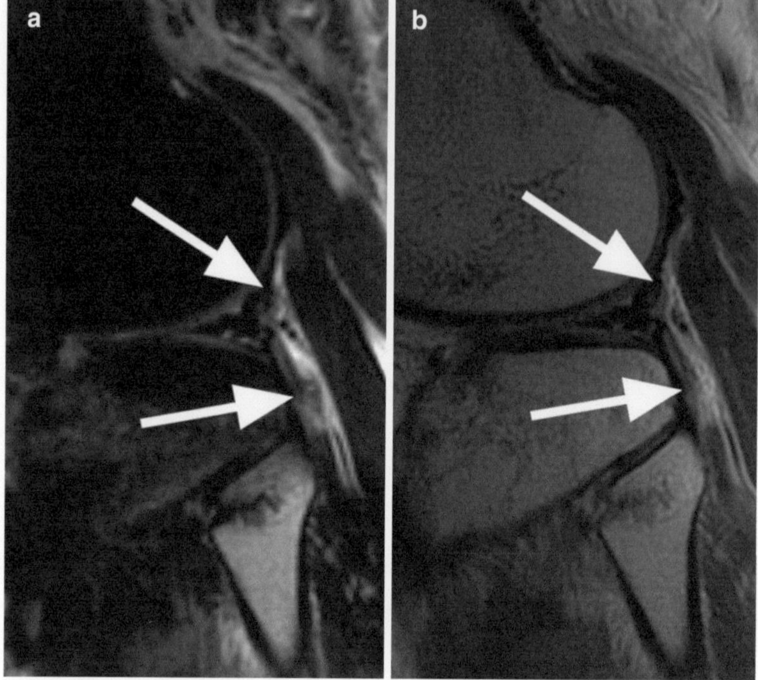

Fig. 4.16 Sagittal T2-weighted fat-suppressed image (**a**) and sagittal proton-density (PD) FSE image (**b**) show signal abnormalities around the capsule (edema) and the lack of visualization of the small posterolateral ligaments (*arrows* in **a**, **b**) suggestive for popliteomeniscal fascicles tears

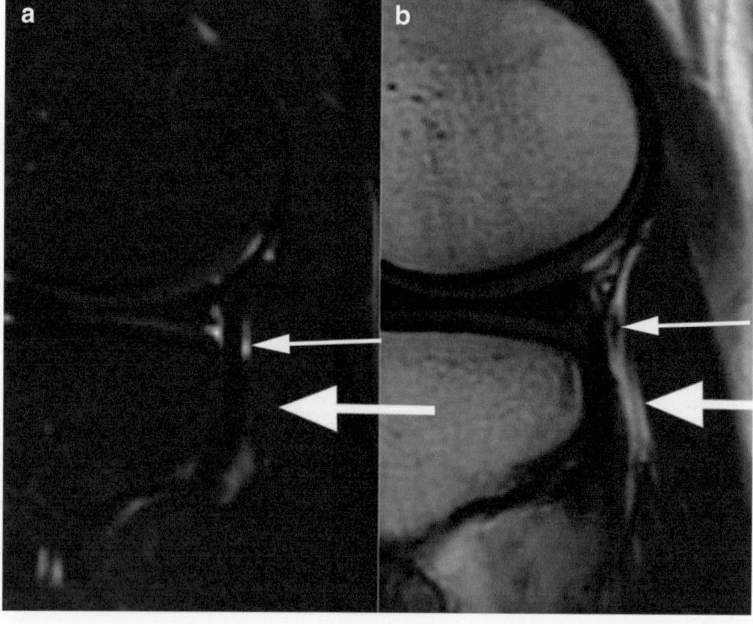

Fig. 4.17 Normal appearance of the postero-lateral capsular region in a 30 year old male. Sagittal T2-weighted fat-suppressed image (**a**) and sagittal proton-density (PD) FSE image (**b**) show the presence of homogeneous fat behind the popliteal tendon (PT) hypointense on fat-suppressed image (*large arrow* in **a**) and hyperintense on proton-density (PD) FSE image (*large arrow* in **b**). Note the presence of a small vessel adjacent to the posterior margin of the popliteal tendon (PT) (*small arrow* in **a**, **b**) which should not be interpreted as edema

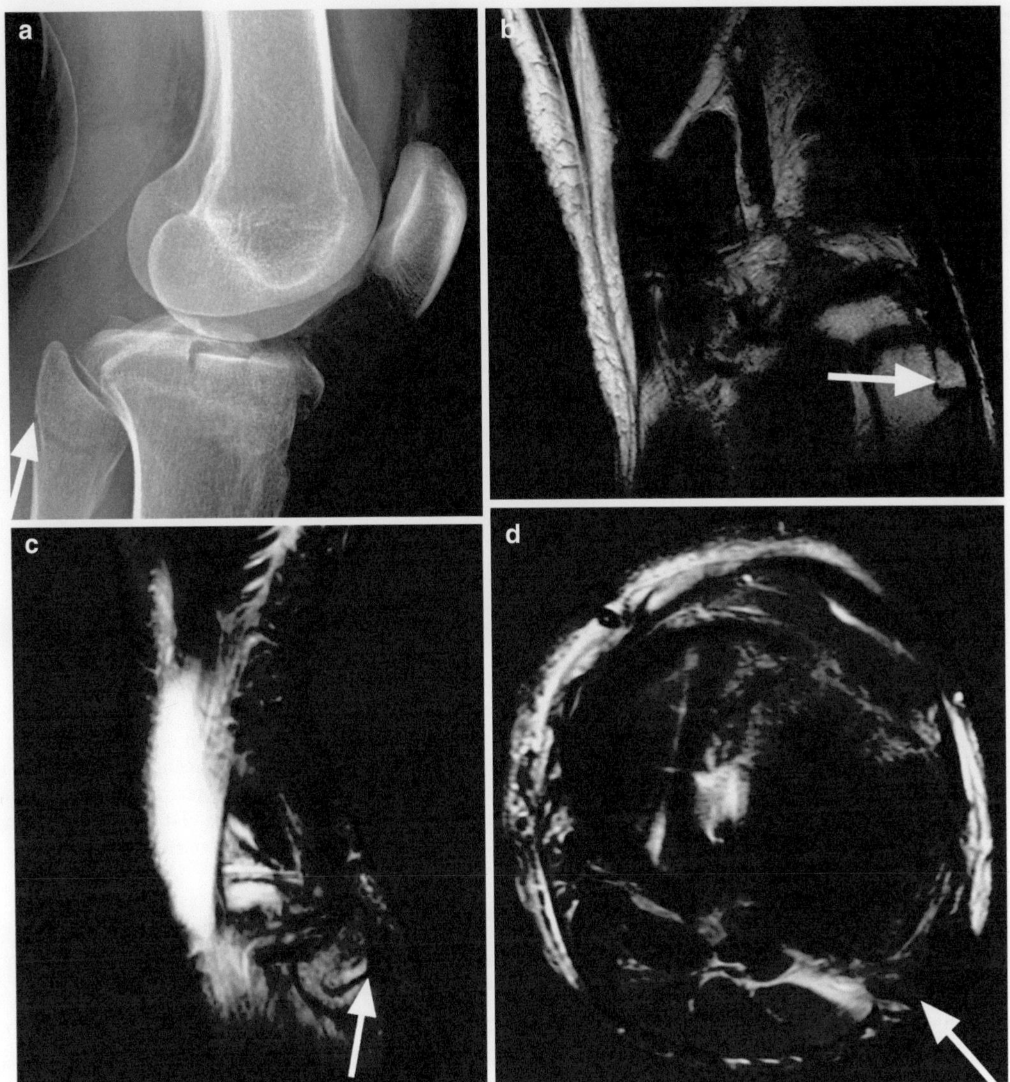

Fig. 4.18 The arcuate sign in a 34 year old male. Plain radiography (**a**) shows a fracture of the fibular head (*arrow*). Coronal proton-density (PD) FSE image (**b**), sagittal T2-weighted fat-suppressed image (**c**), and axial proton-density (PD) FSE fat-suppressed image (**d**) show partial detachment of the bone fragment (*arrow* in **b–d**) at the insertion of the lateral collateral ligament and biceps tendon

4.2.3   The "Arcuate" Sign and the Segond Fracture

The presence of a small bone fragment detached from the proximal head of fibula on radiography is known as the "arcuate" sign (Fig. 4.18). The sign may indicate avulsion of lateral collateral ligament (LCL), biceps tendon (BT), arcuate ligament (AL) (Fig. 4.19), popliteofibular ligament (PFL), or fabellofibular ligament (FFL) from the fibular insertion, and MR imaging is necessary for complete evaluation [1].

The Segond fracture is an avulsion of the lateral capsule from the lateral tibial plateau and may be an indicator of an isolated posterolateral corner injury (Fig. 4.20) [23–25]. The lesion may be also associated with anterior cruciate ligament and posterior cruciate ligament tears.

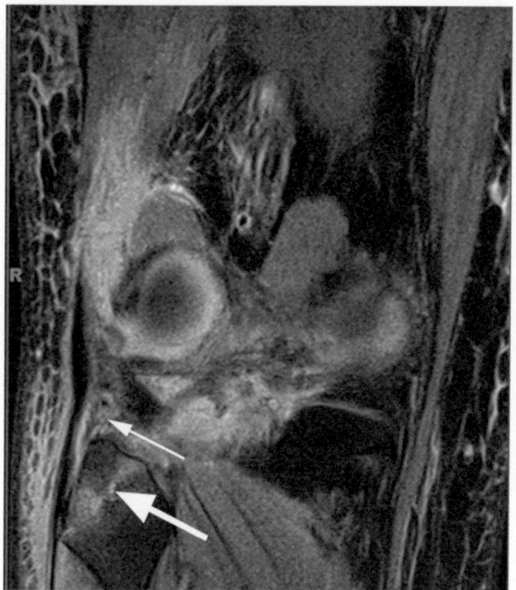

Fig. 4.19 The arcuate sign in a 40 year old female. Coronal proton-density (PD) FSE fat-suppressed image shows the fracture of the fibular head (*large arrow*) with extensive edema in the posterolateral corner. Note the absence of visualization of any band-like structure. In this case, the aspect suggests a tear of the arcuate ligament (AL) (*small arrow*) with loss of its Y shape

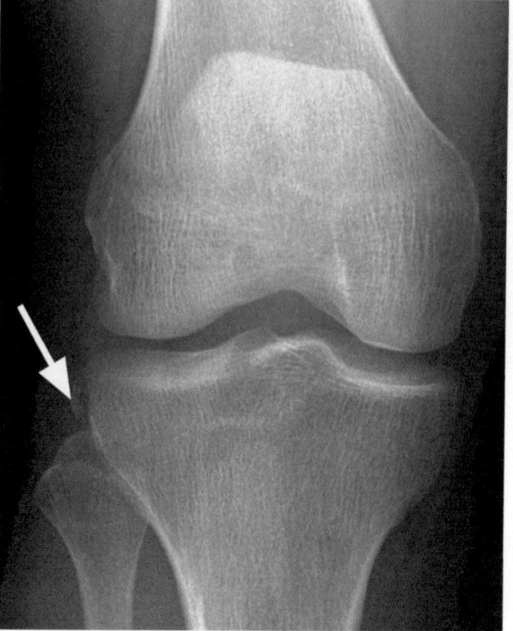

Fig. 4.20 Segond fracture. Plain radiography shows a small bone fragment detached from the lateral tibial plateau from the area of the insertion of the lateral capsule (*arrow*). The MR imaging examination is mandatory in all cases because the Segond fracture may be an indicator of posterolateral corner injuries and always suggest an anterior cruciate ligament involvement

4.3 Role of Preoperative MRI

The structures that need to be identified on the lateral and posterolateral side of the knee on preoperative MRI are the iliotibial band (ITB), lateral collateral ligament (LCL), biceps femoris tendon, popliteus tendon, and capsular structures. Injury may occur to all or a portion of these structures. It is critical, however, to recognize injury to the key stabilizers, such as the lateral collateral ligament, the conjoined tendon of the biceps femoris, and the popliteofibular ligament.

The iliotibial band, the terminal extension of the tensor fascia lata, inserts distally onto Gerdy's tubercle. It is uncommon to injure the iliotibial band. However, any discontinuity or significant injury is indicator for a high-energy injury, and one should look for associated injuries of other structures.

It is more common to injure the structures of the posterolateral corner in combination rather than in isolation [26]. The most frequent combination of injury is a lateral collateral ligament-popliteus injury (52 %) followed by a lateral collateral ligament-popliteus-biceps tendon injury (33 %). It is important to identify the location of the lateral collateral ligament rupture, whether it is at the femoral origin, the midsubstance, or at the proximal fibula. It is also important to identify and describe an avulsion of the biceps femoris tendon, particularly if there is retraction. Failure to recognize and repair an avulsed and retracted conjoined tendon early on may have serious consequences because it is often impossible to reattach a retracted biceps femoris in a delayed surgery or in a chronic rupture.

Meniscal injuries are important to recognize in the context of multiligamentous knee injuries. The high energy involved in this injury pattern frequently results in meniscal damage, including root avulsions [27]. The presence of a displaced meniscal tear may dictate that early intervention is warranted. Meniscal root avulsions may also be overlooked given the complexity of the injury; however, failure to recognize these and address them at the time of surgery may have a negative effect on outcome.

4.4 MRI Postoperative Findings

4.4.1 Indications for Posterolateral Corner Repair/Reconstruction

The indications for treatment of posterolateral corner (PLC) injuries are based on a multitude of factors, including the specific anatomical structures of the posterolateral corner (PLC) that are injured, the grade of injury, the presence of concomitant injuries of the knee, and the period of time since the injury. The indications for treatment and methods of treatment are not universally accepted and remain somewhat controversial. The complexity of this issue is further compounded by the difficulty of establishing a clear diagnosis of posterolateral corner (PLC) injury [28–31]. Failure to recognize an injury to the posterolateral corner (PLC) in the context of a multiligament knee injury has been reported to cause a significant loss of function and, e.g., to contribute to cruciate ligament reconstruction graft failure [21, 28, 32–35]. In contrast, early treatment of these injuries has been shown to be associated with improved objective, subjective, and functional outcomes [10, 32]. This further emphasizes the importance of establishing the diagnosis by early MR imaging.

An accurate diagnosis is achieved by a combination of a detailed history of the injury mechanism, a comprehensive physical examination, and a variety of imaging examinations, including radiographs, CT (in case of fractures of the tibia), and MR imaging. It is of critical importance to investigate for the presence of a vascular injury, which takes precedence in terms of treatment. Following this, any associated nerve injury, in particular damage to the common peroneal nerve, should be ruled out. Next, the grade of the injury according to the International Knee Documentation Committee (IKDC) classification, the specific structures that are damaged including any bony injury, and the chronicity of the injury need to be ascertained. An understanding of the true incidence of posterolateral corner injuries in the context of acute knee injuries is also critical to heighten the awareness and suspicion of this serious injury pattern [34].

4.4.2 Operative Versus Nonoperative Management (Table 4.1)

The treatment of knee dislocations in the literature remains controversial. However, the current evidence-based medicine, although limited to a few level III studies, does support operative management. Surgical treatment of knee dislocations showed improved overall knee function, stability, and patient satisfaction compared to the nonoperative treatment [36].

The best *surgical treatment* of an unstable posterolateral corner (PLC) remains unclear [22, 37]. A number of authors have proposed

Table 4.1 Posterolateral corner injuries – indications for treatment

Grade of injury	Treatment	
Grade I[a]	Conservative management	
Grade II[b]		
	Acute	Chronic
Grade III[c]	Repair ± reconstruction	Reconstruction ± corrective osteotomy

[a]Injuries with minimal instability (either varus 0–5 mm opening or rotational instability 0–5°)
[b]Injuries with moderate instability (either varus 6–10 mm opening or rotational instability 6–10°)
[c]Injuries with significant instability (either varus >10 mm opening or rotational instability >10°)

acute repair of tears of the posterolateral corner if the tissue quality of the torn structures is adequate [22, 38]. If the tissue quality is insufficient or with chronic posterolateral corner (PLC) instability, a wide variety of reconstructive procedures have been advocated to achieve stability. Stannard et al. [39], in a cohort study comparing acute repair versus reconstruction, demonstrated superior results with reconstruction versus repair in the acute setting for high-energy posterolateral corner injuries. The authors recommended that repairs be reserved to treat avulsion fractures with good quality tissue [39]. In reality, a combination of reconstruction and repair is required in most cases of acute high-grade posterolateral corner (PLC) injuries [40].

The timing of surgery may be acute (<3 weeks) or chronic (>6 weeks). In general, operating acutely has been shown by a number of authors to yield better results [41–43]. In patients with bony avulsions or impaction fractures, the earlier the treatment is performed, the easier it is to achieve an anatomical repair or correct the bony deformity. The repair may incorporate reconstruction procedures as well if necessary. The advantages of early, definitive treatment include avoiding the need for multiple procedures, allowing healing of the soft tissue injury, fracture, and reconstruction at the same time, and reducing the potential rehabilitation time. However, it should be considered that early reconstruction is not always possible due to the presence of other significant comorbidities. Injury and retraction of the biceps femoris is a relative indication for early surgical intervention, as delayed treatment may be extremely difficult due to retraction and contracture of the avulsed conjoined tendon of the short and long heads of biceps femoris to the fibular head. Given that multiligamentous injuries are complex and involve a spectrum of injury, some surgeons advocate "staged" surgery. In this setting, the posterolateral corner injuries may be dealt initially, followed by delayed intervention to address the cruciate ligaments [39].

4.4.3 Posterolateral Corner Structures Typically Repaired/Reconstructed

The aim of surgical repair is to reattach any avulsed ligaments or capsular structures to their anatomic location. Avulsion fractures or capsular avulsions are reduced and held in place with a variety of technique, including suture anchors, trans-osseous sutures, and screw fixation. The structures that most frequently require reconstruction are the lateral collateral ligament, the popliteus tendon unit, and the popliteofibular ligament. The choice to proceed with an isolated fibular-based reconstruction or a combined, "two-tailed," reconstruction involving both the fibular head and the proximal tibia is based on whether the proximal tibiofibular joint has been disrupted and the presence of a hyperextension external rotation recurvatum deformity.

There are a number of different surgical techniques described. Fanelli et al. [44] described a combine PCL and PLC reconstruction involving biceps tenodesis with a posterolateral capsular shift and demonstrated significant improvement in knee stability at 2–10-year follow-up. However, Fanelli et al. [45] has reported that this technique is not as effective at controlling posterolateral instability as a fibular-based free graft. Some authors have described a fibular-based reconstruction technique, which is frequently combined with capsular repair or plication [37]. In the recent past, the combination of tibial and fibular reconstruction with the goal of reconstructing the LCL, the popliteus tendon, and the popliteofibular ligament has been proposed and is being increasingly used [39, 46, 47]. Each technique differs slightly in the position of the femoral tunnels and the orientation of the grafts, but with the mutual aim of restoring the tibiofibular joint stability.

4.4.4 Role of Postoperative MRI

Postoperatively, MR imaging is important to identify the integrity of the reconstruction and the presence of any concomitant intra-articular pathology.

In the context of multiligamentous injury, the reconstruction frequently necessitates a number of tunnels in both the femur and tibia. Postoperative graft rupture may occur. Additionally, it is important to take into account other injuries, especially to the menisci, which may have been overlooked acutely because of the extent of soft tissue damage. One should also be aware of the possibility of iatrogenic injury to the meniscal root, which may occur because of aberrant tunnel placement. As with any soft tissue graft reconstruction, tunnel widening may occur over time. Although this may be possible to see on MRI, CT scans may also be required to investigate the location and extent of widening. It is important to be cognizant that in the setting of a failed reconstruction, mechanical malalignment may be a causative factor. Therefore, additional imaging modalities such as three-foot standing films may also be helpful in selected cases.

4.5 MRI Impression

4.5.1 Nonoperative Lateral Collateral Ligament and Posterolateral Corner

Lesions involving well-defined and well-delineated structures:
1. Lateral collateral ligament (LCL) lesions:
   (a) Sprain with intact fibers
   (b) Partial tear of lateral collateral ligament with or without posterolateral corner lesions
   (c) Complete tear of lateral collateral ligament with or without posterolateral corner lesions
2. Popliteus tendon (PT) lesions:
   (a) Partial tear of PT with or without posterolateral corner lesions involving the musculotendinous junction
   (b) Complete tear of PT with or without posterolateral corner lesions
   (c) Avulsion of the femoral insertion of PT
3. Avulsion of the head of fibula ("arcuate" sign) with or without lesions of posterolateral corner (PLC)
4. Segond fracture with or without lesion of posterolateral corner (PLC)

Lesions involving small structures that are inconsistently present and that are part of the capsule
1. Probably torn based on indirect signs (edema, hemorrhage, lack of visualization)

4.5.2 Postoperative Lateral Collateral Ligament and Posterolateral Corner

1. Normal postoperative MRI – normal positioning of the tunnels without any signs of postoperative complications
2. Postoperative graft tears
3. Tunnel or tunnel widening
4. Normal menisci or postoperative meniscal injuries (iatrogenic meniscal root injuries)

References

1. Bolog N, Hodler J. MR imaging of the posterolateral corner of the knee. Skeletal Radiol. 2007;36(8):715–28.
2. Wang CJ, Walker PS. The effects of flexion and rotation on the length patterns of the ligaments of the knee. J Biomech. 1973;6(6):587–96.
3. LaPrade RF, Hamilton CD. The fibular collateral ligament-biceps femoris bursa. An anatomic study. Am J Sports Med. 1997;25(4):439–43.
4. Meister BR, et al. Anatomy and kinematics of the lateral collateral ligament of the knee. Am J Sports Med. 2000;28(6):869–78.
5. De Maeseneer M, et al. Posterolateral supporting structures of the knee: findings on anatomic dissection, anatomic slices and MR images. Eur Radiol. 2001;11(11):2170–7.
6. Sugita T, Amis AA. Anatomic and biomechanical study of the lateral collateral and popliteofibular ligaments. Am J Sports Med. 2001;29(4):466–72.
7. Davies H, Unwin A, Aichroth P. The posterolateral corner of the knee. Anatomy, biomechanics and management of injuries. Injury. 2004;35(1):68–75.
8. Munshi M, et al. MR imaging, MR arthrography, and specimen correlation of the posterolateral corner of the knee: an anatomic study. AJR Am J Roentgenol. 2003;180(4):1095–101.
9. Brinkman JM, et al. The insertion geometry of the posterolateral corner of the knee. J Bone Joint Surg Br. 2005;87(10):1364–8.
10. DeLee JC, Riley MB, Rockwood Jr CA. Acute posterolateral rotatory instability of the knee. Am J Sports Med. 1983;11(4):199–207.

11. Beall DP, et al. Magnetic resonance imaging of the collateral ligaments and the anatomic quadrants of the knee. Radiol Clin North Am. 2007;45(6):983–1002, vi.
12. Diamantopoulos A, et al. The posterolateral corner of the knee: evaluation under microsurgical dissection. Arthroscopy. 2005;21(7):826–33.
13. Recondo JA, et al. Lateral stabilizing structures of the knee: functional anatomy and injuries assessed with MR imaging. Radiographics. 2000;20(Spec No): S91–102.
14. De Maeseneer M, et al. Normal anatomy and pathology of the posterior capsular area of the knee: findings in cadaveric specimens and in patients. AJR Am J Roentgenol. 2004;182(4):955–62.
15. Vincent JP, et al. The anterolateral ligament of the human knee: an anatomic and histologic study. Knee Surg Sports Traumatol Arthrosc. 2012;20(1):147–52.
16. Sussmann PS, et al. Development of the popliteomeniscal fasciculi in the fetal human knee joint. Arthroscopy. 2001;17(1):14–8.
17. Huang GS, et al. Avulsion fracture of the head of the fibula (the "arcuate" sign): MR imaging findings predictive of injuries to the posterolateral ligaments and posterior cruciate ligament. AJR Am J Roentgenol. 2003;180(2):381–7.
18. Stannard JP, et al. Reconstruction of the posterolateral corner of the knee. Arthroscopy. 2005;21(9):1051–9.
19. Terry GC, LaPrade RF. The posterolateral aspect of the knee. Anatomy and surgical approach. Am J Sports Med. 1996;24(6):732–9.
20. Watanabe Y, et al. Functional anatomy of the posterolateral structures of the knee. Arthroscopy. 1993;9(1): 57–62.
21. O'Brien SJ, et al. Reconstruction of the chronically insufficient anterior cruciate ligament with the central third of the patellar ligament. J Bone Joint Surg Am. 1991;73(2):278–86.
22. Covey DC. Injuries of the posterolateral corner of the knee. J Bone Joint Surg Am. 2001;83-A(1):106–18.
23. Seebacher JR, et al. The structure of the posterolateral aspect of the knee. J Bone Joint Surg Am. 1982;64(4):536–41.
24. Dietz GW, Wilcox DM, Montgomery JB. Segond tibial condyle fracture: lateral capsular ligament avulsion. Radiology. 1986;159(2):467–9.
25. Robertson A, Nutton RW, Keating JF. Dislocation of the knee. J Bone Joint Surg Br. 2006;88(6):706–11.
26. Becker EH, Watson JD, Dreese JC. Investigation of multiligamentous knee injury patterns with associated injuries presenting at a level I trauma center. J Orthop Trauma. 2013;27(4):226–31.
27. Koenig JH, et al. Meniscal root tears: diagnosis and treatment. Arthroscopy. 2009;25(9):1025–32.
28. Hughston JC, et al. Classification of knee ligament instabilities. Part I. The medial compartment and cruciate ligaments. J Bone Joint Surg Am. 1976;58(2):159–72.
29. DeHaven KE. Diagnosis of acute knee injuries with hemarthrosis. Am J Sports Med. 1980;8(1):9–14.
30. Hughston JC, Jacobson KE. Chronic posterolateral rotatory instability of the knee. J Bone Joint Surg Am. 1985;67(3):351–9.
31. LaPrade RF, Terry GC. Injuries to the posterolateral aspect of the knee. Association of anatomic injury patterns with clinical instability. Am J Sports Med. 1997; 25(4):433–8.
32. Baker Jr CL, Norwood LA, Hughston JC. Acute posterolateral rotatory instability of the knee. J Bone Joint Surg Am. 1983;65(5):614–8.
33. LaPrade RF, et al. The effects of grade III posterolateral knee complex injuries on anterior cruciate ligament graft force. A biomechanical analysis. Am J Sports Med. 1999;27(4):469–75.
34. LaPrade RF, et al. The magnetic resonance imaging appearance of individual structures of the posterolateral knee. A prospective study of normal knees and knees with surgically verified grade III injuries. Am J Sports Med. 2000;28(2):191–9.
35. Noyes FR, Barber-Westin SD. Revision anterior cruciate surgery with use of bone-patellar tendon-bone autogenous grafts. J Bone Joint Surg Am. 2001;83-A(8):1131–43.
36. Wong CH, et al. Knee dislocations-a retrospective study comparing operative versus closed immobilization treatment outcomes. Knee Surg Sports Traumatol Arthrosc. 2004;12(6):540–4.
37. Veltri DM, Warren RF. Operative treatment of posterolateral instability of the knee. Clin Sports Med. 1994;13(3):615–27.
38. Clancy Jr WG, Shepard MF, Cain Jr EL. Posterior lateral corner reconstruction. Am J Orthop (Belle Mead NJ). 2003;32(4):171–6.
39. Stannard JP, et al. The posterolateral corner of the knee: repair versus reconstruction. Am J Sports Med. 2005;33(6):881–8.
40. Geeslin AG, LaPrade RF. Outcomes of treatment of acute grade-III isolated and combined posterolateral knee injuries: a prospective case series and surgical technique. J Bone Joint Surg Am. 2011;93(18):1672–83.
41. Ibrahim SA. Primary repair of the cruciate and collateral ligaments after traumatic dislocation of the knee. J Bone Joint Surg Br. 1999;81(6):987–90.
42. Wang CJ, et al. Outcome of surgical reconstruction for posterior cruciate and posterolateral instabilities of the knee. Injury. 2002;33(9):815–21.
43. Liow RY, et al. Ligament repair and reconstruction in traumatic dislocation of the knee. J Bone Joint Surg Br. 2003;85(6):845–51.
44. Fanelli GC, Edson CJ. Combined posterior cruciate ligament-posterolateral reconstructions with Achilles tendon allograft and biceps femoris tendon tenodesis: 2- to 10-year follow-up. Arthroscopy. 2004;20(4):339–45.
45. Fanelli GC, et al. Treatment of combined anterior cruciate-posterior cruciate ligament-medial-lateral side knee injuries. J Knee Surg. 2005;18(3):240–8.
46. LaPrade RF, et al. An analysis of an anatomical posterolateral knee reconstruction: an in vitro biomechanical study and development of a surgical technique. Am J Sports Med. 2004;32(6):1405–14.
47. Noyes FR, Barber-Westin SD. Posterolateral knee reconstruction with an anatomical bone-patellar tendon-bone reconstruction of the fibular collateral ligament. Am J Sports Med. 2007;35(2):259–73.

Meniscus

5

Nicolae Bolog, Gustav Andreisek, and Erika Ulbrich

5.1 Anatomy and Normal MRI Appearance

The menisci and their insertions into bone represent a fibrocartilaginous functional unit [1]. Their function is to distribute loads and to protect the cartilage and the subchondral bone. They measure approximately 35 mm in diameter and are divided into anterior horn, posterior horn, and body of meniscus. Both menisci are hypovascular and contain mainly water and a dense elaborate type I collagen network with a predominantly circumferential alignment [1]. The vascular supply is provided by branches of lateral, medial, and middle genicular arteries. A perimeniscal capillary plexus originating in the capsular and synovial tissues of the joint supplies the peripheral 10–33 % of the menisci [2, 3]. Both menisci are interconnected and are separately attached to the capsule and anchored to the adjacent bone structures. The tibial attachment of the menisci are known as the meniscal root ligaments. On MR images menisci are seen as homogeneous low-signal intensity structures on all sequences (Fig. 5.1).

5.1.1 Medial Meniscus

The medial meniscus has a more open C-shaped structure than the lateral meniscus, covers approximately 60 % of the corresponding tibial plateau and is wider posteriorly than anteriorly (Fig. 5.1) [1]. In a loaded, in vitro situation, 50% of the axial load in the medial compartment is absorbed by the medial meniscus [4].

Capsular Attachments

The medial meniscus is intimately attached to the knee capsule along its entire circumference. The meniscofemoral, the meniscotibial, and the meniscopatellar ligaments are the structures that defines the deep layer (layer 3) of the medial collateral ligament. *The meniscofemoral ligament* is seen on MR images as a thin band that originates from the superior margin of the body of the medial meniscus and inserts on the femoral condyle 1–2 cm above the joint line (Fig. 5.2) [5]. *The meniscotibial ligament* is shorter and connects the inferior margin of the medial meniscus to tibial cortex inferior to the joint line (Fig. 5.2) [5]. The meniscotibial ligament extends along the entire circumference of the posteromedial edge of the meniscus and further form the deepest layer of the capsule and is also called the coronary ligament or the meniscocapsular ligament. *The patellomeniscal ligament* is seen on MR images anteriorly from the medial meniscus to the patellar margin (Fig. 5.3) [6]. A small bursa, known as medial posterior femoral recess or medial gastrocnemius bursa separates the posterior horn of the medial meniscus from the joint capsule [7].

Bone Attachments

The anterior and posterior horns are firmly attached to bone through the insertional ligaments known as the meniscal root ligaments. The tibial

N.V. Bolog et al., *MRI of the Knee: A Guide to Evaluation and Reporting*,
DOI 10.1007/978-3-319-08165-6_5, © Springer International Publishing Switzerland 2015

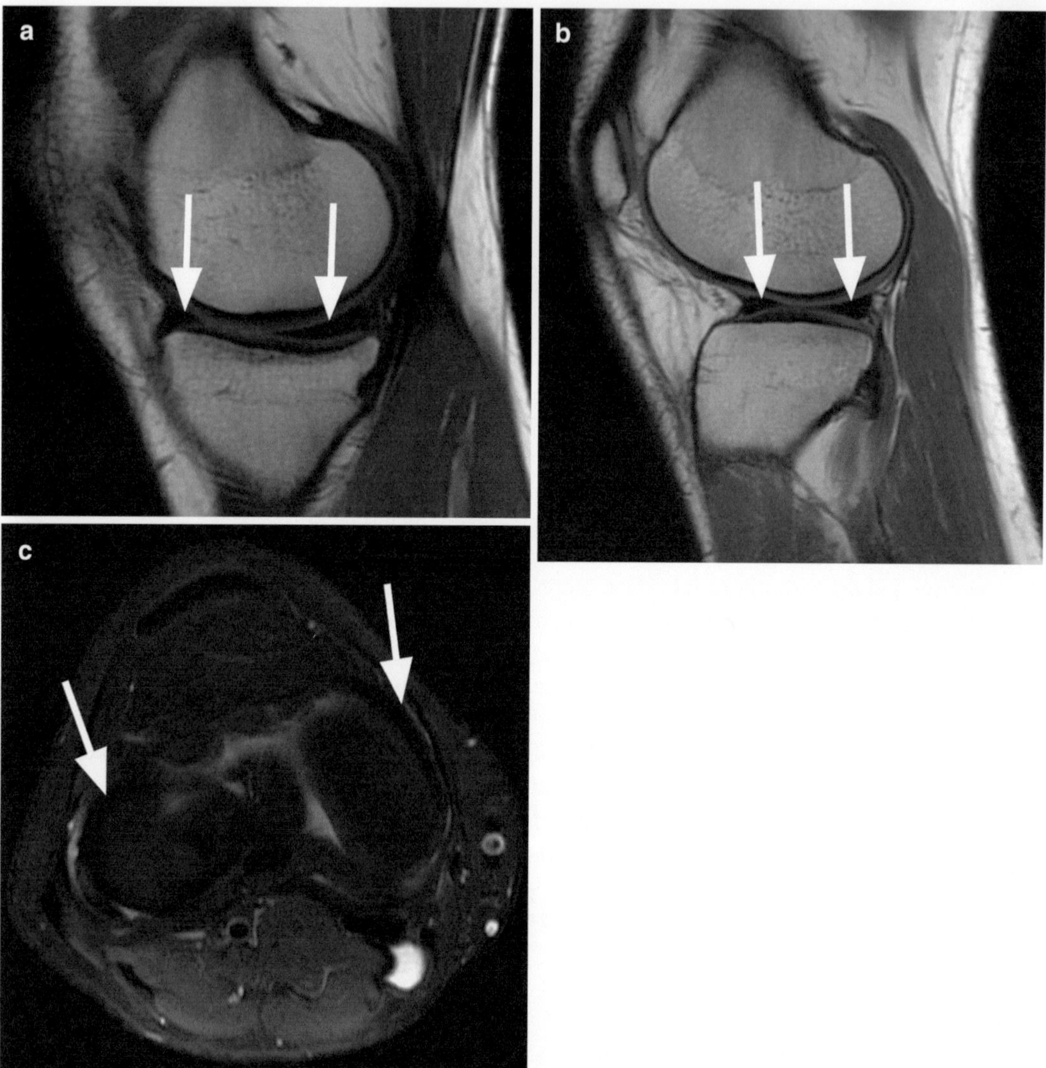

Fig. 5.1 Normal menisci in a 19 year old female. Sagittal proton-density (PD) FSE image through the medial compartment (**a**) shows the medial meniscus which is wider posteriorly than anteriorly (*arrows*). Sagittal proton-density (PD) FSE image through the lateral compartment (**b**) shows the normal homogeneous hypointense anterior and posterior horn of the lateral meniscus (*arrows*). A complete evaluation of the meniscus should include axial images as shown in the axial proton-density (PD) FSE fat-suppressed image (*arrows* in **c**)

attachment of the anterior horn of the medial meniscus or the anterior medial root ligament is situated at the intercondylar fossa, 6–7 mm anteriorly to the anterior cruciate ligament (ACL) attachment (Fig. 5.4) [8]. The posterior medial root ligament attaches the posterior horn of the medial meniscus with the posterior intercondylar tibial fossa (Fig. 5.4). The attachment site is situated between the insertion of the posterior lateral root ligament and the insertion of posterior cruciate ligament (PCL) (Fig. 5.4) [1]. Both, the anterior and posterior ligaments, are larger that those of the lateral meniscus. The meniscal roots are defined on MR imaging as the last few millimeters of meniscal tissue angling down to the tibial plateau attachment in the intercondylar notch and are visible on axial, sagittal, and coronal planes (Figs. 5.4 and 5.5) [9].

Inconsistently, a medial anterior meniscofemoral ligament may be present connecting the anterior horn of the medial meniscus to the lateral wall of the intercondylar fossa of the femur [10].

Intermeniscal Connections

The anterior transverse ligament, also known as *the geniculate ligament*, connects the anterior horns of the medial and lateral meniscus. Medially the transverse ligament blends with the posterior attachment of the anterior medial root ligament. There is an association between the presence of a transvers ligament's attachment and the presence of tears in the medial meniscus [11]. The ligament is inconsistently present and is best seen on sagittal and coronal MR images

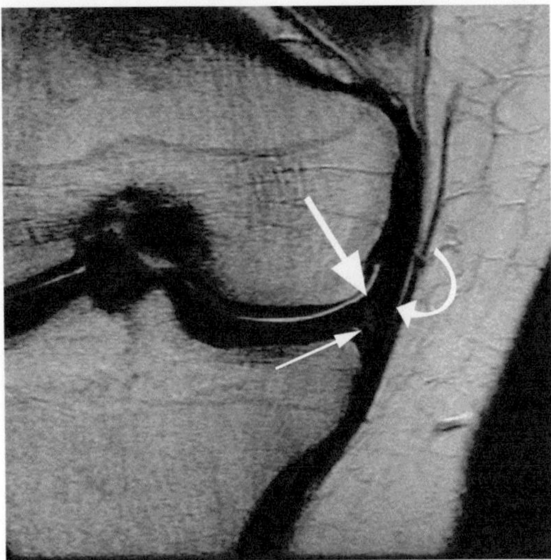

Fig. 5.2 Meniscofemoral and meniscotibial ligaments in a 22 year old male. Coronal proton-density (PD) FSE image shows the meniscofemoral ligament inserting on the femoral condyle and the superior margin of the body of the medial meniscus (*large arrow*) and the shorter meniscotibial ligament (*small arrow*) which connects the inferior margin of the medial meniscus to tibia. Both ligaments are structures of the deep layer of medial collateral ligament (*curved arrow*)

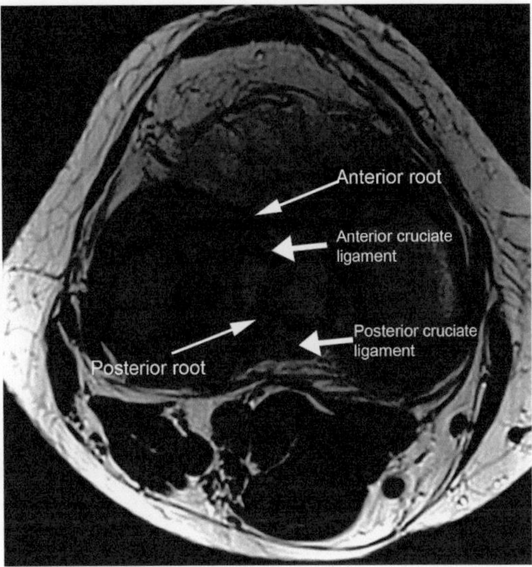

Fig. 5.4 Axial (PD) FSE image shows the anterior medial root ligament anteriorly to the anterior cruciate ligament. The posterior root of the medial meniscus is situated between the insertion of anterior cruciate ligament and the insertion of posterior cruciate ligament

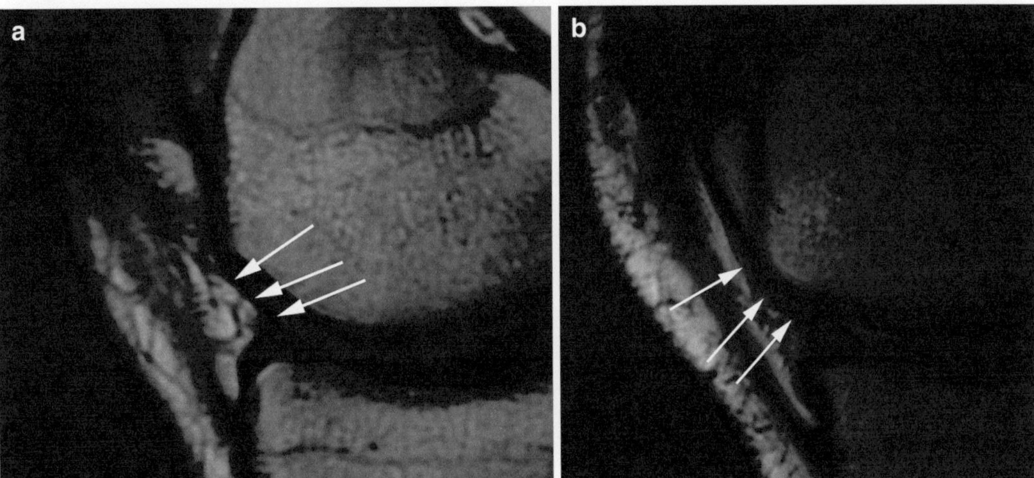

Fig. 5.3 Patellomeniscal ligament. Sagittal proton-density (PD) FSE images in a 22 year old male (**a**) and 19 year old female (**b**) show the patellomeniscal ligament (*arrows*) anteriorly, connecting the medial meniscus to the patellar margin. The ligament is hard to see on one image. Usually, dynamic view over multiple images is needed

(Fig. 5.6) [12]. *The posterior transverse ligament* is much more rarely present than the anterior transverse ligament. It connects the posterior horns of the medial and lateral meniscus and is seen on MR images, when present, on coronal plane in front of the posterior cruciate ligament. Inconsistently, *two oblique meniscomeniscal ligaments* may be recognized on MR images [13]. The oblique ligaments extends from the anterior horn of the medial meniscus to the posterior horn

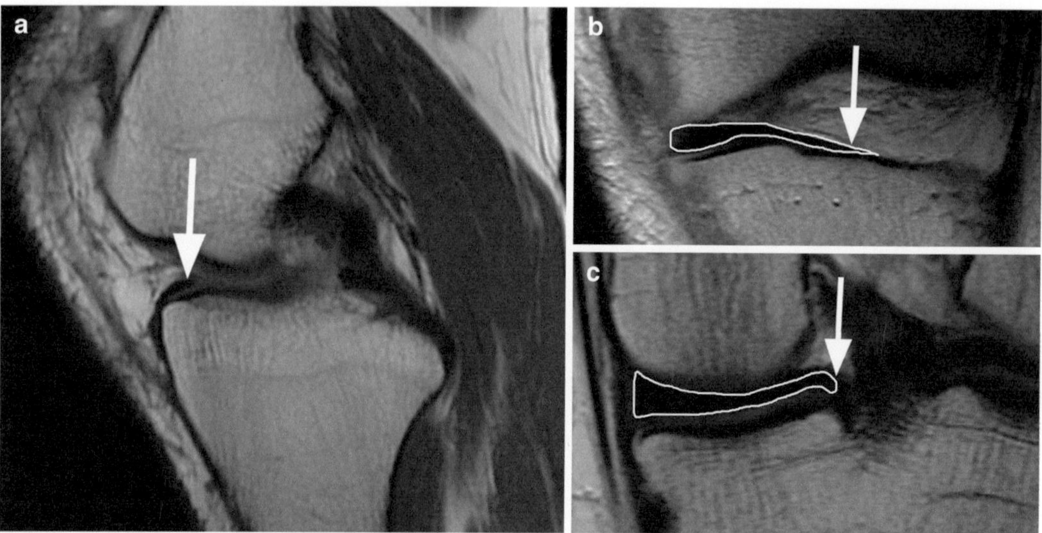

Fig. 5.5 The anterior and posterior medial roots ligaments. Sagittal proton-density (PD) FSE image (**a**) shows the anterior root ligament of the medial meniscus (*arrow*). Coronal proton-density (PD) FSE image (**b**) shows the most anterior segment of the anterior horn of the medial meniscus and enables the evaluation of its anterior root ligament (*arrow*). Coronal proton-density (PD) FSE image through the posterior knee joint (**c**) shows the posterior horn of the medial meniscus and its posterior root ligament (*arrow*)

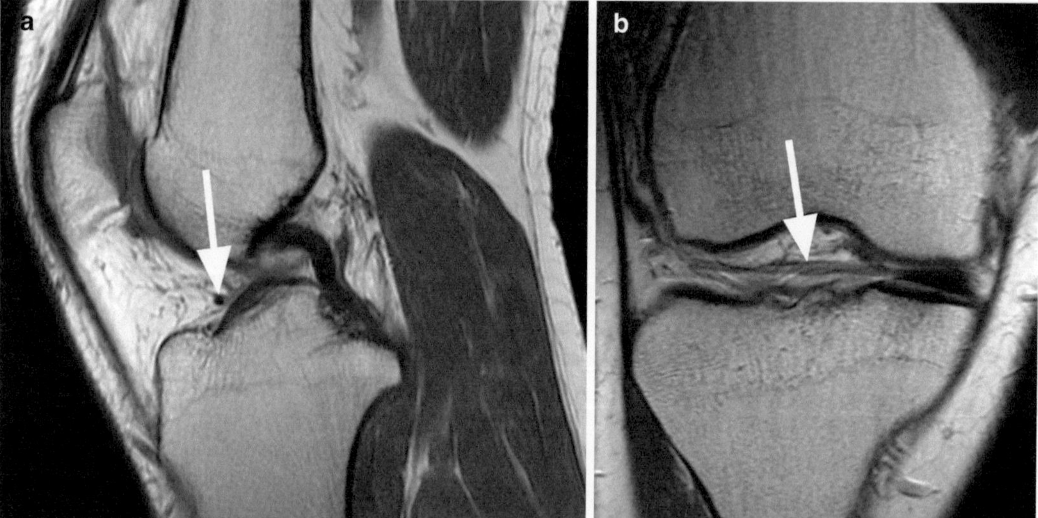

Fig. 5.6 The anterior transverse ligament or the geniculate ligament. Sagittal proton-density (PD) FSE image (**a**), coronal proton-density (PD) FSE image (**b**), and axial (PD) FSE fat-suppressed image (**c**) show the ligament which connects the anterior horns of the medial and lateral meniscus (*arrows*)

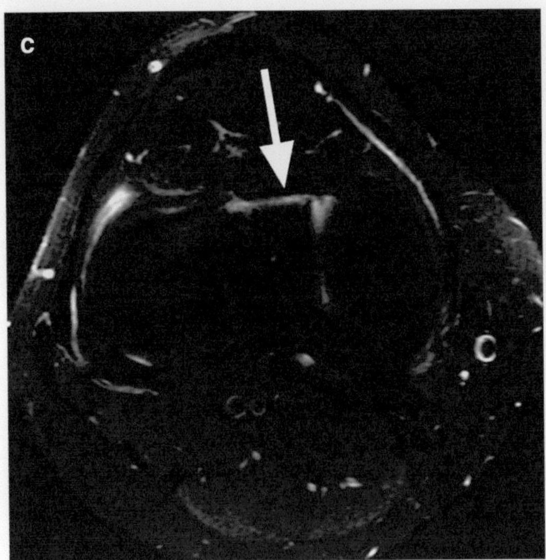

Fig. 5.6 (continued)

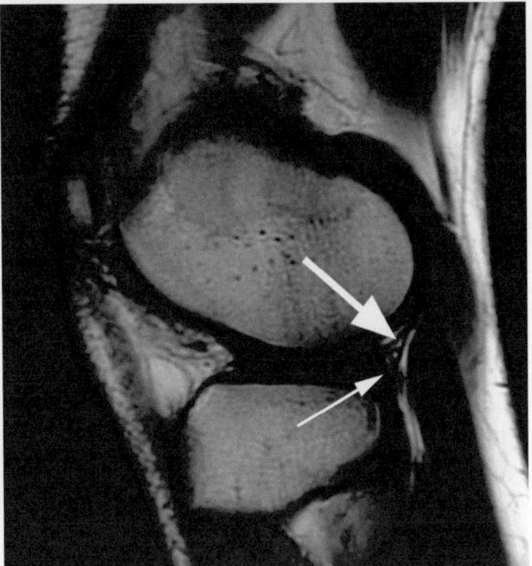

Fig. 5.8 The popliteomeniscal fascicles (PMF). Sagittal (PD) FSE image shows both ligaments. The posterosuperior PMF extends from the posterolateral aspect of the lateral meniscus to the popliteus tendon (*large arrow*). The anteroinferior PMF extends from the middle third of the lateral meniscus to the popliteus tendon (*small arrow*)

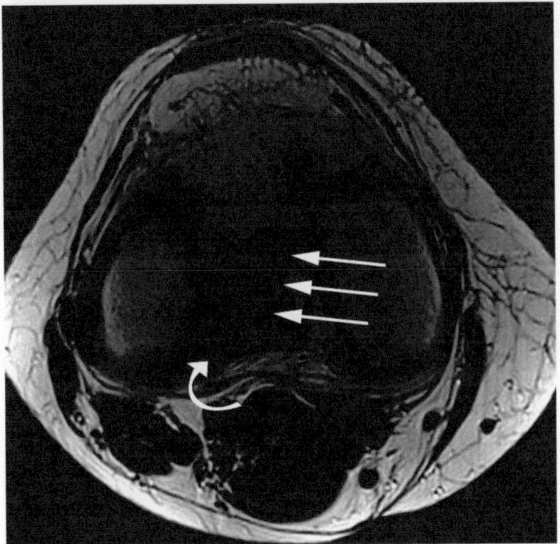

Fig. 5.7 Axial (PD) FSE image shows the lateral oblique ligament (*arrows*) which connects the posterior horn of the medial meniscus (*curved arrow*) with the anterior horn of the lateral meniscus

of the lateral meniscus (medial oblique ligament) and from the anterior horn of the lateral meniscus to the posterior horn of the medial meniscus (lateral oblique ligament) (Fig. 5.7) [13].

5.1.2 Lateral Meniscus

The lateral meniscus is more circular O-shaped than the medial meniscus and covers 80 % of the corre-

sponding tibial plateau [1]. Its width is constant from anterior to posterior. In a loaded, in vitro situation, 70% of the axial load in the lateral compartment is absorbed by the lateral meniscus [4]. The lateral meniscus is more mobile than the medial meniscus and, compared to the medial meniscus, has a loose attachment to the knee capsule and no attachment to the lateral collateral ligament.

Popliteomeniscal Fascicles (PMF)

The lateral meniscus is strongly attached to the popliteus tendon (PT) through the two popliteomeniscal fascicles (PMF) that are part of the posterolateral corner of the knee. On MR images the PMF are inconsistently seen as hypointense structures on sagital planes (Fig. 5.8) [14]. The posterosuperior PMF extends from the posterolateral aspect of the lateral meniscus to the PT (Fig. 5.8) and the anteroinferior PMF extends from the middle third of the lateral meniscus to the PT (Fig. 5.8). The anteroinferior PMF is stronger and shorter than the posterosuperior PMF [15, 16]. The PMF are situated around the popliteus bursa which is a synovial space adjacent to the posterior horn of the lateral meniscus [17, 18].

Bone and Capsular Attachments

The lateral meniscotibial ligament also known as *the coronary ligament or the meniscocapsular ligament* connects the lateral meniscus to the tibia along the entire circumference of the lateral meniscus.

The posterior horn of the lateral meniscus attaches to the medial femoral condyle through *the meniscofemoral ligaments*. The posterior meniscofemoral ligament (Wrisberg ligament) extends from the posterior horn of the meniscus to the medial femoral condyle proximal to the posterior cruciate (PCL) insertion (Fig. 5.9). The anterior meniscofemoral ligament (Humphrey ligament) attaches on the medial femoral condyle, inferior to the PCL insertion (Fig. 5.10). Many variations of these ligaments have been reported and the incidence of the presence of one or the other ligament is 70–100 % [19].

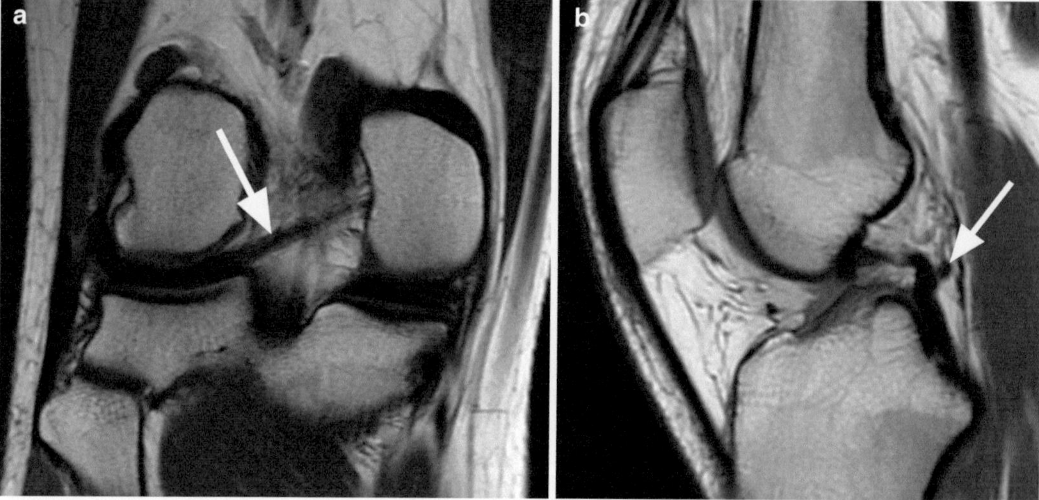

Fig. 5.9 Posterior meniscofemoral ligament (Wrisberg ligament). Coronal proton-density (PD) FSE image (**a**) and sagittal proton-density (PD) FSE image (**b**) show the posterior meniscofemoral ligament (*arrow*). On the coronal image (**a**) the entire length of the ligament is visualised

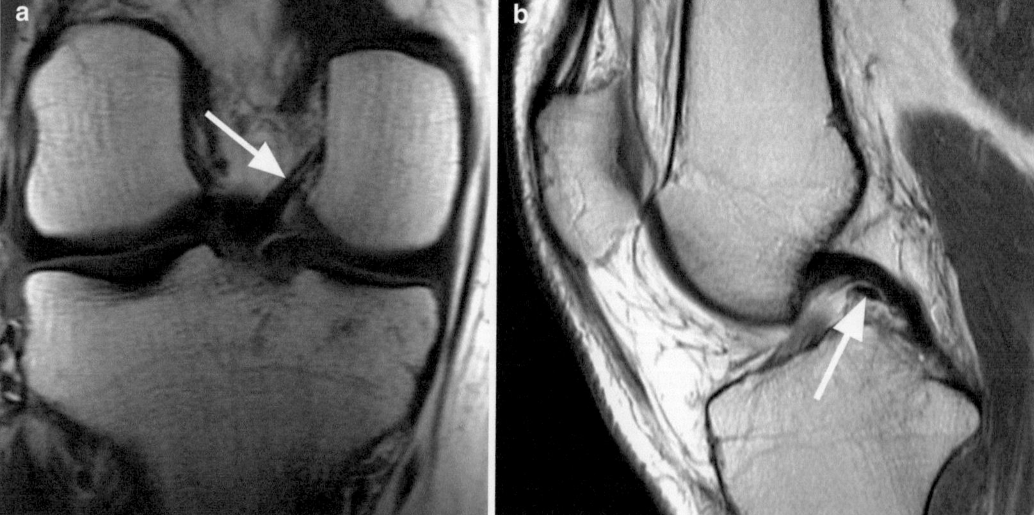

Fig. 5.10 Anterior meniscofemoral ligament (Humphrey ligament). Coronal proton-density (PD) FSE image (**a**) and sagittal proton-density (PD) FSE image (**b**) show the anterior meniscofemoral ligament (*arrow*)

The lateral meniscus is attached to the tibia by *the lateral root ligaments*. The anterior lateral meniscal root ligament attaches the anterior horn of the lateral meniscus to the lateral intercondylar tibial eminence just behind the anterior cruciate ligament (ACL) insertion (Figs. 5.11 and 5.12) [1]. The posterior root ligament of the lateral meniscus attaches posterior to the lateral intercondylar tibial eminence anterior to the posterior root ligament of the posterior horn of the medial meniscus (Figs. 5.11 and 5.12).

A *meniscofibular ligament* was described connecting the lateral meniscus to the proximal fibula [20]. This ligament is located anterior to the popliteus tendon and is intra-capsular.

Intermeniscal Connections
See Sect. 5.1.1.

5.1.3 Normal Variants – Meniscal Flounce

The medial meniscal flounce is a normal positional variant characterized by a single symmetric fold along the free edge of the meniscus [21, 22]. The flounce is less commonly seen on MRI

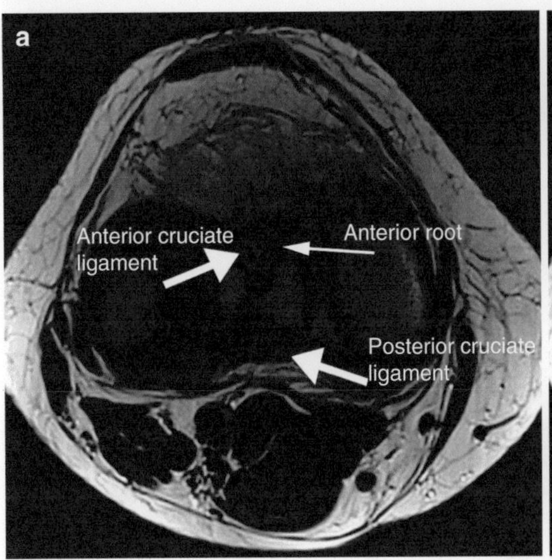

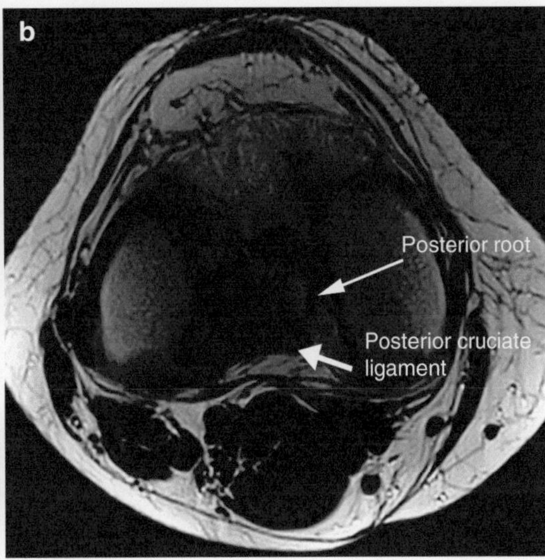

Fig. 5.11 Two consecutive axial (PD) FSE images show the anterior lateral root ligament which inserts posteriorly to the anterior cruciate ligament (**a**) and the posterior root of the lateral meniscus which inserts near the posterior cruciate ligament (**b**)

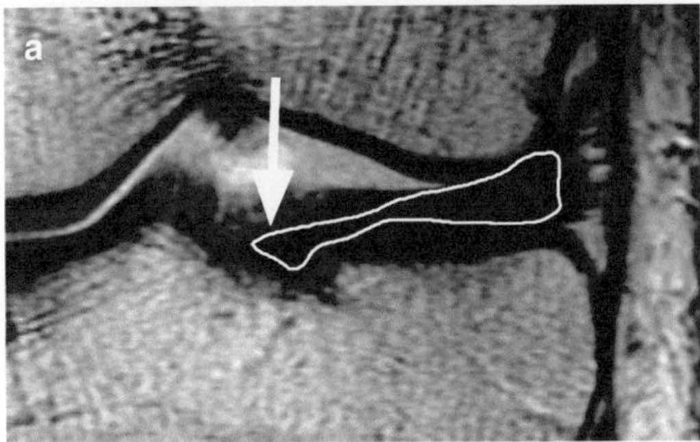

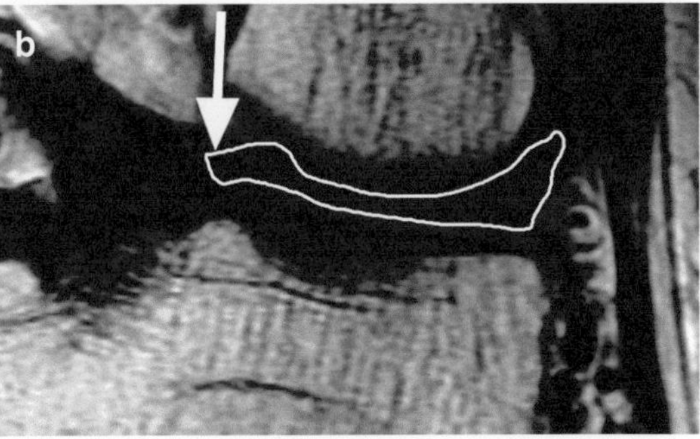

Fig. 5.12 The anterior and posterior lateral roots ligaments. Coronal proton-density (PD) FSE image (**a**) shows the most anterior segment of the anterior horn of the lateral meniscus and enables the evaluation of its anterior root ligament (*arrow*). Coronal proton-density (PD) FSE image through the posterior knee joint (**b**) shows the posterior horn of the lateral meniscus and its posterior root ligament (*arrow*)

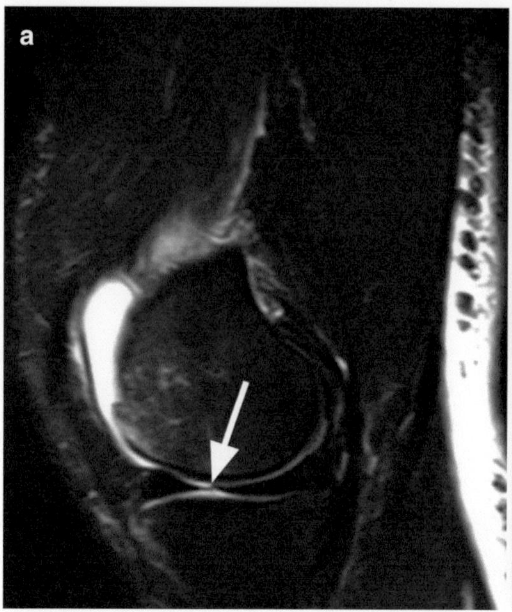
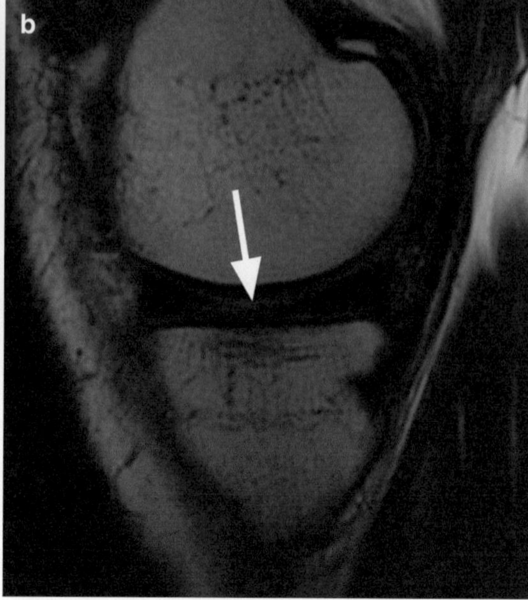

Fig. 5.13 Two different patients with internal meniscal flounce. Sagittal proton-density (PD) FSE fat-suppressed image (**a**) in a 23 year old patient and sagittal proton-density (PD) FSE image (**b**) in a 22 year old patient show in both cases a wavy, irregular meniscal contour of the meniscus (*arrows*)

compared to arthroscopy and is considered it to be the result of traction of the medial meniscus during tibial rotation [22]. In these cases, the flounce is a transient finding and it may disappear during maximal knee extension or flexion [22]. On MR images the body of the medial meniscus shows a wavy, irregular S-shaped along the free margin of the meniscus on sagittal planes (Fig. 5.13). A similar appearance may be seen in patients with knee instability or joint effusion when the flounce can be also seen in the lateral meniscus. Although, the meniscal flounce is a rare anatomic variant, its presence should be recognised since a meniscal tear or a discoid meniscus may resemble same appearance (Fig. 5.14). However, meniscal flounce and meniscal tears may coexist.

5.2 MRI Pathological Findings

5.2.1 Discoid Meniscus

A discoid meniscus is a congenitally tall and elongated meniscus that can be symmetrically or asymmetrically increased in size [23]. The lateral discoid meniscus is more common (incidence of 0.4–16.6 %) than the medial discoid meniscus

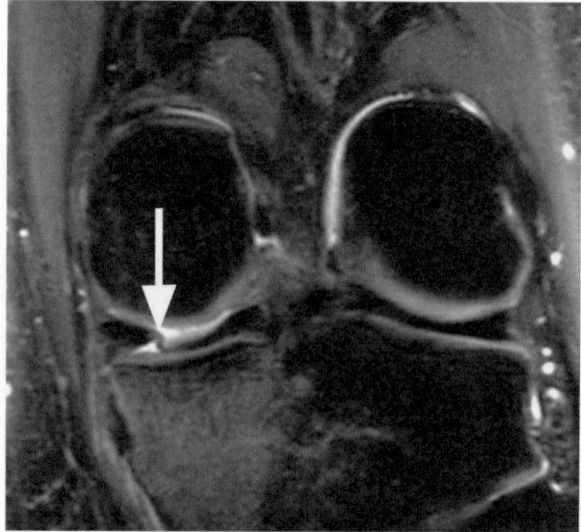

Fig. 5.14 Differential diagnosis between meniscal flounce and meniscal tear. In the cases of irregular margins of the meniscus on sagittal images a meniscal tear can be easily mistaken for meniscal flounce. Therefore the coronal images should be carefully evaluated. Coronal proton-density (PD) FSE fat-suppressed image in a 18 year old male shows a bucket-handle tear of the medial meniscus (*arrow*) which presents with a wavy contour of the meniscus

(incidence of 0.3 %) [24]. There are three types of discoid meniscus: complete, incomplete, and the Wrisberg type [25]. The complete and incomplete variants describe the shape of the meniscus with the incomplete type having a more semilunar shape. Both types, complete and incomplete discoid meniscus, are stable due to a normal posterior capsular and tibial attachment. The Wrisberg discoid meniscus is unstable and the only posterior attachment is the posterior meniscofemoral ligament of Wrisberg with a deficient posterior root meniscotibial ligament [26]. Clinically, patients can be asymptomatic or may complain of pain, swelling, clicking, and snapping especially in Wrisberg type due to the hypermobility of the meniscus. The MR imaging diagnosis of discoid meniscus is mainly based on the meniscus width and not on the meniscus height since it has been demonstrated that the accuracy of the meniscus height of the discoid meniscus is low [24]. Taking into consideration that the normal meniscus width is 14 mm measured on central slices, the diagnosis of discoid meniscus is suggestive when on sagittal images a continuity between the anterior and posterior horn is seen on four or more continuous slices (3 mm slice thickness) (Fig. 5.15) [27, 28].

The coronal images through the middle joint are more accurate and show an abnormally wide meniscus (>15 mm) (Fig. 5.16) [28]. The discoid meniscus may extend into the intercondylar notch in the complete type (Fig. 5.17) or may be seen in a normal position in the incomplete discoid type [29]. In the Wrisberg type, in the absence of the meniscotibial and posterior capsular attachment, an increased T2 signal intensity may be present between the capsule and the meniscus, simulating a peripheral tear [26]. Regardless the type, a discoid meniscus is prone to degeneration and tears (Figs. 5.18 and 5.19).

5.2.2 Meniscal Avulsion

Meniscal avulsion or the "floating" meniscus is defined as the detachment of the meniscus from the tibial plateau without separating completely from the capsule [30]. Typically, the lesion is limited to the meniscotibial ligaments (coronary

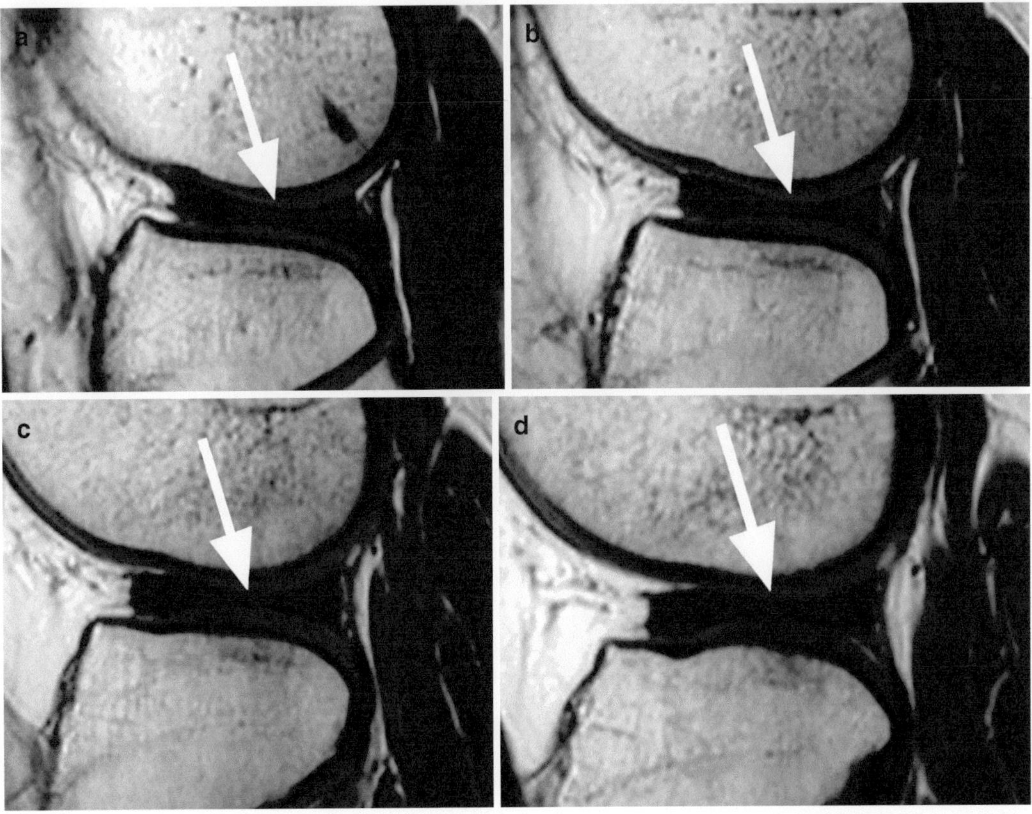

Fig. 5.15 Lateral discoid meniscus in a 39 year old female. Five consecutive sagittal proton-density (PD) FSE image (**a–e**) using 3 mm slice thickness show a continuity between the anterior and posterior horn (*arrow*)

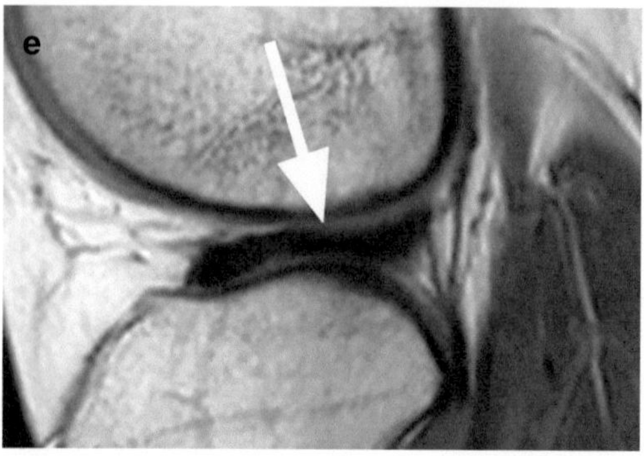

Fig. 5.15 (continued)

ligaments) while the meniscofemoral ligaments remain intact [31]. In the setting of acute trauma the meniscotibial ligaments may become disrupted and the meniscus is avulsed from the tibial plateau without evidence of tear within the substance of the meniscus [31]. The medial meniscus is more frequently involved than the lateral meniscus [30]. On MRI, the meniscal avulsion is best evaluated on sagittal and coronal T2-weighted images and on MR arthrography. The presence of high-intensity fluid of greater than 3 mm

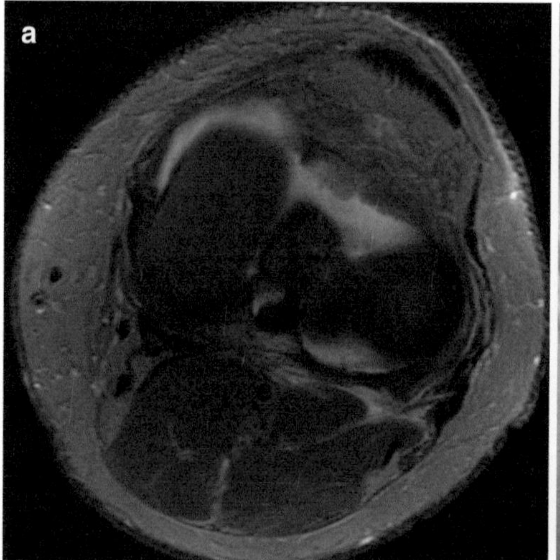

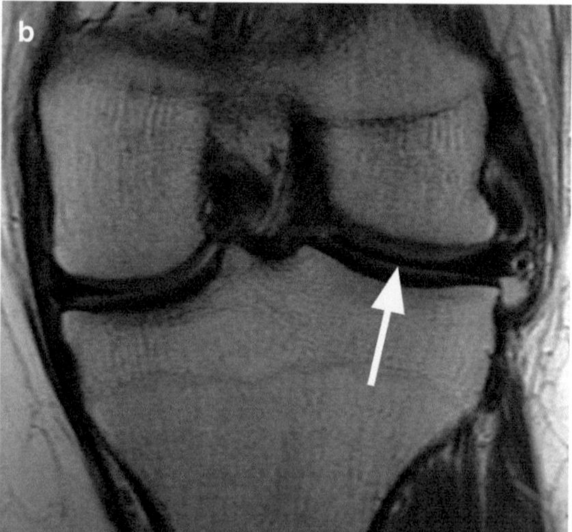

Fig. 5.16 Discoid meniscus – stable type. Axial (PD) FSE fat-suppressed image (**a**) shows an enlarged meniscus that can be identified entirely on axial plane (*circles*). Coronal proton-density (PD) FSE image (**b**) through the meniscus (*line* in **a**) shows an abnormally wide meniscus (>15 mm) at this level (*arrow* in **b**)

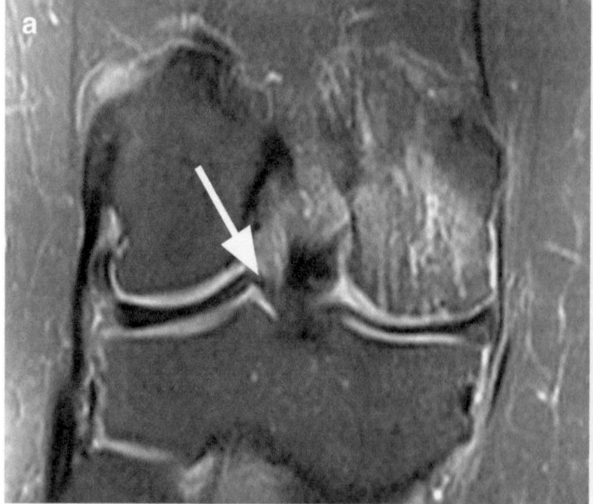

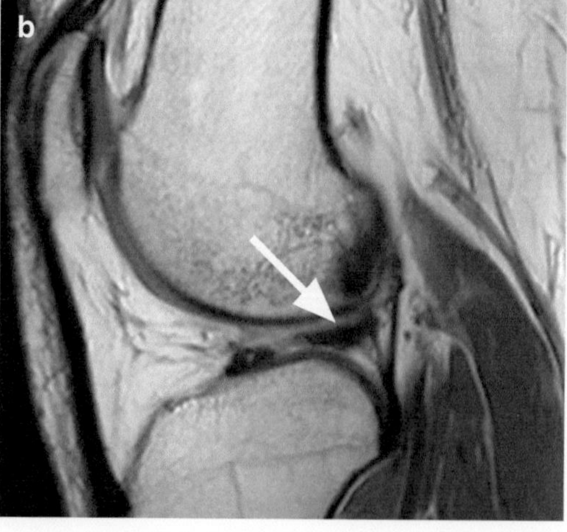

Fig. 5.17 Discoid meniscus in the intercondylar notch in a 39 year old female. Coronal proton-density (PD) FSE fat-suppressed image (**a**) and sagittal proton-density (PD) FSE image (**b**) show an enlarged meniscus extending into the intercondylar notch (*arrow*)

thickness in the long axis between the meniscus and the tibial plateau is suggestive for meniscal avulsion (Fig. 5.20) [31].

5.2.3 Meniscal Extrusion

Meniscal extrusion is considered when the meniscus is displaced beyond the tibial margin [32]. Meniscal radial and oblique tears, meniscal roots tears, meniscal degeneration, cartilage defects and the absence of the meniscofemoral ligaments are the most common causes of the radial expansion of the meniscus from the joint space. The meniscal tears as well as the meniscal roots tears alter the circumferential margin of the meniscus that resists radial displacement and permit the meniscal extrusion from the joint space [33]. The meniscal roots tears are strongly associated with meniscal extrusion especially in the medial compartment. There is also a significant association between all grades of meniscal degeneration and cartilage damage of the medial compartment and the medial meniscal extrusion (Fig. 5.21) [34]. A rare cause of meniscal extrusion may be the knee effusion when the extrusion is seen in the medial compartment as a result of the distention of the capsule that is firmly attached to the medial meniscus [35]. Recognising the meniscal extrusion is of clinical importance since it may lead to development of osteoarthritis. On coronal MR images the extrusion is assessed between the tibial margins (excluding osteophytes) and the outer margin of the lateral or medial meniscus (Fig. 5.21) [34]. A distance of more than 3 mm for the medial meniscus and more than 1 mm for the lateral meniscus is considered abnormal [9].

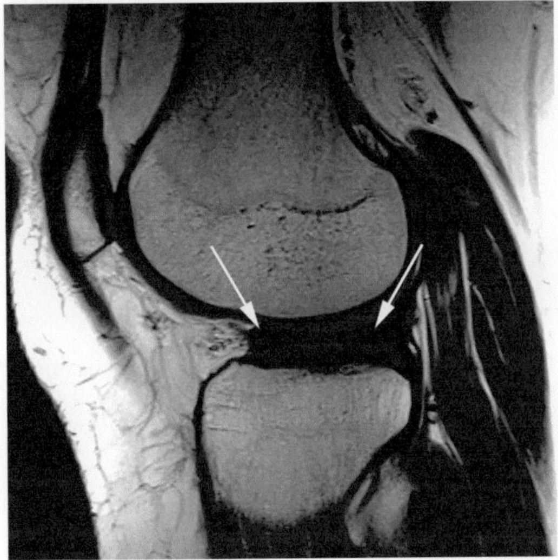

Fig. 5.18 Degenerative changes of lateral discoid meniscus in a 41 year old female. Sagittal proton-density (PD) FSE image show intrameniscal diffuse degenerative changes of the anterior and posterior horn (*arrows*)

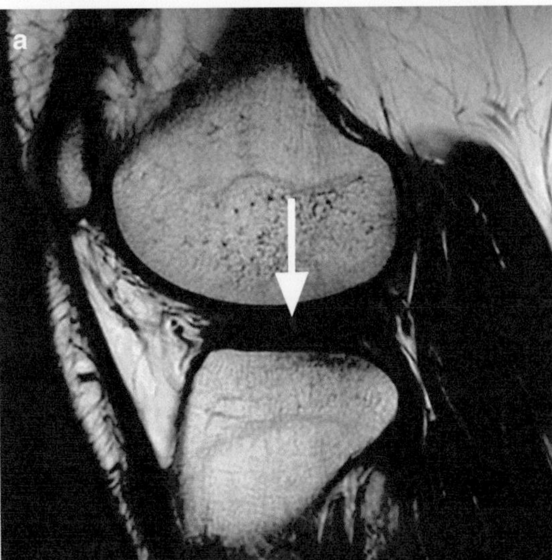

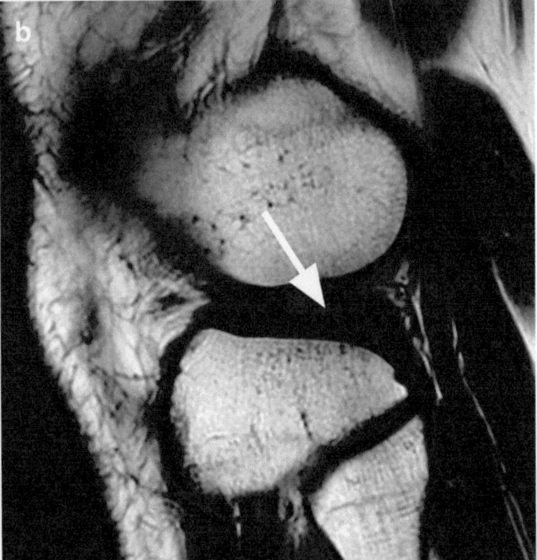

Fig. 5.19 Multiple tears of lateral discoid meniscus in a 31 year old female. Two consecutive sagittal proton-density (PD) FSE images (**a**, **b**) show vertical longitudinal tear (*arrow* in **a**) as well as horizontal tear (*arrow* in **b**)

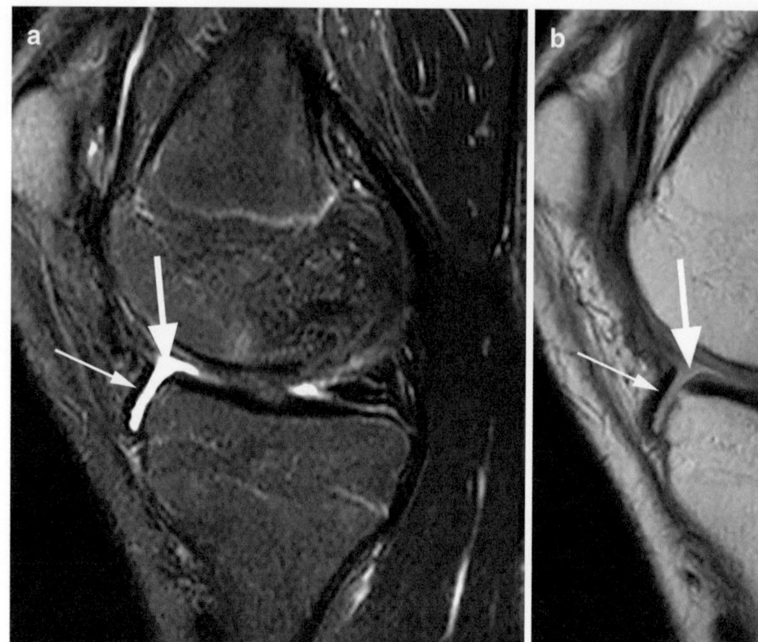

Fig. 5.20 Meniscal avulsion in a 19 year old male with acute trauma. Sagittal T2-weighted fat-suppressed image (**a**) and sagittal proton-density (PD) FSE image (**b**) show the presence of an abnormal volume of fluid anteriorly between tibia and femur (*large arrows*) with the anterior horn of the meniscus displaced anteriorly (*small arrows*)

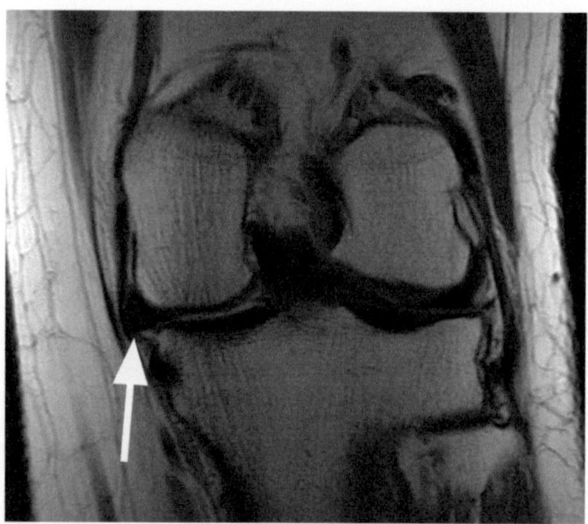

Fig. 5.21 Medial meniscal extrusion in a 56 year old female with osteoarthritis. Coronal proton-density (PD) FSE image shows that the meniscal margin is beyond the tibial plateau (*arrow*). Note the intrameniscal degenerative changes

5.2.4 Meniscocapsular Separation

Meniscocapsular separation is the result of the disruption of the capsular attachment of meniscus. The lesion can occur at the meniscocapsular junction or within the peripheral zone of the meniscus. Because of the strong fixation of the medial meniscus, tears of the meniscotibial or the coronary ligaments, especially of the posterior horn, are more frequently compared to the lateral meniscus. Coronal and sagittal T2-weighted MR images are particularly useful in demonstrating the lesion (Figs. 5.22 and 5.23). The presence of fluid with an increased distance between medial collateral ligament and medial meniscus, the displacement of meniscus from tibia, tear within the peripheral zone of meniscus, and irregular meniscal margins are the best predictors of medial meniscocapsular separation (Fig. 5.22) [36]. Laterally, a displaced meniscus and the disruption of the popliteomeniscal fascicles with high-signal intensity edema in the posterolateral corner of the knee are suggestive for lateral meniscocapsular separation [37]. Perimeniscal fluid may be also present in medial or lateral meniscocapsular separation (Fig. 5.23).

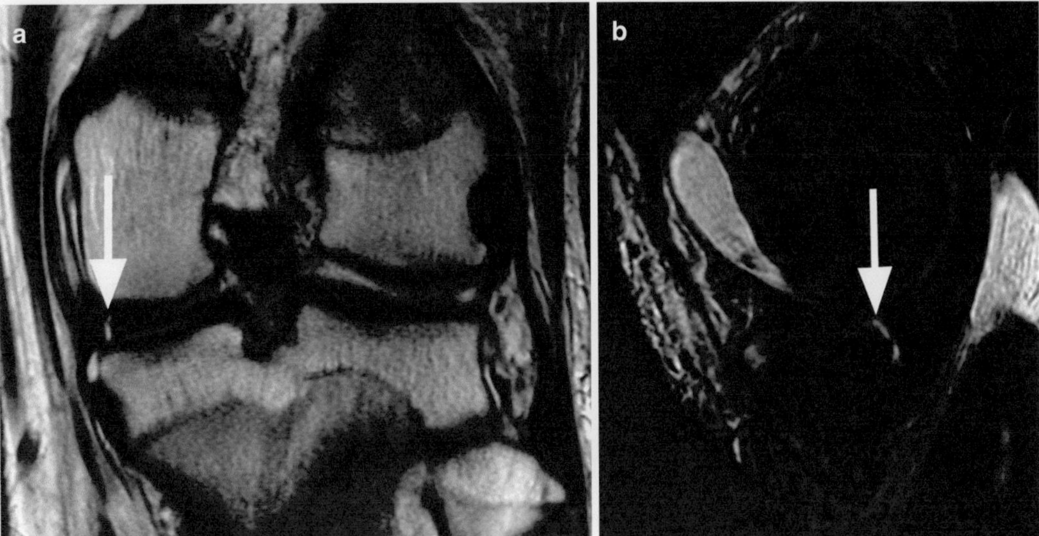

Fig. 5.22 Medial meniscocapsular separation in an 18 year old male. Coronal proton-density (PD) FSE image (**a**) and sagittal proton-density (PD) FSE fat-suppressed (**b**) images show a linear high-signal intensity separation between the peripheral zone of meniscus and the medial collateral ligament (*arrow* in **a**). The lesion is also visible on the sagittal image as a peripheral vertical tear of the posterior medial meniscus (*arrow* in **b**)

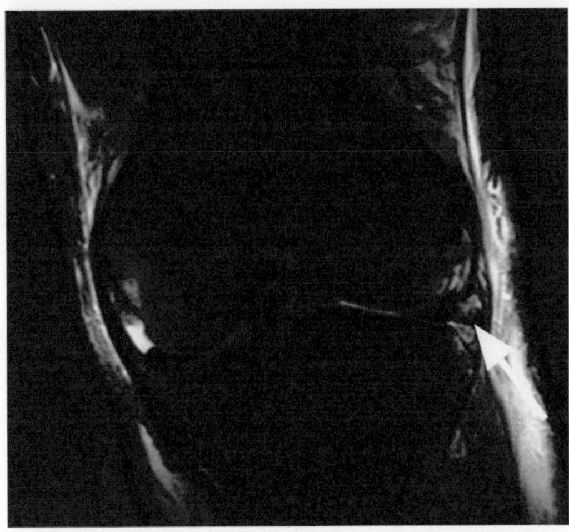

Fig. 5.23 Lateral meniscocapsular separation in a 51 year old male. Coronal proton-density (PD) FSE fat-suppressed image shows perimeniscal hematoma (*arrow*) between the lateral meniscus and the lateral collateral ligament suggestive for meniscocapsular separation

5.2.5   Degenerative Changes

The degenerative meniscal changes are the result of the internal derangement of the normal meniscal architecture followed by intrasubstance mucoid degeneration. It is frequently seen in elderly but it can appear at younger ages in response to high mechanical loading. The degenerative changes involve more frequently the posterior horn of the medial meniscus and are usually asymptomatic. On MR images the lesion appears as diffuse or focal increased signal intensity changes surrounded by normal low-signal intensity of the normal meniscal substance (Fig. 5.24). The degenerative lesions do not extend to the articular surfaces of the meniscus [29]. However, in some cases the free margin may display irregularities and the mucoid changes may progress to horizontal tears. When the linear changes do not convincingly extend to the articular surface, it is better to be descriptive rather than overdiagnose an equivocal finding [29].

5.2.6   Meniscal Contusion

Meniscal contusion appears in the setting of acute trauma and it usually involves the meniscal surface [38]. Bone injury adjacent to the menis-cal contusions have been described in these

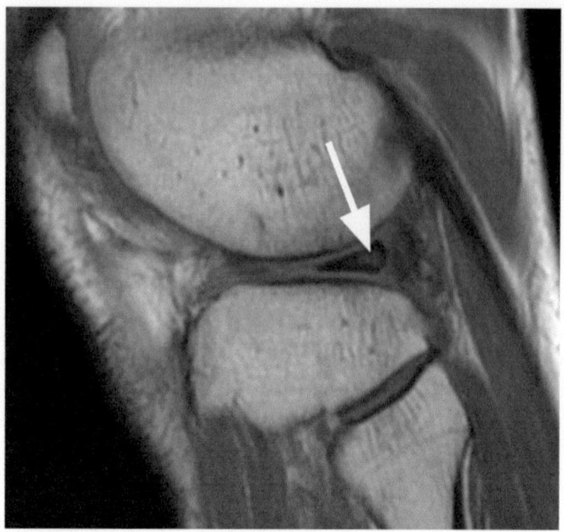

Fig. 5.24 *Degenerative intrasubstance mucoid degenera-tion of the posterior horn of the lateral meniscus in a 54 year old male. Sagittal proton-density (PD) FSE image shows a focal signal-intensity change within the meniscus (arrow). The lesion does not extend to the articular sur-faces of the meniscus*

patients suggesting that the mechanism of these lesions may be a compressive injury [38]. Meniscal contusion is seen on MR images as a diffuse, amorphous area of abnormal signal intensity that extends to the articular surface (Fig. 5.25). The signal does not meet the definite linear pattern of a meniscal tear neither the well-defined intrameniscal signal of the mucoid degeneration. At arthroscopy these lesions do not have the appearance of typical meniscal tears [38]. On MR imaging follow-up the meniscal contusion may resolve or improve suggesting the transient character of the contusion [38].

5.2.7 Meniscal Tears

The meniscal tear is described as a linear increased signal intensity within the meniscus. The MR report should not only identify the presence of a

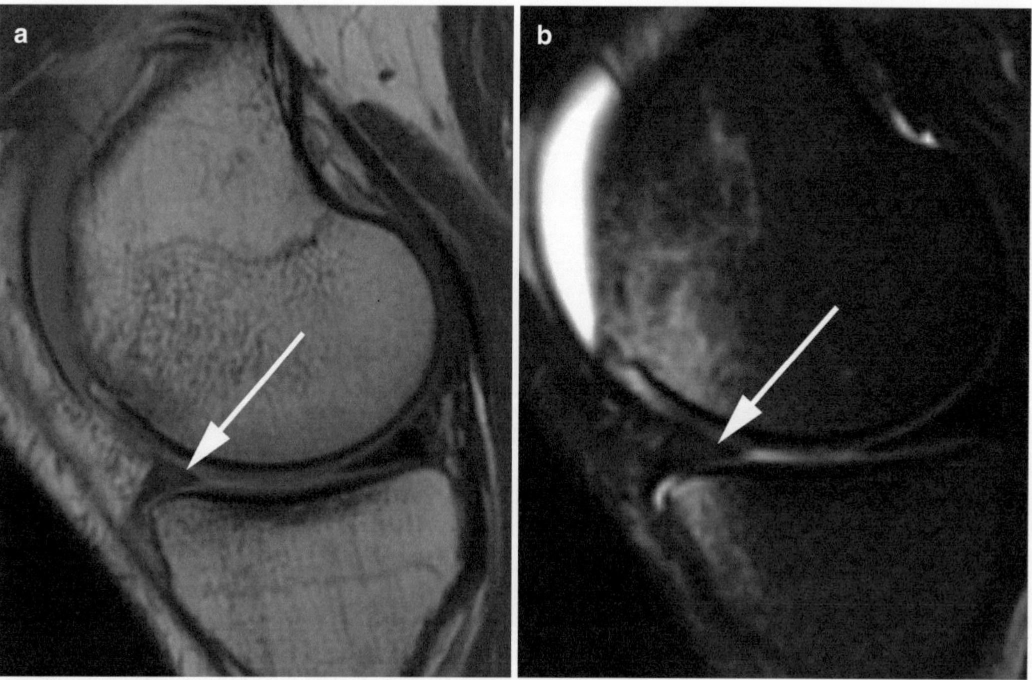

Fig. 5.25 Meniscal contusion in a 32 year old male with knee injury. Sagittal proton-density (PD) FSE image (**a**) and sagittal proton-density (PD) FSE fat-suppressed image (**b**) show diffuse signal intensity changes in the anterior horn of the medial meniscus that extends to the articular surface (*arrows*). Note the bone marrow contu-sion of the medial femoral condyle

Table 5.1 Classification of meniscal tears and the clinical significance [29, 39, 40]

Meniscal tear	**Vertical**	Longitudinal	Incomplete		Stable	Low clinical relevance, not always correlated with symptoms = "leave alone" lesion
			Complete		Unstable when meniscocapsular separation is present or in extensive lesion	High clinical relevance
		Radial	Without meniscal root involvement		Usually unstable	High clinical relevance
			Radial meniscal root tear			
	Horizontal or oblique-horizontal	Incomplete			Stable	Low clinical relevance, not always correlated with symptoms = "leave alone" lesion
		Complete			Unstable/stable	Different clinical relevance depending on associated lesions
	Complex	Horizontal and vertical tear, complex linear pattern			Unstable	High clinical relevance
		Bucket-handle				
		Flap tears (including parrot- beak tears)				
		Free meniscal fragment				

linear meniscal tear but also should accurately describe the orientation, location, length and stability, because these criteria are important and may influence the choice of operative or nonoperative treatment. The classifications of meniscal tears is based on different criteria (Table 5.1). According to the orientation, a meniscal tear can be vertical, horizontal, or complex. Vertical tears are further subdivided into radial (perpendicular to the long axis of the meniscus), which includes the tears of the meniscal root and longitudinal (parallel to the long axis of the meniscus) [29]. The complex tears refer either to a combination of more orientations (vertical and horizontal) including the parrot beak tear and tears with displaced fragments (bucket-handle tear, flap meniscus tear, or free meniscus fragment). Meniscal grading (grade I–III) that has been widely used in the past is now considered obsolete in the clinical routine imaging [41].

The tear may be complete (full thickness tear) when the linear signal changes extend to one or both meniscal articular surfaces, or incomplete. Linear signal changes that are not in contact or those which are only possibly in contact with the meniscal surface should be considered incomplete tears. The definition of complete or incomplete meniscal tear is appropriately used for horizontal or oblique-horizontal tears. In the case of vertical longitudinal tears an incomplete tear is considered when the linear signal change is in contact with only one meniscal surface. However, the vertical radial tears may not be classified in complete or incomplete. The horizontal, oblique-horizontal, as well as the incomplete longitudinal tears may be encountered in both symptomatic and asymptomatic patients [39]. According to the location, length, and stability these lesions may have a low, moderate or high clinical relevance. The vertical longitudinal complete tears, the vertical radial tears and the complex tears should be considered of high clinical relevance [39].

The meniscal tear may be in contact with the inferior (tibial) articular surface, the superior (femoral) articular surface, or both. This information is valuable for arthroscopists because the inferior surface of the meniscus is the most difficult region to visualize directly at arthroscopy [42].

The MR imaging description of the meniscal tears should also include the location of the tear within the anterior, body, or posterior horn and within the peripheral or central zone. The posterior horn of the medial meniscus is the most frequently involved, followed by the posterior horn of the lateral meniscus, the anterior horn of the lateral meniscus and the anterior horn of the medial meniscus [43]. The location within the periphery or the central zone of the meniscus is also important because a tear located in the rich vascular peripheral zone is more likely to heal conservatively [29].

The size (length and depth) of the meniscal tear can be evaluated on MR examination and should be reported because it may influence the treatment choice. Finally, the meniscal tears can be classified in stable and unstable tears. The stable tears have potential for healing conservatively and include the incomplete tears and the small complete simple tears. The complex lesions with different orientations of the lesion, the displaced fragments, the presence of fluid in the tear, and the peripheral meniscal separation may be considered unstable meniscal tears [40].

Vertical Longitudinal Tear

The vertical longitudinal tears are parallel to the long axis of the meniscus. This type of lesions appears in young active patients and are located more frequently in the peripheral zone of the meniscus. The peripheral location of the vertical longitudinal tear may be a cause of meniscocapsular separation (Fig. 5.22) and is commonly associated with anterior cruciate ligament deficiency [44]. Usually, they involve the posterior horn and may extend anteriorly. If the tear extends over a long enough distance it may transform into a bucket-handle tear with displacement of the inner fragment [29]. On MR images the lesion is best seen on sagittal planes (Fig. 5.26).

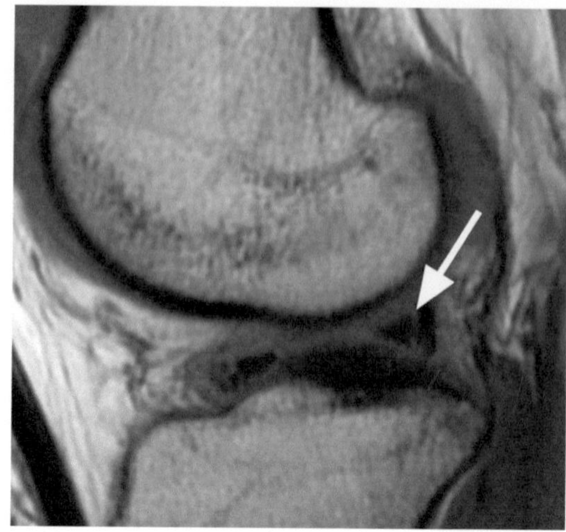

Fig. 5.26 Vertical longitudinal tear of the posterior horn of the lateral meniscus in a 27 year old male. Sagittal proton-density (PD) FSE image shows the vertical tear typically located in the peripheral zone of the meniscus (*arrow*)

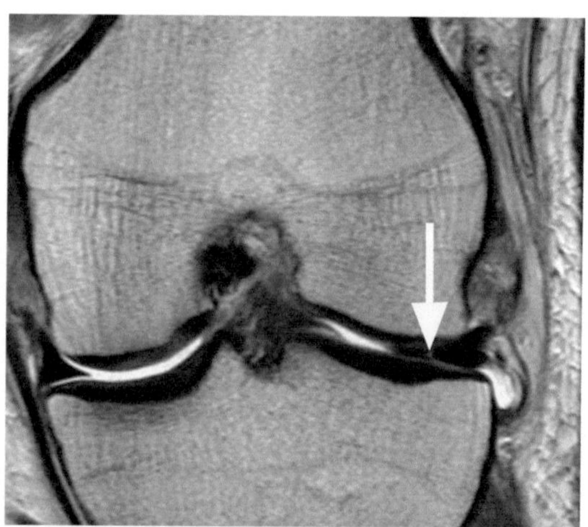

Fig. 5.27 The cleft sign revealing vertical radial tear of the lateral meniscus in a 44 year old male. Coronal proton-density (PD) FSE image shows the vertical high-signal extending through meniscus (*arrow*)

Vertical Radial Tear and Radial Meniscal Root Tear

In vertical radial tears the linear signal change within the meniscus is oriented perpendicularly to the long axis of the meniscus. Compared to the longitudinal tears, radial tears involves more frequently the central zone and the free margin of the meniscus. Because of orientation, radial tears are best depicted on coronal MR images as a linear defect in sagittal plane (also known as "the cleft" sign) (Figs. 5.27, 5.28, and 5.29) [45].

On sagittal MR images there is a truncation of the free edge of the meniscus or a replacement of the low-signal intensity meniscus with high intensity signal area on one sagittal image when the MR slice is through the radial tear (the "ghost" meniscus sign) (Fig. 5.30) [45].

The radial tears may involve the meniscal root ligaments and they are called in these cases *radial meniscal root tears*. The lesions are difficult to be recognised on MR imaging and they have a different clinical implication from a usual radial tear [46]. Posterior medial meniscus root tear is strongly associated with degenerative joint disease, cartilage defect of the medial femoral condyle, and medial meniscal extrusion [47]. The posterior lateral meniscus root tear might have a better prognosis for degenerative changes development and meniscal extrusion, especially if the meniscofemoral ligaments are present and are intact [48]. In the case of

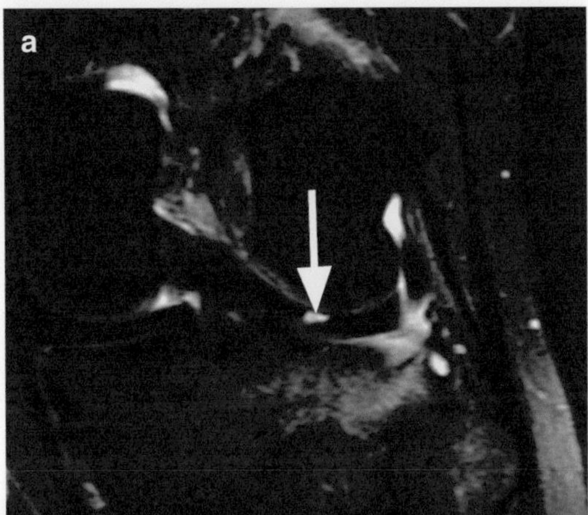

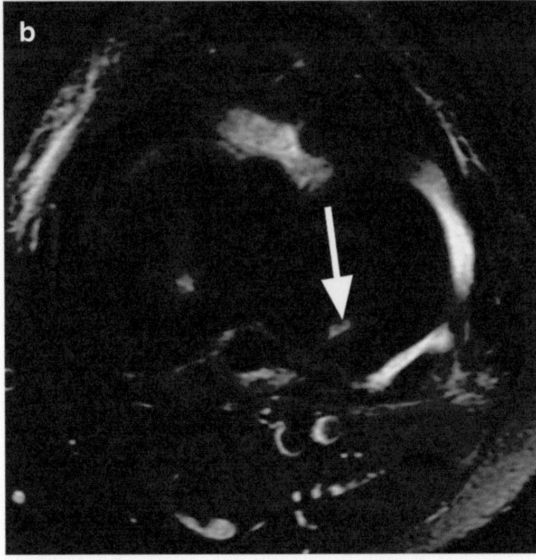

Fig. 5.28 The cleft sign revealing vertical radial tear of the lateral meniscus in a 28 year old female. Coronal proton-density (PD) FSE fat-suppressed image (**a**) and axial proton-density (PD) FSE fat-suppressed image (**b**) show the vertical high-signal intensity within the meniscus (*arrow* in **a**) and a focal high-signal intensity lesion (*arrow* in **b**) representing the same radial tear on axial plane

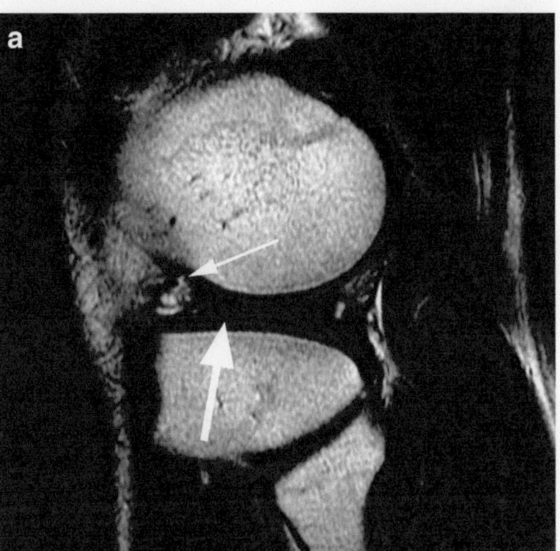

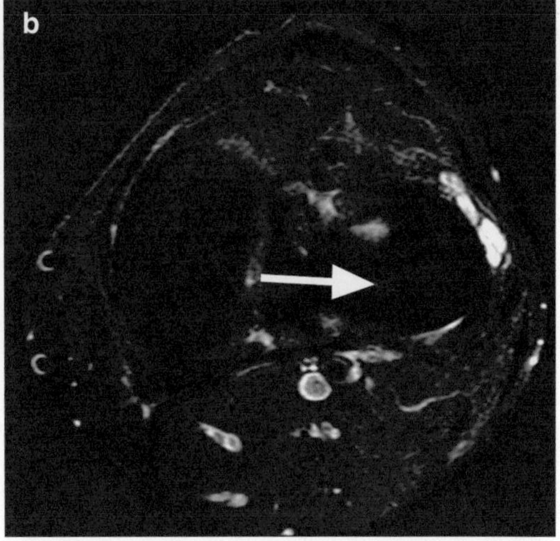

Fig. 5.29 Radial vertical tear in evolution in a 28 year old male. Sagittal proton-density (PD) FSE image (**a**) and axial proton-density (PD) FSE fat-suppressed image (**b**) at the first presentation of the patient show a typical radial tear of the lateral meniscus (*arrows* in **a**, **b**). Note the anterior meniscal cyst (*small arrow* in **a**). Although, most of the radial tears are usually unstable, the patient was treated conservatively. Two years after the first examination sagittal proton-density (PD) FSE image (**c**) shows that the lesion has the same dimension with a discrete degenerative transformation (*arrow* in **c**)

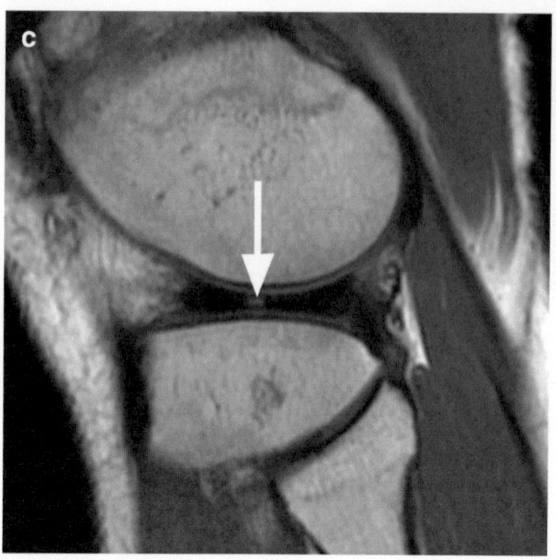

Fig. 5.29 (continued)

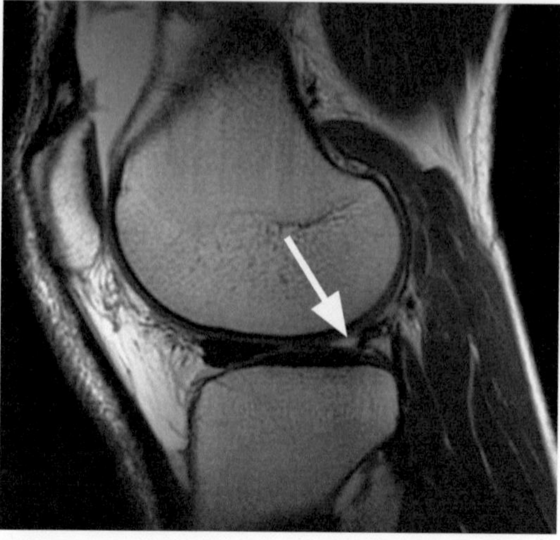

Fig. 5.30 The "ghost" meniscus sign in a 28 year old male. Sagittal proton-density (PD) FSE image shows high-signal intensity area (*arrow*) replacing the normal low-signal intensity of the free margin of the meniscus. The sign appears when the sagittal image is through the radial tear and, usually, appears only on one image

posterior medial meniscus root tears the MR imaging characteristic finding is the absence of the normal medial meniscus tibial insertion near the posterior cruciate ligament insertion (Fig. 5.31) [41]. On coronal images a cleft of high-signal intensity on T2-weighted images is seen between the posterior cruciate ligament and posterior medial meniscus (Fig. 5.31) [41]. The lateral meniscus root tear is more difficult to diagnose and may be suggested on coronal MR images when the posterior horn of the lateral meniscus does not cover the most medial aspect of the posterior lateral tibial plateau on at least one image (Fig. 5.32) [49].

Horizontal Tear

The horizontal meniscal tear is often present in old adults and is seen as a linear signal intensity change within the meniscus substance parallel or oblique-parallel to the tibial plateau. It may be classified as complete or incomplete and it divides the meniscus into upper and lower segments (Fig. 5.33) [46]. In complete tears, the inferior segment might be displaced with a subluxation of the meniscus and becomes an inferior flap tear. Horizontal tears may be seen in symptomatic and asymptomatic patients and may be not always related to symptoms [39]. The preferred location of the

lesion is the posterior horn of the medial meniscus (Fig. 5.34) and is frequently related to degeneration of the meniscus and meniscal cyst formation.

Bucket-Handle Tear

The bucket-handle tear is a complex and unstable lesion that results from an extensive vertical longitudinal tear. The tear divides the meniscus into a central and a peripheral segment that are still connected anteriorly and posteriorly with the central fragment displaced in the intercondylar notch with resultant mechanical locking of the knee. The lesion is more common medially than laterally [50]. The diagnosis of bucket-handle tears requires identification of the displaced segment because the peripheral nondisplaced peripheral segment may have only a subtle truncated shape [51].

There are several MRI signs that refers to the displaced segment and are suggestive for bucket-handle tear. The double-PCL sign is seen when the meniscal fragment is displaced anteriorly and parallel to the posterior cruciate ligament and is best identified on coronal and sagittal MR images

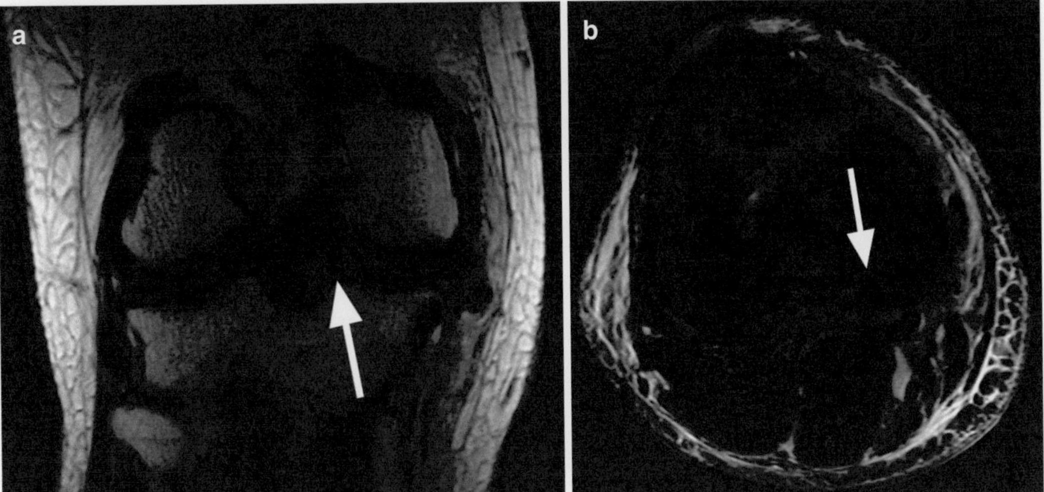

Fig. 5.31 Posterior lateral meniscus root tear in a 36 year old male. Coronal proton-density (PD) FSE image (**a**) and axial (PD) FSE fat-suppressed image (**b**) show a diffuse lesion between the medial meniscus and the posterior cruciate ligament (*arrow* in **a**). The lesion is typically located at the tibial insertion of the posterior meniscal root. On the axial image alone, the lesion is difficult to diagnose (*arrow* in **b**). However, the lesion is more easily identified when interpreted with the coronal image

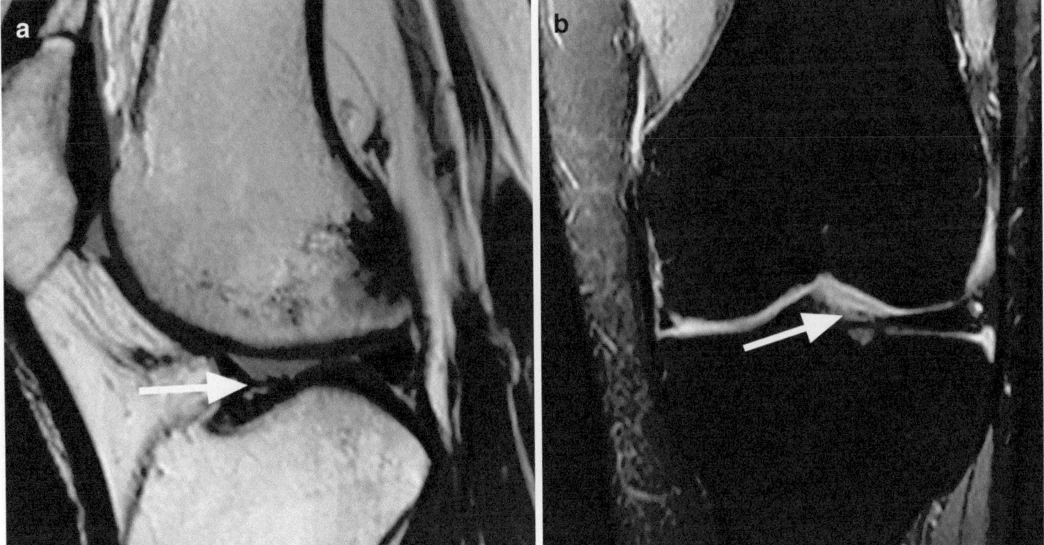

Fig. 5.32 Lateral meniscal roots injury in a 48 year old female. Sagittal proton-density (PD) FSE image (**a**) and coronal proton-density (PD) FSE fat-suppressed image (**b**) show a tear of the anterior lateral meniscal root (*arrow*)

(Fig. 5.35). The sign has demonstrated a specificity of 100 % for bucket-handle tears [52]. On sagittal images the absent bow-tie sign is suggestive for bucket-handle tears with a sensitivity of 88.4 % and is defined as the absence of visualization of the meniscus body on three or more adjacent slices of 3 mm thickness (Fig. 5.35) [52, 53]. Another sign that may suggest the bucket-handle tear is the truncated meniscus sign with the loss of the normal triangular meniscal shape [51].

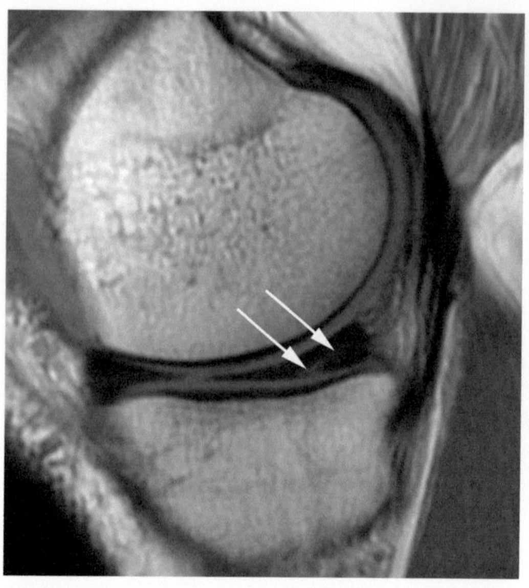

Fig. 5.33 Horizontal meniscal tear in a 36 year old male. Sagittal proton-density (PD) FSE image shows a linear signal intensity lesion oblique-horizontal with the tibial plateau in the posterior horn of the medial meniscus (*arrows*). It is a complete lesion and divides the menisci into an upper and a lower segment. The tear is in contact with the tibial articular surface of the meniscus and this orientation should be mentioned in the MR impression

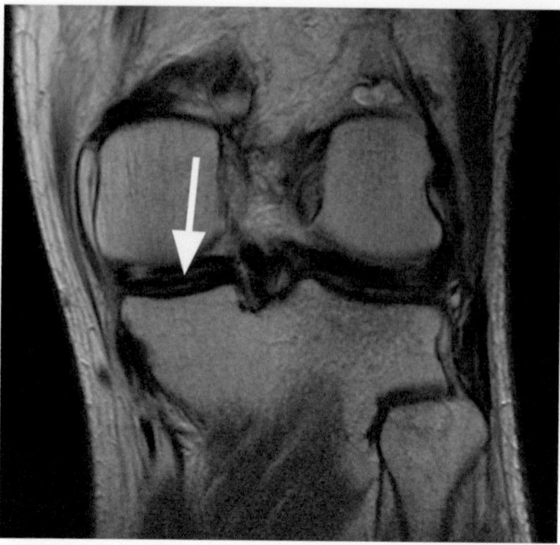

Fig. 5.34 Horizontal meniscal tear in a 46 year old male. Coronal proton-density (PD) FSE image shows an horizontal lesion of the posterior horn of the medial meniscus (*arrow*)

Flap Tear

The flap tears are complex unstable lesions that are of high clinical relevance. They result from horizontal, oblique or vertical tears and they typically present a displaced fragment. The meniscal fragment may be dislocated adjacent to the meniscus horns or to the synovial recesses [54]. *The flipped meniscus fragment* may be seen on MR imaging either anteriorly or posteriorly lying to the intact posterior or anterior horn resulting into a disproportionate posterior horn sign (Fig. 5.36) or into a double-anterior horn appearance or the flipped meniscus sign having the appearance of an abnormally large anterior horn (Fig. 5.37) [55].

On the medial site, a complete horizontal tear of the medial meniscus may displace the inferior segment into the adjacent synovial recesses, usually deep to the medial collateral ligament [54]. The lesion is called an *inferior flap tear* and the coronal MR images are most useful in identification of the meniscal fragment which in most

cases is situated inferior to the body of meniscus between tibial cortex and medial collateral ligament.

The parrot-beak tear is an unstable vertical tear that combines radial and horizontal patterns [29]. The lesion involves in most of the cases the free margin of the posterior horn of the lateral meniscus and results in a flap of unstable fragment. Rarely, the fragment may be displaced into the intercondylar notch having a similar aspect to the bucket-handle tear. However, the MR diagnosis of the parrot-peak tear is difficult an may be suggested on sagittal, coronal and axial images by a triangular signal intensity change extending to the free margin of the meniscus (Fig. 5.38).

Free Meniscal Fragment

A complete detached meniscal fragment may be displaced in any of the joint recesses, in the intercondylar notch, or in the suprapatellar pouch. The clinical symptoms and the MRI appearance depends on the location and the mobility of the sequestrated fragment. Usually, the meniscal fragment has the same signal intensity as the normal meniscus and it is easily identified when is surrounded by joint effusion or intraarticular contrast (Fig. 5.39). Nevertheless, the fragment should not

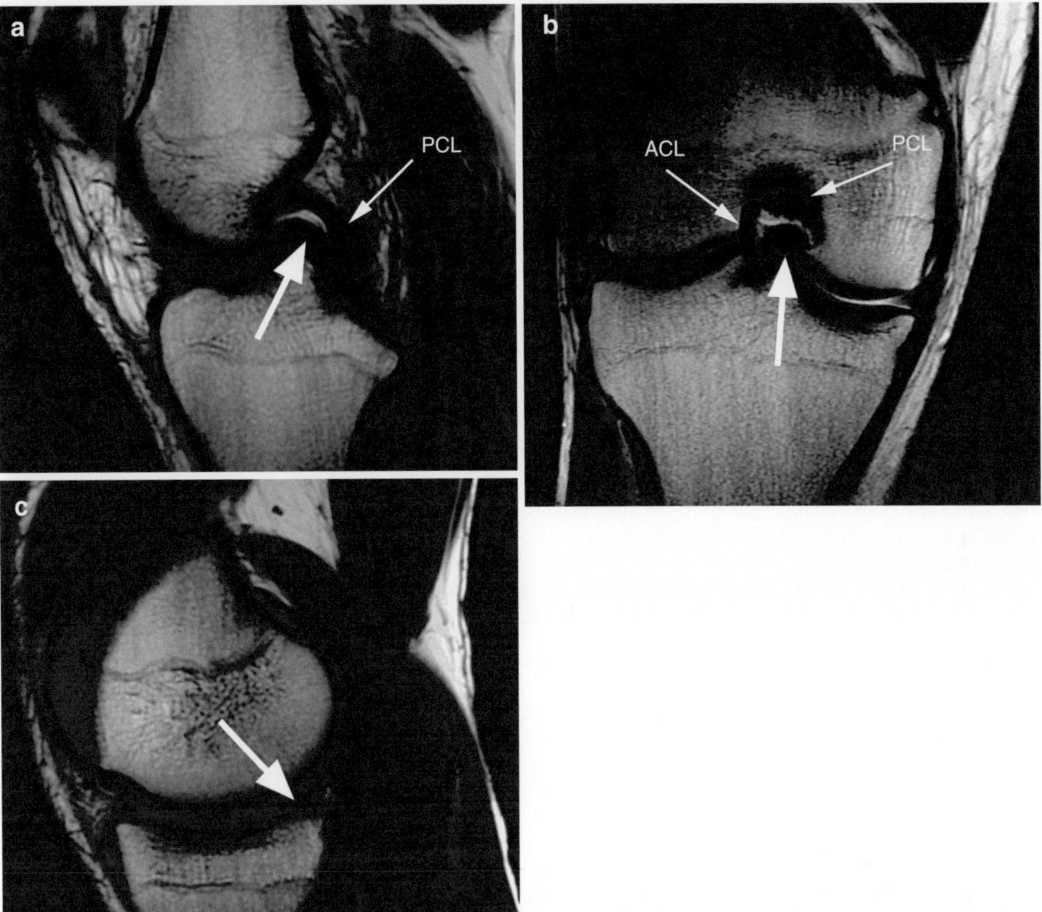

Fig. 5.35 Bucket-handle tear of the medial meniscus in a 27 year old male. Sagittal proton-density (PD) FSE image (**a**) shows the central meniscal fragment (*large arrow*) displaced parallel to the posterior cruciate ligament (*PCL*)=double-PCL sign. Coronal proton-density (PD) FSE image (**b**) shows the central fragment in the intercondylar notch (*large arrow*) inferiorly to the posterior cruciate ligament (*PCL*) and medially to the anterior cruciate ligament (*ACL*). Sagittal proton-density (PD) FSE image (**c**) more medially from the first sagittal image shows the absent bow-tie sign defined as the absence of visualization of the meniscus body (*arrow*)

be confused with other possible detached structures such as cartilage and ostechondral fragments. Both menisci should be carefully evaluated in order to identify the origin of the fragment which is suggested when a portion of meniscus is not seen [29].

5.2.8   Meniscal Cysts

Meniscal cysts may be classified into intrameniscal and parameniscal cysts. Both types of meniscal cysts are the result of a microscopic or macroscopic meniscal tear and meniscal degeneration. Horizontal tears are most frequently associated with cysts formation. The intrameniscal cysts are very rare and are located at the site of the meniscal tear or within the degenerative mucoid area.

The parameniscal cysts are lobulated lesions with or without internal septa that contain mucinous material communicating with the intrameniscal substance (Fig. 5.40). They are located adjacent to the meniscal tear and, therefore, they may be present in any compartment at the periphery of the meniscus (Fig. 5.41). Clinically, the patients may be asymptomatic or they may

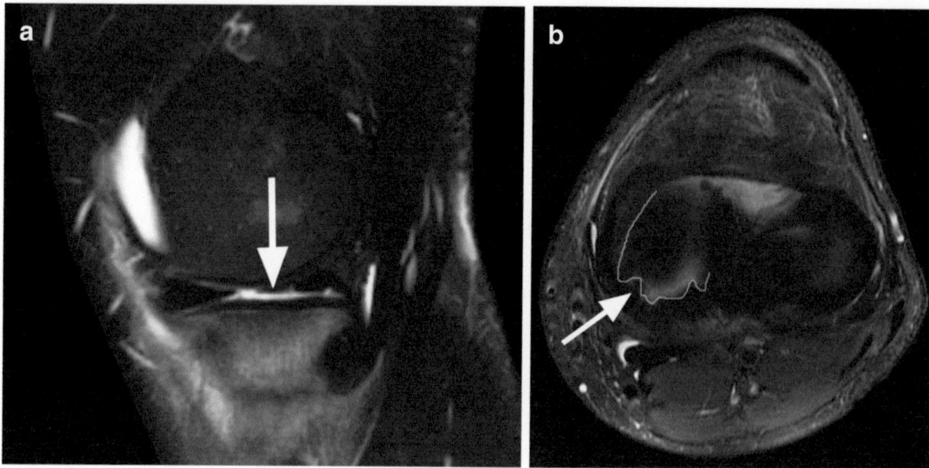

Fig. 5.36 Flap tear (flipped meniscus) of the medial meniscus in a 32 year old male. Sagittal T2-weighted fat-suppressed image (**a**) shows a flipped meniscus fragment (*arrow*) lying to the intact posterior meniscal horn result-ing into a disproportionate posterior horn sign. Axial (PD) FSE fat-suppressed image (**b**) shows the entire length of the tear which involves the body and the posterior horn (*line drawn*)

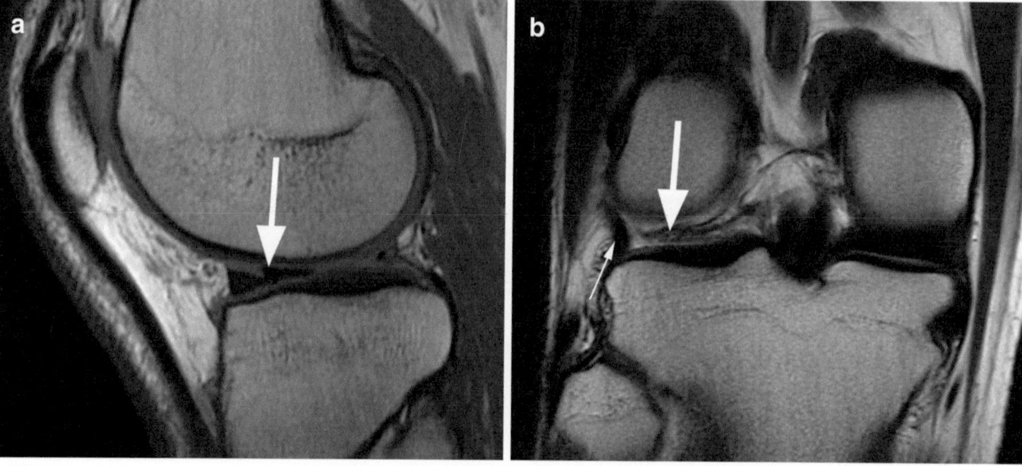

Fig. 5.37 Flap tear (flipped meniscus) of the lateral meniscus in a 26 year old male. Sagittal proton-density (PD) FSE image (**a**) shows the double anterior horn sign (*large arrow*) which is the result of the anterior dislocation of a fragment of the posterior horn after a vertical longitudinal tear. The dislocation of the posterior meniscus is demonstrated on coronal proton-density (PD) FSE image (**b**) in which the meniscus is absent (missing menis-cus sign) (*large arrow*). The popliteal tendon (*small arrow* in **b**) should not be misinterpreted as a meniscal fragment

present with swelling, palpable mass, and pain. Intrameniscal calcifications and bone erosions are rare and present in large parameniscal cysts [56]. Special attention should be given to the posterior lateral parameniscal cysts. These lesions should be differentiated from a posterior cruciate ligament (PCL) ganglion cyst because the treatment option is different. The parameniscal cyst communicates with a meniscal tear and is located posterior and around the posterior cruciate ligament (PCL) in comparison with a posterior cruciate ligament (PCL) ganglion cyst which rarely surrounds the ligament [57].

On MR images parameniscal cysts are seen as well delineated lobulated cystic lesions with or without a distinct communication with a meniscal

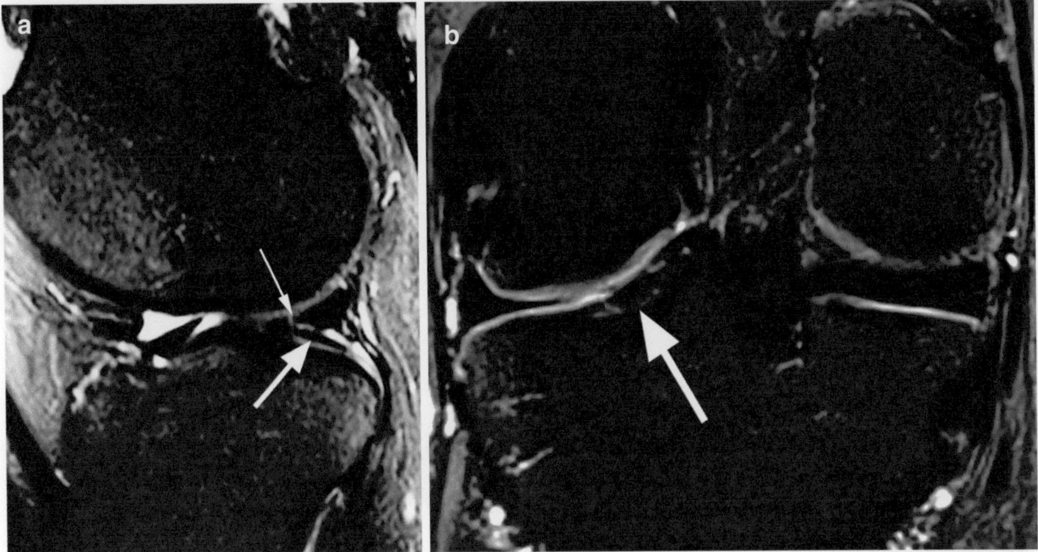

Fig. 5.38 Parrot-beak tear of the lateral meniscus in a 21 year old male. Sagittal T2-weighted fat-suppressed FSE image (**a**) shows a tear with complex pattern of the posterior horn. There is a vertical longitudinal tear (*small arrow*) combined with an horizontal component (*large arrow*). Coronal proton-density (PD) fat-suppressed image (**b**) shows the displaced fragment medially and inferiorly (*large arrow* in **b**)

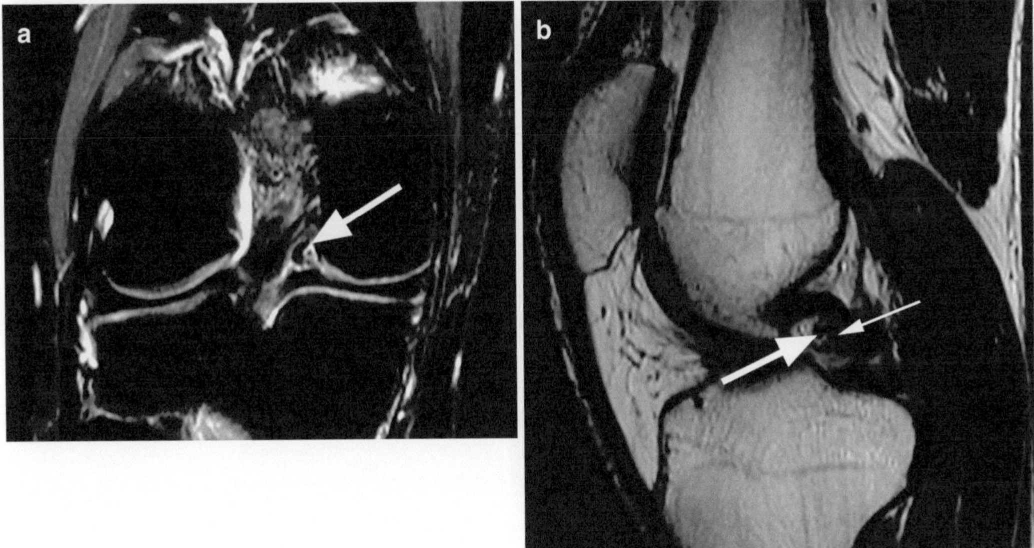

Fig. 5.39 Free meniscal fragment in a 21 year old male. Coronal proton-density (PD) fat-suppressed image (**a**) and sagittal proton-density (PD) image (**b**) show a small meniscal fragment (*large arrow* in **a**, **b**) detached from the medial meniscus and displaced anteriorly to the posterior cruciate ligament (PCL). On sagittal image the free meniscal fragment may be misdiagnosed as a normal anterior meniscofemoral ligament (*small arrow*)

tear. The lesions are low- or intermediate-signal intensity on T1-weighted images due to their mucinous content and high-signal intensity on T2-weighted images (Figs. 5.40 and 5.41).

5.2.9 Meniscal Calcifications

Foci of calcifications within the meniscus may be seen in meniscal ossicles and in chondrocalcinosis.

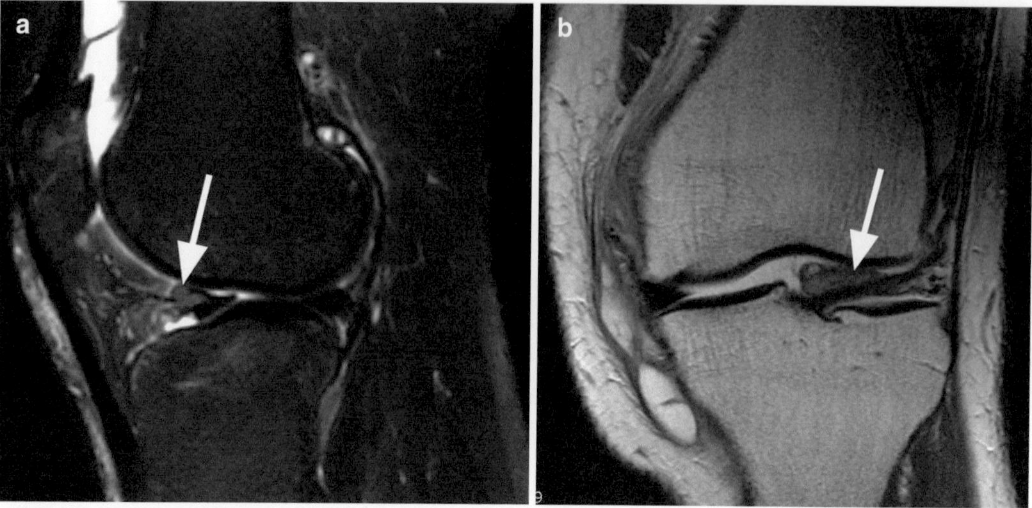

Fig. 5.40 Parameniscal cysts in a 58 year old male. Sagittal T2-weighted fat-suppressed FSE image (**a**) and coronal proton-density (PD) FSE image (**b**) show a lobulated cystic lesion (*arrow*) of intermediate signal intensity adjacent to the anterior horn of the lateral meniscus

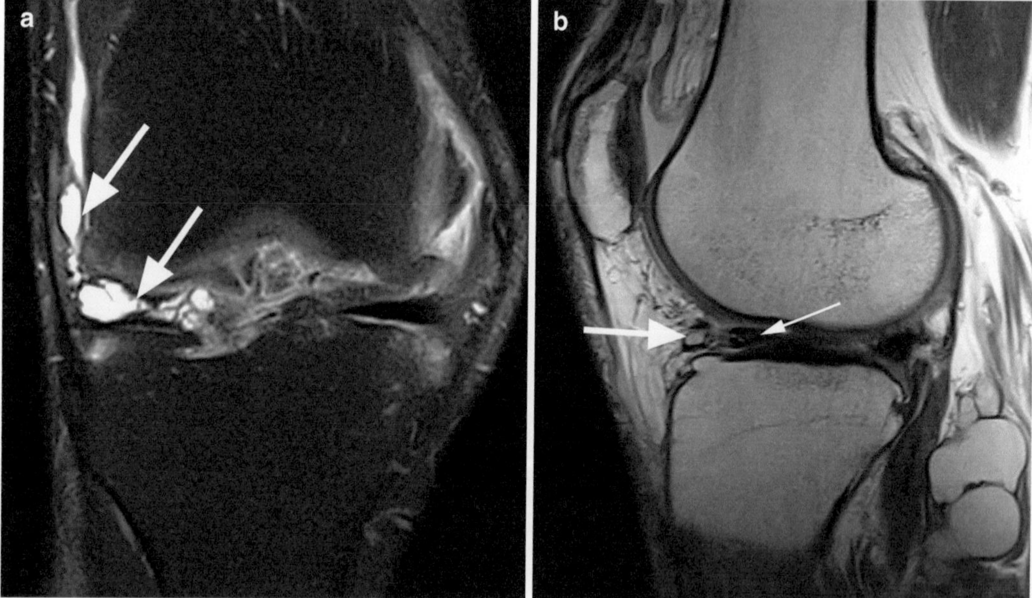

Fig. 5.41 Parameniscal cyst in a 43 year old male with horizontal tear of the anterior horn of the lateral meniscus. Coronal proton-density (PD) fat-suppressed image (**a**) and sagittal proton-density (PD) image (**b**) show a lobulated anterior parameniscal cyst (*large arrows* in **a** and **b**) communicating with an horizontal tear of the meniscus (*small arrow* in **b**)

Meniscal ossicles are foci of calcification surrounded by hyaline cartilage of different shapes that range from millimeters to 1 cm [58]. They are more frequently seen in the posterior horns of the medial meniscus and they are located in the meniscal substance without contact with the meniscal surface. The etiology is unknown but a previous trauma may be related to the calcifications. The patients may be asymptomatic or they may present locking and pain [58]. On MR

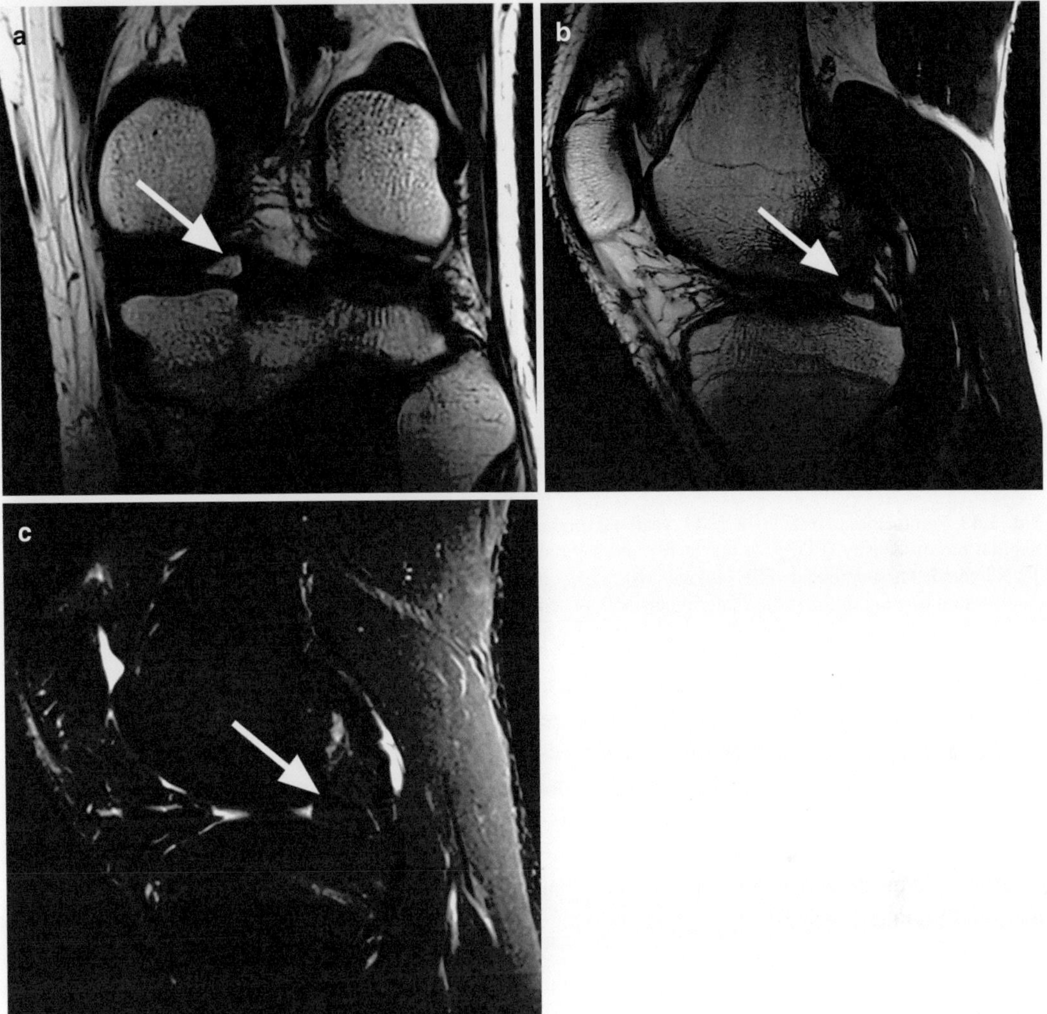

Fig. 5.42 Meniscal ossicle in a 26 year old male. Coronal T1-weighted FSE image (**a**), sagittal proton-density (PD) FSE image (**b**), and sagittal T2-weighted FSE fat-suppressed image (**c**) show an intrameniscal calcification of 1 cm (*arrow*)

images the signal intensity is that of the bone marrow within the substance of the meniscus (Figs. 5.42 and 5.43).

Chondrocalcinosis is a general term that refers to cartilage and meniscal calcification. Different diseases such as calcium pyrophosphate dihydrate crystal (pseudogout), dicalcium phosphate dihydrate or calcium hydroxyapatite crystals depositions may be responsible for meniscal chondrocalcinosis [59]. On MRI the meniscus may appear enlarged with intrameniscal high-signal intensity changes on T1- and T2-weighted images. This high signal alteration pattern decreases the accuracy for meniscal tears detection making the correlation with radiography necessary [59].

5.3   MRI Postoperative Findings

The main role of the menisci is to transmit the loading forces by increasing the contact area between femur and tibia and, therefore, any change in shape and dimension may be followed by long term undesirable effects. Any intervention should be focused on maintaining, as closely

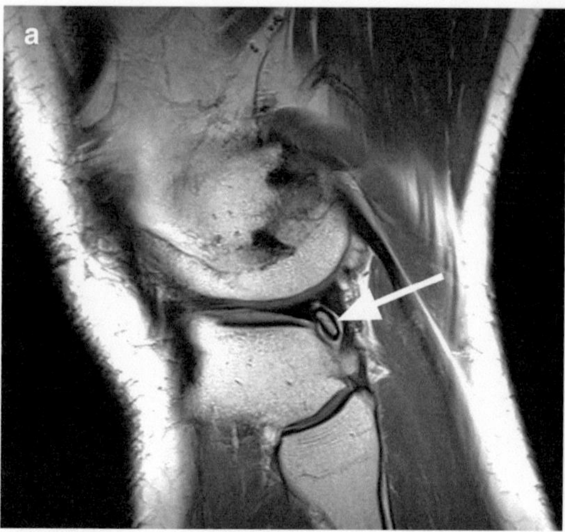
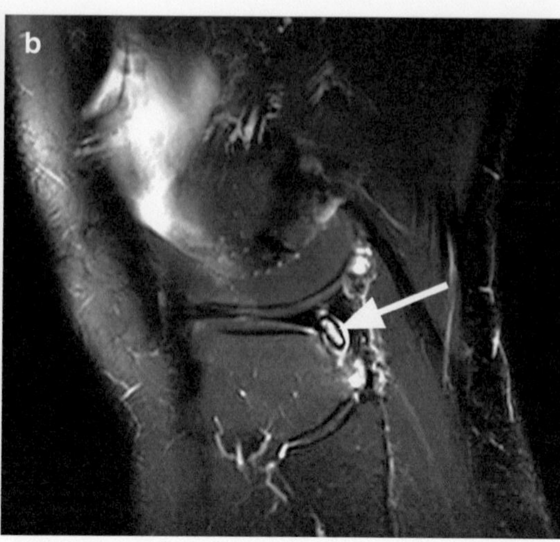

Fig. 5.43 Parameniscal ossicle in a 44 year old male. Sagittal proton-density (PD) FSE image (**a**) and sagittal T2-weighted fat-suppressed FSE image (**b**) show a calcification (*arrow*) in the posterolateral corner between the posterior horn of the lateral meniscus and the popliteal tendon. Note the high signal intensity edema of the calcified lesion

as possible, the normal triangular and semilunar shape of the normal meniscus [60]. There are three major types of interventions (meniscectomy, primary repair, and transplantation) and the choice depends on the patient age, on the meniscus pathology (degenerative or tear), and on the location, extension, and stability of the meniscal tear. Interpretation of MRI findings is challenging after any type of meniscal surgery and the radiologists should be aware of the particular type of intervention that have been performed.

5.3.1 Meniscectomy and Meniscal Repair

Meniscectomy is the preferred modality of treatment of unstable tears (see Table 5.1) and tears associated with degenerative changes. Meniscectomy may be total or partial with two types of partial resection: segmental or circumferential [61]. As a general rule, tears of the avascular zone of the meniscus, being incapable of repair with conservative treatment (immobilization, physical therapy) due to its lack of vascularisation, are often treated by partial meniscectomy. Meniscus repair (internal fixation and suturing of the tear) implies several surgical techniques that

preserve the meniscus. Meniscal tears suitable for repair are the longitudinal and oblique-horizontal tears of the periphery of the meniscus (the vascular zone). Meniscal replacement after total meniscectomy is a rarely performed procedure and indications are usually limited to young and active patients where the knee joint shows no or minimal degenerative changes.

The MRI of the postoperative meniscus is based on the evaluation of the meniscus shape, contour, and volume and the intrameniscal changes. The MRI appearance of the meniscus after partial meniscectomy may vary from a normal meniscus shape and size (after minimal meniscectomy) to a diminished meniscal volume with or without truncation of the free edge (after mid- to large-volume meniscectomy) (Fig. 5.44). Total meniscectomy implies the total removal of the meniscus and is followed by fibrous regeneration within 3 weeks to 3 months [62]. In this case, the "new meniscus" is seen as a thin and small inhomogeneous signal intensity structure.

The classic signs of a tear of a non-operative meniscus cannot be applied with the same confidence after surgery because of the "normal postoperative" intrameniscal changes [63]. The presence of a globular or linear signal intensity change that extends to the meniscal surface is a

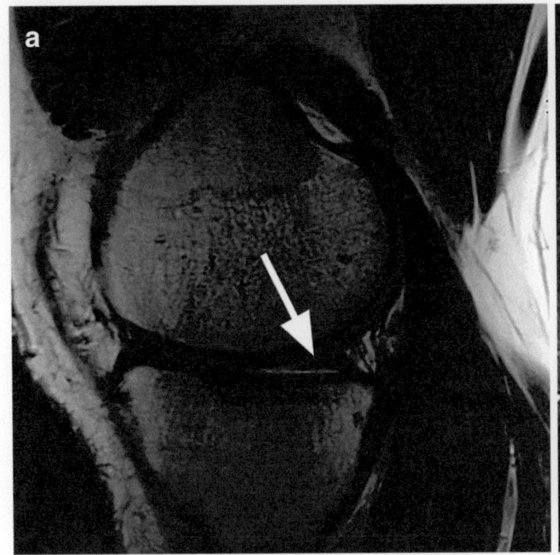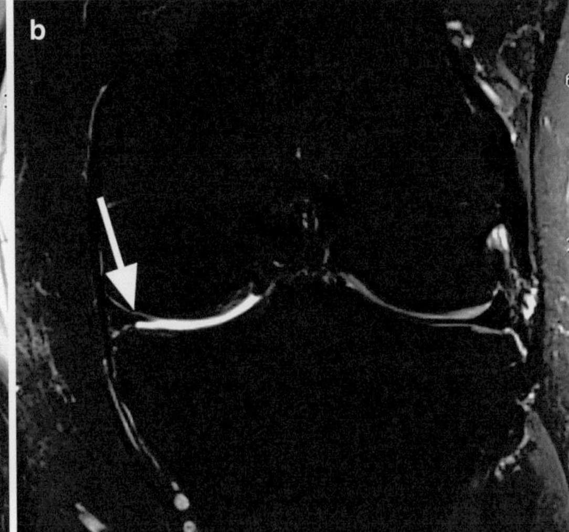

Fig. 5.44 Postoperative medial meniscus in a 45 year old male 5 years after partial meniscectomy. Sagittal proton-density (PD) FSE image (**a**) and coronal proton-density (PD) FSE fat-suppressed image (**b**) show a small posterior horn of the medial meniscus without truncation of the free edge (*arrow*). No pathological intrameniscal changes are noted

common sign that may persist for years and may represent healing process, myxomatous changes, or a persistent residual cleft with synovial fluid (Fig. 5.45) [64]. However, a linear high signal intensity lesion on different MR sequences - proton-density, T1- and T2-weighted - is a more accurate sign of retear than the high signal intensity on T2-weighted images only [65, 66]. The T2-weighted images alone have high sensitivity (88–92 %) but low specificity (41–69 %) [65, 66].

Direct MR arthrography might be helpful in these situations as the intraarticular gadolinium-based contrast agent would nicely outline graft tears. However, to the author's knowledge, so far, there has been no prospective study evaluating the value of direct MR arthrography for meniscal allograft evaluation. Overall however, direct MR arthrography has proven to be more accurate than conventional MRI in diagnosing a repeat tear or an unhealed meniscus repair after surgery and some authors consider this technique the first imaging modality choice in the evaluation of postoperative meniscus.

It needs to be noted that there is only limited value for indirect MR arthrography with i.v. application of contrast agent in the evaluation of

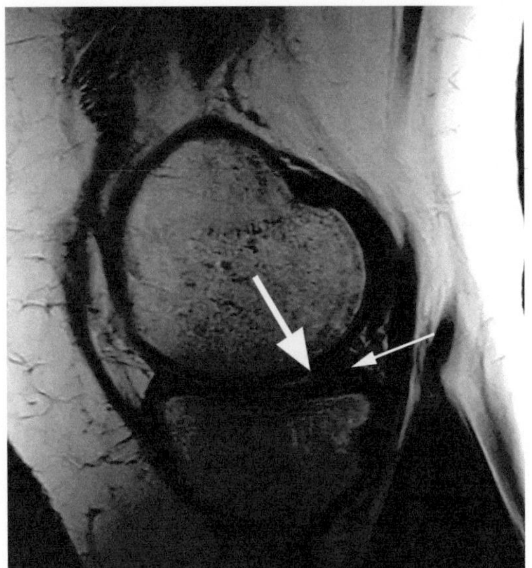

Fig. 5.45 Postoperative intrameniscal changes in a 25 year old male 3 months after partial meniscectomy. Sagittal proton-density (PD) FSE image shows truncation of the free edge of the medial meniscus (*large arrow*) and normal intrameniscal linear changes after meniscectomy (*small arrow*)

postoperative menisci as there will be enhancement of the repair tissue which hampers the diagnosis of re-tears.

5.3.2 Transplantation

Autologous meniscal transplantation may be used in young patients with irreparable tears or with failed prior meniscectomy [67].

Literature is spare on postoperative imaging of meniscal allografts and the role of MR imaging in evaluating allografts is not defined clearly [63, 68, 69]. The "normal" signal intensity of meniscal allografts was described as greyish or patchy rather which means that the typical hypointens signal of normal native menisci may no bee seen in allografts. This may cause difficulties in the detection of tears of the meniscal allograft, as a tear is usually defined as a linear increase in signal intensity. On postoperative MR images susceptibility artefacts along the capsular margins and small linear defects in tibia are present. The altered intrameniscal signal may be normally present 6–12 month after transplantation [70]. Most meniscal transplants show degeneration of the posterior horn and, in the case of allograft failure, fragmentation, meniscal detachment and extrusion, and cartilage defects are the most suggestive MR findings [68, 71, 72].

5.3.3 Complications After Surgery

Accelerated osteoarthritis is the most common complication after total or large partial meniscal resection. Other postoperative complications are arthrofibrosis, inflammations and infections, postoperative free meniscal fragments, meniscal extrusion, subchondral tibial fractures and osteonecrosis (post-meniscectomy osteonecrosis) [73, 74].

5.4 MRI Impression

5.4.1 Nonoperative Meniscus

1. Discoid meniscus (lateral/medial)
   - With/without degenerative changes
   - Tear (to mention the tear type)
2. Meniscal avulsion (medial/lateral) involving the anterior, body, or posterior horn
3. Meniscal extrusion (medial/lateral) involving the anterior, body, or posterior horn; to mention the distance from the tibial plateau in mm
4. Degenerative changes of the anterior, body, or/and posterior horn (medial/lateral)
5. Meniscal contusion with or without subchondral bone changes (ostechondral lesion, bone edema, fracture)
6. Meniscal tear – should be classified based on Table 5.1
7. Parameniscal cyst: location, size
   - With/without distinct communication with a meniscal lesion
8. Intrameniscal cyst: location, size
9. Meniscal calcifications (ossicles/chondrocalcinosis) - must be correlated with radiography

5.4.2 Postoperative Meniscus

1. Normal postoperative: shape, size, and morphology accordingly to the type of intervention; without MR signs of complications
   - Normal size and shape after minimal resection
   - Diminished in size with or without truncation of the free margin of the remnant meniscus
   - Absent or with the visualization of a fibrous tissue ("new meniscus")
   - Normal linear signal intensity change after meniscus repair
   - Normal altered signal intensity changes after meniscus repair or transplantation
   - Susceptibility artifacts (transplantation)
2. MRI appearance suggestive for tear of the remnant meniscus (location, orientation)
3. Extrusion of the remnant meniscus
4. Degeneration of the transplanted meniscus
5. MRI appearance suggestive for transplant failure (fragmentation, extrusion, cartilage defects)
6. Post-operative arthrofibrosis
7. Complications
   - Free meniscal fragment or meniscal extrusion
   - MR appearance suggestive for inflammatory or infectious arthritis

- With/without suggestive MR signs of osteoarthritis
- Subchondral tibial fracture with or without subchondral osteonecrosis

References

1. Messner K, Gao J. The menisci of the knee joint. Anatomical and functional characteristics, and a rationale for clinical treatment. J Anat. 1998;193(Pt 2):161–78.
2. Arnoczky SP, Warren RF. Microvasculature of the human meniscus. Am J Sports Med. 1982;10(2):90–5.
3. Gray JC. Neural and vascular anatomy of the menisci of the human knee. J Orthop Sports Phys Ther. 1999;29(1):23–30.
4. Ahmed AM, Burke DL. In-vitro measurement of static pressure distribution in synovial joints–part I: tibial surface of the knee. J Biomech Eng. 1983;105(3):216–25.
5. De Maeseneer M, et al. Three layers of the medial capsular and supporting structures of the knee: MR imaging-anatomic correlation. Radiographics. 2000; 20(Spec No):S83–9.
6. Starok M, et al. Normal patellar retinaculum: MR and sonographic imaging with cadaveric correlation. AJR Am J Roentgenol. 1997;168(6):1493–9.
7. Fenn S, Datir A, Saifuddin A. Synovial recesses of the knee: MR imaging review of anatomical and pathological features. Skeletal Radiol. 2009;38(4):317–28.
8. Johnson DL, et al. Insertion-site anatomy of the human menisci: gross, arthroscopic, and topographical anatomy as a basis for meniscal transplantation. Arthroscopy. 1995;11(4):386–94.
9. Brody JM, et al. Lateral meniscus root tear and meniscus extrusion with anterior cruciate ligament tear. Radiology. 2006;239(3):805–10.
10. Anderson AF, Awh MH, Anderson CN. The anterior meniscofemoral ligament of the medial meniscus: case series. Am J Sports Med. 2004;32(4):1035–40.
11. de Abreu MR, et al. Anterior transverse ligament of the knee: MR imaging and anatomic study using clinical and cadaveric material with emphasis on its contribution to meniscal tears. Clin Imaging. 2007;31(3):194–201.
12. Sintzoff Jr SA, et al. Transverse geniculate ligament of the knee: appearance at plain radiography. Radiology. 1991;180(1):259.
13. Sanders TG, et al. Oblique meniscomeniscal ligament: another potential pitfall for a meniscal tear–anatomic description and appearance at MR imaging in three cases. Radiology. 1999;213(1):213–6.
14. Bolog N, Hodler J. MR imaging of the posterolateral corner of the knee. Skeletal Radiol. 2007;36(8):715–28.
15. Sussmann PS, et al. Development of the popliteomeniscal fasciculi in the fetal human knee joint. Arthroscopy. 2001;17(1):14–8.
16. Diamantopoulos A, et al. The posterolateral corner of the knee: evaluation under microsurgical dissection. Arthroscopy. 2005;21(7):826–33.
17. Johnson RL, De Smet AA. MR visualization of the popliteomeniscal fascicles. Skeletal Radiol. 1999;28(10): 561–6.
18. Recondo JA, et al. Lateral stabilizing structures of the knee: functional anatomy and injuries assessed with MR imaging. Radiographics. 2000;20(Spec No): S91–102.
19. Heller L, Langman J. The menisco-femoral ligaments of the human knee. J Bone Joint Surg Br. 1964;46:307–13.
20. Bozkurt M, et al. An anatomical study of the meniscofibular ligament. Knee Surg Sports Traumatol Arthrosc. 2004;12(5):429–33.
21. Chew FS. Medial meniscal flounce: demonstration on MR imaging of the knee. AJR Am J Roentgenol. 1990;155(1):199.
22. Park JS, Ryu KN, Yoon KH. Meniscal flounce on knee MRI: correlation with meniscal locations after positional changes. AJR Am J Roentgenol. 2006;187(2):364–70.
23. Silverman JM, Mink JH, Deutsch AL. Discoid menisci of the knee: MR imaging appearance. Radiology. 1989;173(2):351–4.
24. Samoto N, et al. Diagnosis of discoid lateral meniscus of the knee on MR imaging. Magn Reson Imaging. 2002;20(1):59–64.
25. Rosenberg TD, et al. Discoid lateral meniscus: case report of arthroscopic attachment of a symptomatic Wrisberg-ligament type. Arthroscopy. 1987;3(4): 277–82.
26. Singh K, et al. MRI appearance of Wrisberg variant of discoid lateral meniscus. AJR Am J Roentgenol. 2006;187(2):384–7.
27. Mesgarzadeh M, et al. MR imaging of the knee: expanded classification and pitfalls to interpretation of meniscal tears. Radiographics. 1993;13(3):489–500.
28. Yaniv M, Blumberg N. The discoid meniscus. J Child Orthop. 2007;1(2):89–96.
29. Anderson MW. MR imaging of the meniscus. Radiol Clin North Am. 2002;40(5):1081–94.
30. El-Khoury GY, Usta HY, Berger RA. Meniscotibial (coronary) ligament tears. Skeletal Radiol. 1984;11(3): 191–6.
31. Bikkina RS, et al. The "floating" meniscus: MRI in knee trauma and implications for surgery. AJR Am J Roentgenol. 2005;184(1):200–4.
32. Costa CR, Morrison WB, Carrino JA. Medial meniscus extrusion on knee MRI: is extent associated with severity of degeneration or type of tear? AJR Am J Roentgenol. 2004;183(1):17–23.
33. Jones RS, et al. Direct measurement of hoop strains in the intact and torn human medial meniscus. Clin Biomech (Bristol, Avon). 1996;11(5):295–300.
34. Crema MD, et al. Factors associated with meniscal extrusion in knees with or at risk for osteoarthritis: the Multicenter Osteoarthritis study. Radiology. 2012;264(2): 494–503.
35. Miller TT, et al. Meniscal position on routine MR imaging of the knee. Skeletal Radiol. 1997;26(7):424–7.
36. De Maeseneer M, et al. Medial meniscocapsular separation: MR imaging criteria and diagnostic pitfalls. Eur J Radiol. 2002;41(3):242–52.

37. LaPrade RF, Konowalchuk BK. Popliteomeniscal fascicle tears causing symptomatic lateral compartment knee pain: diagnosis by the figure-4 test and treatment by open repair. Am J Sports Med. 2005;33(8): 1231–6.
38. Cothran Jr RL, et al. MR imaging of meniscal contusion in the knee. AJR Am J Roentgenol. 2001;177(5): 1189–92.
39. Zanetti M, et al. Patients with suspected meniscal tears: prevalence of abnormalities seen on MRI of 100 symptomatic and 100 contralateral asymptomatic knees. AJR Am J Roentgenol. 2003;181(3):635–41.
40. Vande Berg BC, et al. Lesions of the menisci of the knee: value of MR imaging criteria for recognition of unstable lesions. AJR Am J Roentgenol. 2001;176(3):771–6.
41. Barber BR, McNally EG. Meniscal injuries and imaging the postoperative meniscus. Radiol Clin North Am. 2013;51(3):371–91.
42. Quinn SF, Brown TF. Meniscal tears diagnosed with MR imaging versus arthroscopy: how reliable a standard is arthroscopy? Radiology. 1991;181(3):843–7.
43. De Smet AA, et al. Diagnosis of meniscal tears of the knee with MR imaging: effect of observer variation and sample size on sensitivity and specificity. AJR Am J Roentgenol. 1993;160(3):555–9.
44. Ahn JH, et al. Longitudinal tear of the medial meniscus posterior horn in the anterior cruciate ligament-deficient knee significantly influences anterior stability. Am J Sports Med. 2011;39(10):2187–93.
45. Harper KW, et al. Radial meniscal tears: significance, incidence, and MR appearance. AJR Am J Roentgenol. 2005;185(6):1429–34.
46. Jung JY, et al. Meniscal tear configurations: categorization with 3D isotropic turbo spin-echo MRI compared with conventional MRI at 3 T. AJR Am J Roentgenol. 2012;198(2):W173–80.
47. Lee YG, et al. Magnetic resonance imaging findings of surgically proven medial meniscus root tear: tear configuration and associated knee abnormalities. J Comput Assist Tomogr. 2008;32(3):452–7.
48. Forkel P, et al. Biomechanical consequences of a posterior root tear of the lateral meniscus: stabilizing effect of the meniscofemoral ligament. Arch Orthop Trauma Surg. 2013;133(5):621–6.
49. Tuckman GA, et al. Radial tears of the menisci: MR findings. AJR Am J Roentgenol. 1994;163(2):395–400.
50. Watt AJ, Halliday T, Raby N. The value of the absent bow tie sign in MRI of bucket-handle tears. Clin Radiol. 2000;55(8):622–6.
51. Singson RD, et al. MR imaging of displaced bucket-handle tear of the medial meniscus. AJR Am J Roentgenol. 1991;156(1):121–4.
52. Dorsay TA, Helms CA. Bucket-handle meniscal tears of the knee: sensitivity and specificity of MRI signs. Skeletal Radiol. 2003;32(5):266–72.
53. Vande Berg BC, et al. Meniscal tears with fragments displaced in notch and recesses of knee: MR imaging with arthroscopic comparison. Radiology. 2005;234(3): 842–50.
54. Lecas LK, et al. Inferiorly displaced flap tears of the medial meniscus: MR appearance and clinical significance. AJR Am J Roentgenol. 2000;174(1): 161–4.
55. Haramati N, et al. The flipped meniscus sign. Skeletal Radiol. 1993;22(4):273–7.
56. Al-Khateeb H, Ruiz A. Lateral meniscal cyst producing lesion of the tibial plateau and literature review. Int J Surg. 2008;6(5):412–4.
57. Lektrakul N, et al. Pericruciate meniscal cysts arising from tears of the posterior horn of the medial meniscus: MR imaging features that simulate posterior cruciate ganglion cysts. AJR Am J Roentgenol. 1999; 172(6):1575–9.
58. Rohilla S, et al. Meniscal ossicle. J Orthop Traumatol. 2009;10(3):143–5.
59. Kaushik S, et al. Effect of chondrocalcinosis on the MR imaging of knee menisci. AJR Am J Roentgenol. 2001;177(4):905–9.
60. Newman AP, Daniels AU, Burks RT. Principles and decision making in meniscal surgery. Arthroscopy. 1993;9(1):33–51.
61. Cannon Jr WD, Morgan CD. Meniscal repair: arthroscopic repair techniques. Instr Course Lect. 1994;43:77–96.
62. Doyle JR, Eisenberg JH, Orth MW. Regeneration of knee menisci: a preliminary report. J Trauma. 1966; 6(1):50–5.
63. Toms AP, et al. Imaging the post-operative meniscus. Eur J Radiol. 2005;54(2):189–98.
64. Arnoczky SP, et al. Magnetic resonance signals in healing menisci: an experimental study in dogs. Arthroscopy. 1994;10(5):552–7.
65. Farley TE, et al. Meniscal tears: MR and arthrographic findings after arthroscopic repair. Radiology. 1991;180(2):517–22.
66. Lim PS, et al. Repeat tear of postoperative meniscus: potential MR imaging signs. Radiology. 1999;210(1): 183–8.
67. Milachowski KA, Weismeier K, Wirth CJ. Homologous meniscus transplantation. Experimental and clinical results. Int Orthop. 1989;13(1):1–11.
68. van Arkel ER, et al. Meniscal allografts: evaluation with magnetic resonance imaging and correlation with arthroscopy. Arthroscopy. 2000;16(5):517–21.
69. Verdonk PC, et al. Meniscal allograft transplantation: long-term clinical results with radiological and magnetic resonance imaging correlations. Knee Surg Sports Traumatol Arthrosc. 2006;14(8):694–706.
70. Siegel MG, Roberts CS. Meniscal allografts. Clin Sports Med. 1993;12(1):59–80.
71. Potter HG, et al. MR imaging of meniscal allografts: correlation with clinical and arthroscopic outcomes. Radiology. 1996;198(2):509–14.
72. Verstraete KL, et al. Current status and imaging of allograft meniscal transplantation. Eur J Radiol. 1997;26(1):16–22.
73. Johnson TC, et al. Osteonecrosis of the knee after arthroscopic surgery for meniscal tears and chondral lesions. Arthroscopy. 2000;16(3):254–61.
74. MacDessi SJ, et al. Subchondral fracture following arthroscopic knee surgery. A series of eight cases. J Bone Joint Surg Am. 2008;90(5):1007–12.

Articular Cartilage and Subchondral Bone

6

Nicolae Bolog and Gustav Andreisek

6.1 Anatomy and Normal MRI Appearance

The knee articular cartilage is a hyaline cartilage composed of water (65–80 %), collagen (10–20 %, with type II collagen representing 90–95 % of the network), proteoglycans (10–20 %), and chondrocytes (1–5 %) [1]. Morphologically there are four cartilage zones with different composition, structure, and function. *The superficial zone* is the thinnest zone of the cartilage (10–20 % from the cartilage thickness) and is covered by synovial fluid. It is mainly composed of collagen fibers oriented parallel to the articular surface and provides shear strength. *The transitional zone* is the thickest zone (40–60 % from the cartilage thickness) and contains randomly oriented fibers, and its role is to distribute stress uniformly [2]. *The deep or the radial zone* (30 % of the cartilage thickness) contains the largest diameter of collagen fiber. The fibers are oriented perpendicularly to the articular surface, and its role is to anchor the cartilage to the subchondral bone [2]. *The calcified cartilage zone* (5 % of the cartilage thickness), the deepest zone of the cartilage, is a mineralized thin area and represents a shock absorber along the subchondral bone [1].

Hyaline cartilage lacks vascular, neural, and lymphatic networks, as well as local progenitor cells [3]. The sustenance of the cartilage is provided by diffusion from the synovial fluid, by vessels from the synovial membrane, and by vessels of the subchondral bone that are penetrating the calcified cartilage zone. The cartilage and the subchondral bone represent a functional unit with interconnected functions with the subchondral bone providing nourishment and vascularization to the cartilage [4]. The subchondral bone also protects the hyaline cartilage against damages caused by excessive loads [4].

The cartilage thickness depends on the anatomic location, the height, and the weight of the patient. The mean cartilage thickness on histological sections of the knee ranges from 1.65 to 2.98 mm [5] with the mean percentage difference between cartilage thickness in magnetic resonance imaging and direct measurement from histological sections about 10 % [6].

Currently, a vast amount of different MR sequences that enable qualitative, semiquantitative, or quantitative assessment of articular cartilage are available. These techniques can be classified into morphological and compositional techniques [7] (Table 6.1). Despite many promising studies and scientific reports, most of the compositional techniques do not play a role in the clinical routine. The clinical routine is still dominated by morphologic assessment of articular cartilage (Fig. 6.1). Thus, regardless the clinical context (traumatic, inflammatory, or degenerative), the MR knee protocol should include at least one morphologic, high-resolution, cartilage-sensitive MR sequence (Figs. 6.1 and 6.2).

The qualitative evaluation or the morphological evaluation of the cartilage is performed by using different MR sequences that includes all

N.V. Bolog et al., *MRI of the Knee: A Guide to Evaluation and Reporting*,
DOI 10.1007/978-3-319-08165-6_6, © Springer International Publishing Switzerland 2015

Table 6.1 MR imaging sequences for qualitative and quantitative cartilage evaluation [7–15]

Evaluation	MRI sequences	Type of information
Morphological	2-Dimensional T2 fast spin echo (2D T2 FSE)	*Qualitative morphological information:*
	2-Dimensional proton-density (2D PD) FSE	Cartilage signal intensity
	3-Dimensional fast spin echo (3D FSE)	Cartilage thickness
	3-Dimensional fast spin-echo sampling perfection with application-optimized contrast using different flip-angle evolutions (3D FSE SPACE)	Subchondral lesions characterization
	3-Dimensional T1 spoiled gradient-echo (3D SPGR and FLASH)	*Quantitative morphological information:*
	3-Dimensional dual echo steady state (DESS)	Cartilage volume (VC)
	3-Dimensional balanced steady-state free precession pulse sequences (WS-bSSFP)	Area of cartilage surface (AC) Cartilage thickness (ThC) Area of subchondral bone (tAB)
	3-Dimensional driven equilibrium Fourier transform (DEFT)	The denuded area (dAB)
Compositional (mainly used in clinical research for early osteoarthritis detection and cartilage repair)	T1 mapping (2-dimensional or 3-dimensional)	Detects regional variation of collagen network and glycosaminoglycan content
	T2 mapping	Reflects the collagen component of the extracellular matrix (collagen concentration and fibers orientation); water content
	T2 mapping	Quantitative information on collagen fibers integrity and changes in bound water
	Delayed gadolinium-enhanced MRI of cartilage (dGEMRIC)	Glycosaminoglycans depletion
	Sodium imaging	Glycosaminoglycans depletion
	Diffusion weighted	Collagen network and glycosaminoglycans content; more sensitive than T2 mapping and might also provide information on the nutrition of the repair tissue

standard 2-dimensional (2D) MR sequences (2D fast spin-echo sequences) (Figs. 6.1 and 6.2) as well as 3-dimensional (3D) MR sequences [7] (Table 6.1). The morphological evaluation provides information about the structural integrity of the cartilage that refers to thickness and signal intensity, the diffuse or focal cartilage loss, and the subchondral bone changes. The advantages of the so-called "conventional" 2-dimensional (2D) MR sequences result from their relatively short acquisition time and from the practical fact that they are extensively used in the routine clinical MR knee protocol being able to provide in the same time accurate information about all the other structures (e.g., meniscus, ligaments and tendons, bone).

Morphological evaluation may be also used for scoring cartilage damage by using semiquantitative criteria especially in clinical research (assessment of ostearthritis) [8]. WORMS (whole-organ MR imaging score) [16], KOSS (knee osteoarthritis scoring system) [17], and BLOKS (Boston-Leeds osteoarthritis knee score) [18] are such semiquantitative measurements in which the cartilage damage

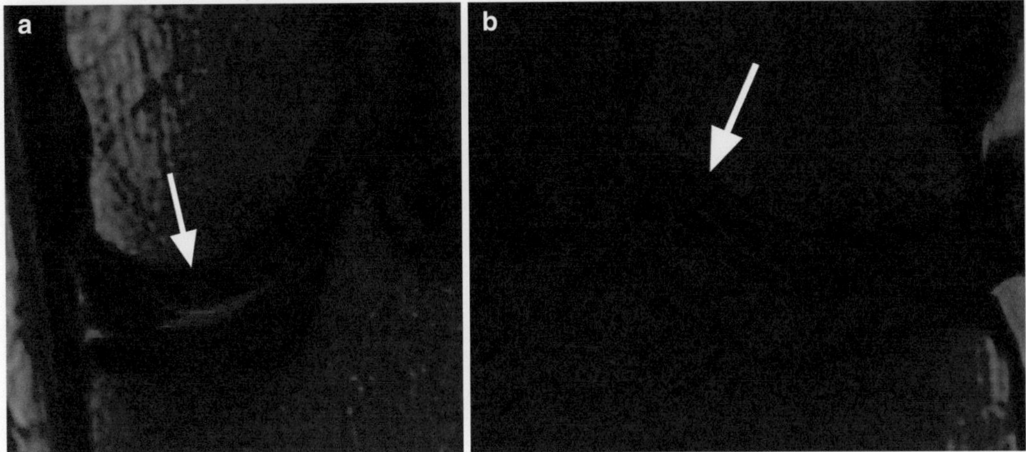

Fig. 6.1 Normal cartilage. Coronal proton-density (PD) FSE images (**a**, **b**) show the normal cartilage appearance in the medial compartment (*arrow* in **a**) and lateral compartment (*arrow* in **b**). This standard 2-dimensional (2D) MR sequence FSE enables the morphological evaluation of the cartilage in clinical routine practice

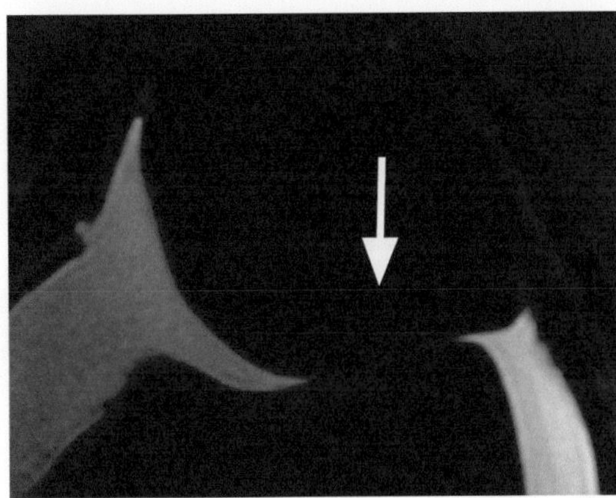

Fig. 6.2 Normal cartilage thickness and normal cartilage signal intensity on axial proton-density (PD) FSE fat-suppressed image (*arrow*)

measurements used in compositional techniques are used for obtaining information regarding the hydration of the cartilage, the glycosamine content, and the orientation of the collagen fibrils (Table 6.1). These MR techniques often need a long scan time, special equipment, and advanced and time-consuming post-processing. Thus, these are mainly used in clinical research especially in monitoring the effects of cartilage-preserving therapies, but not for clinical routine.

6.2 MRI Pathological Findings

The pathological changes of the cartilage and the subchondral bone may be classified based on the etiology in nontraumatic or traumatic lesions. The traumatic lesions may involve only the articular cartilage, only the subchondral bone, or both the articular cartilage and the subchondral bone (Table 6.2).

is assessed concomitant with other structures of the knee (e.g., menisci, subchondral bone, osteophytes, and synovial membrane) [8].

Most of the compositional MRI techniques are relatively new developed MR sequences which include various T2- and T2-mapping techniques, delayed gadolinium-enhanced magnetic resonance imaging of cartilage (dGEMRIC), sodium or natrium imaging, diffusion-weighted imaging, and diffusion tensor imaging, as well as magnetization transfer imaging techniques [7–12] (Table 6.1). The semiquantitative and quantitative

6.2.1 Nontraumatic Cartilage Changes and Subsequently Subchondral Lesions

The cartilage of the knee is involved in osteoarthritis of the joint as well as in inflammatory diseases and may be accompanied by subchon-

Table 6.2 Osteochondral lesions

Type of lesion	Articular cartilage involvement	Subchondral bone involvement
Degenerative	Thinning (due to dehydration and mechanical stress)/denudation	Attrition Edema Subchondral cyst
Inflammatory	Thinning (due to erosions from inflamed synovium)/denudation	Edema Subchondral erosions
Osteonecrosis (idiopathic or secondary)	Often involved	Focal defect Flattening of the surface
Traumatic lesions		
Cartilage fracture	Focal lesion with abrupt margins	No involvement or subchondral edema
Cartilage delamination (Figs. 6.3–6.5)	Linear lesion at the base of the cartilage	No involvement
Osteochondritis dissecans (idiopathic or secondary)	Cartilage and bone involvement: subchondral fracture extending through the cartilage	
Bone bruises	May be affected	Diffuse edema (no fracture line)
Subchondral fracture	With/without involvement	Subchondral linear fracture Surrounding bone edema

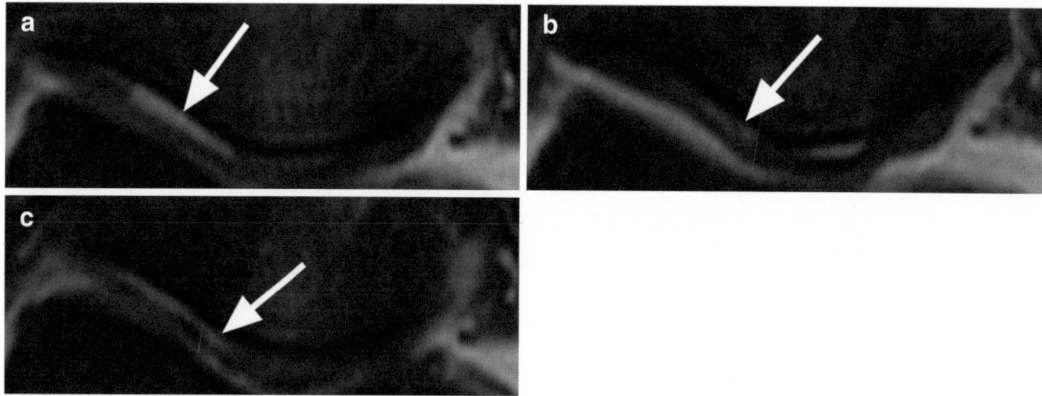

Fig. 6.3 Cartilage delamination in a 31 year old volleyball player after acute knee distortion. Three consecutive axial proton-density (PD) FSE fat-suppressed images (**a–c**) show a typical linear high-signal-intensity change at the base of the patellar cartilage (*arrows*)

dral changes (edema, cysts, erosions). The damaged cartilage is routinely assessed qualitatively based on the thickness changes and signal-intensity alteration. Although cartilage thinning and denudation of subchondral bone are changes that characterize both degenerative and inflammatory diseases, the pathogenesis of these changes is different. Deterioration of the articular cartilage in degenerative disease is the result of dehydration and repetitive microtrauma of the cartilage, while in inflammatory arthritis, the alteration of the cartilage thickness is the result of proliferation of the vascular connective tissue of the synovial membrane (pannus) and the effect of the inflammatory mediators (immunoglobulins, enzymes).

The degenerative changes within the articular cartilage can be divided into an initial phase of superficial degeneration that continues with the phase of basal degeneration [19]. The earliest feature of degeneration starts with discontinuities of the most superficial zone of the cartilage tangential at the articular surface (superficial degeneration), and these changes are not visible on routine MR sequences. Basal degeneration develops in the deep layers of cartilage and manifests as areas of focal softening and swelling attributed to edema and abnormal matrix-protein substances followed by fibrillation, fragmentation that may ultimately denude areas of subchondral bone (Fig. 6.4) [4, 20]. The first basal degeneration changes, also often referred to as chondromalacia, may be seen on MR images as areas of low or high signal intensity (Fig. 6.4) as a result of localized edema without alterations in cartilage thickness and without cartilage surface irregularities

[20]. The clinical significance of these MR findings has not been clearly demonstrated, and moreover, the alteration of the signal intensity within cartilage cannot only be seen in the initial phases of degeneration but also in trauma, as cartilage contusion may have the same MRI appearance (Fig. 6.5).

Regardless the mechanism, degenerative or inflammatory, the MRI report should describe the cartilage thinning or denudation (location and dimension of the affected area) and the presence or absence of subchondral changes. On MR images, thinning of the cartilage is seen as a decreased of normal thickness accompanied by irregularities and high-signal changes at the surface of the cartilage (Fig. 6.4). Cartilage thinning is usually easy to appreciate when present unilaterally (only the medial femoral condyle and/or tibia is affected) but sometimes difficult when present bilaterally because radiologists tend to take the contralateral side for comparison. However, bilateral cartilage thinning is often a sign of severe osteoarthritis of

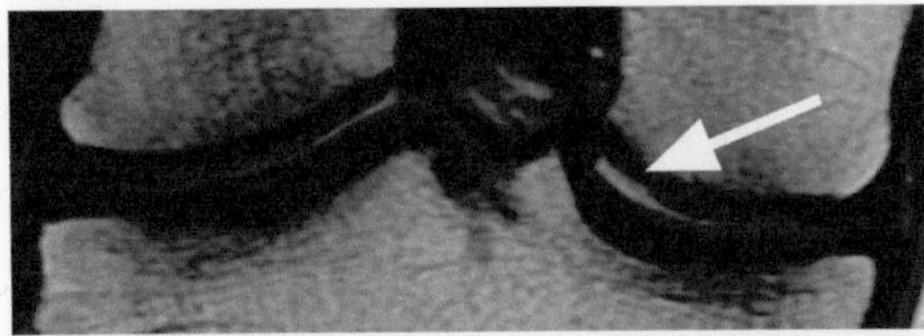

Fig. 6.4 Initial phase of cartilage degeneration. Coronal proton-density (PD) FSE image shows cartilage thinning accompanied by irregularities and high-signal changes at the surface of the cartilage (*arrow*)

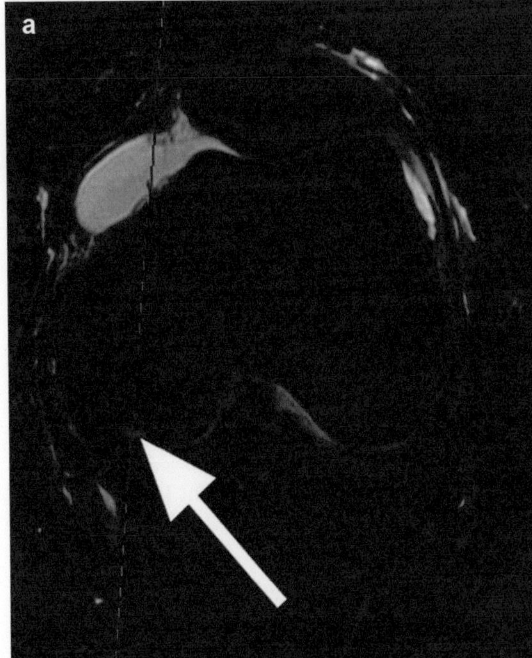

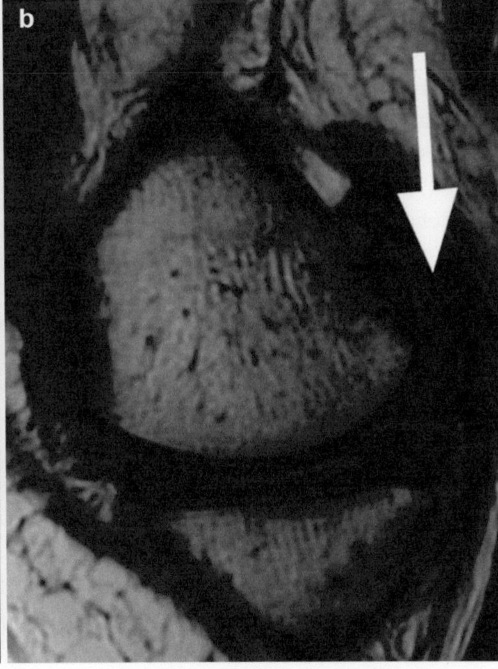

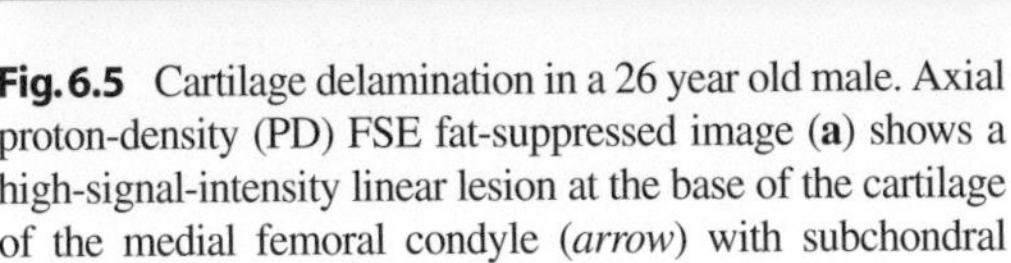

Fig. 6.5 Cartilage delamination in a 26 year old male. Axial proton-density (PD) FSE fat-suppressed image (**a**) shows a high-signal-intensity linear lesion at the base of the cartilage of the medial femoral condyle (*arrow*) with subchondral edema. Sagittal proton-density (PD) FSE image (**b**) at the level of the lesion shows a normal cartilage thickness (*arrow*). Similar cartilage and subchondral changes may be also seen in the initial phases of degeneration

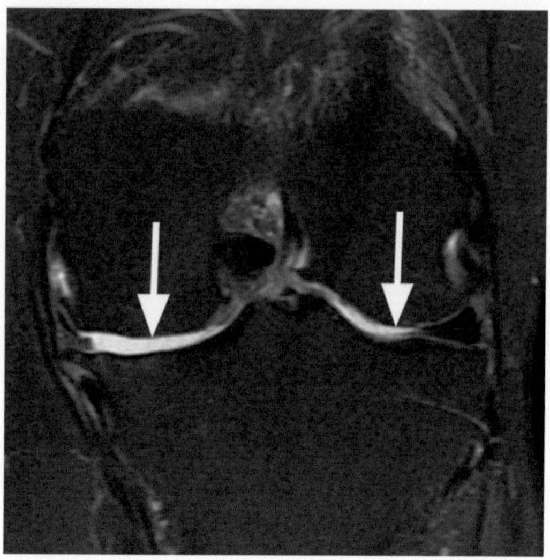

Fig. 6.6 Denuded areas on both femoral condyles. Coronal proton-density (PD) FSE fat-suppressed image shows bilateral femoral areas where the subchondral bone is not covered by articular cartilage (*arrows*). Note the absence of the subchondral changes

the knee or severe inflammation, and often all articular cartilage surfaces including the patellar are involved. Thus, evaluation of cartilage thinning should be considered not only as a search for focal or localized lesions, but one should take a step back and take a "global" view on all cartilage surfaces altogether.

The same rule applies to denuded areas of subchondral bone which are defined as areas where the subchondral bone is not covered by articular cartilage (Fig. 6.6) [21]. Despite the fact that a full cartilage loss seems to be easy to detect, in our clinical practice, we have seen that beginners/first-year residents struggle with this diagnosis especially when the loss is present in the medial and lateral compartment of the femorotibial joint. Difficulties for diagnosis may arise from the fact that when the cartilage is completely lost, beginners tend to misinterpret susceptibility artifacts arising from the subchondral bone which is then exposed directly to the joint fluid. Interestingly, they usually have less diagnostic problems with the patellar cartilage likely because this cartilage is much thicker and complete loss or thinning is therefore better to appreciate.

The specific subchondral changes that appear in degenerative and inflammatory diseases have a different pathogenesis that can be explained through the interconnection between the cartilage and the subchondral bone. In osteoarthritis, the overloading and the vascular obstruction within the subchondral bone leads to subchondral sclerosis, bone marrow edema and bleeding, and subchondral cysts. In the region of subchondral edema, in osteoarthritis the most common pathological changes are necrosis, fibrosis, and trabecular abnormalities [22]. The etiology of subchondral cysts is unknown. Some authors [23] suggest that the intra-articular pressure leads to intrusion of joint fluid into the subchondral bone. Another theory suggests that the bony contusion of two opposing articular surfaces results in subchondral bone necrosis followed by the cyst formation [24]. Pathologically, the subchondral cysts are cavitary lesion with an epithelial lining that is fluid filled [25]. In inflammatory diseases such as rheumatoid arthritis, subchondral edema has special significance. Histologically, it has been shown that edema is the result of osteitis, in which the bone marrow beneath the joint is invaded by an inflammatory and vascular lymphoplasmacytic infiltrate [26]. The inflamed synovium that invades the subchondral bone produces erosions that are defined as cavitary lesions filled with granulation tissue.

On MR imaging, the subchondral edema appears as ill-defined areas of low signal intensity on T1-weighted images and high signal intensity on T2-weighted images (Fig. 6.7). Some confusion exists in the literature about the nomenclature of cysts and erosions. The use of the terms like "cysts" or "erosions" on radiography can be a misnomer because the radiologist is unable to determine whether a radiolucent lesion is a fluid-filled lesion or is filled with solid material [27]. On MR imaging, both lesions are defined as relatively well-defined foci of altered signal intensity which appear hypointense on T1-weighted images and hyperintense on T2-weighted images (Fig. 6.8). Contrast-enhanced T1-weighted images may differentiate fluid-filled cysts from pannus-filled erosions. The latter enhances greatly on gadolinium-enhanced T1-weighted images immediately after contrast administration, while the cysts may enhance only at peripheral margins [28]. However, care needs to be taken when delayed

contrast-enhanced MR imaging (e.g., in indirect MR arthrography) is used since it shows contrast diffusion in fluid-filled spaces causing the bright signal of cystic fluid on T1-weighted sequences similar to erosions [28].

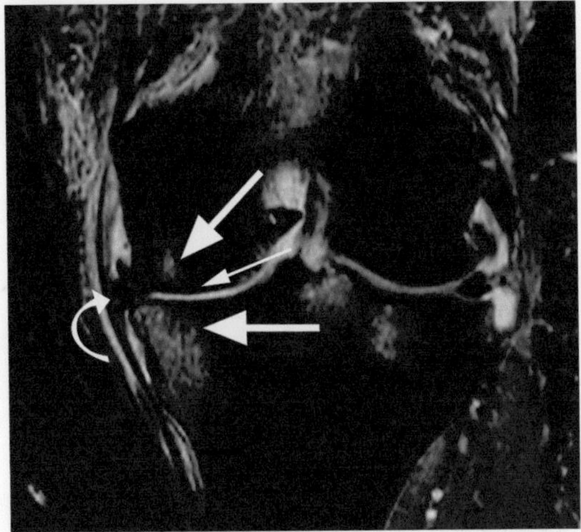

Fig. 6.7 Subchondral tibial and femoral edema in a 62 year old female with advanced medial osteoarthritis. Coronal proton-density (PD) FSE fat-suppressed image shows diffuse high-signal-intensity edema of the subchondral bone (*large arrows*) in the areas of bone denudation (*small arrow*). Note the medial meniscal extrusion (*curved arrow*)

The subchondral bone attrition and the formation of osteophytes are other subchondral changes that may appear in osteoarthritis. Bone attrition is the flattening or depression of the bony surface, and it seems that it is the result of subchondral microfractures and remodeling (Figs. 6.9 and 6.10) [29]. Osteophytes are hypertrophic ossifications that are the result of mechanical instability of the joint, proliferative response caused by adjacent synovial membrane, and tissue response from mechanical stress at the insertion of the capsule [30]. Although the osteophytes occur typically at marginal locations, they may occur also in central location within the articular cartilage [31, 32]. On MR imaging, the osteophytes are identified as abnormal marginal or central ossifications with similar signal intensity as the subchondral bone (Figs. 6.10 and 6.11). The central osteophytes are better depicted and evaluated on MR imaging than on radiographs [32].

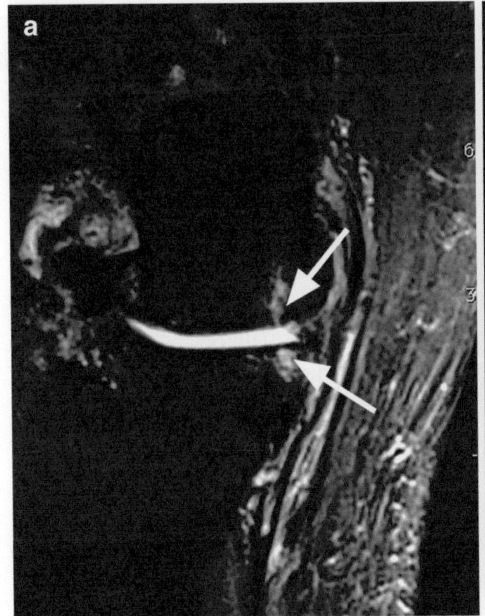
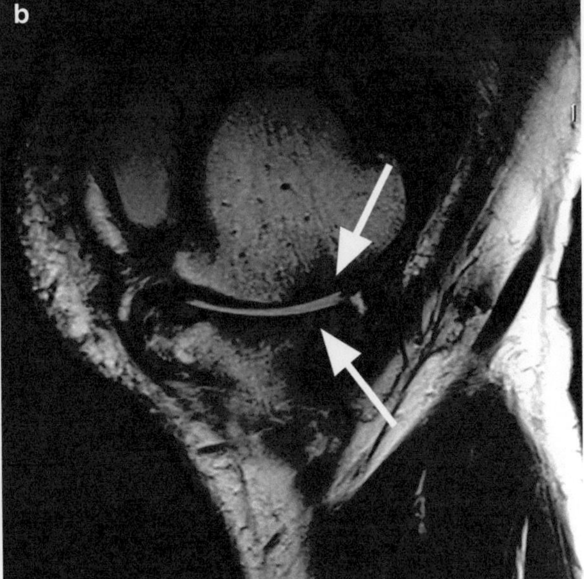

Fig. 6.8 Subchondral cysts in a 74 year old male with osteoarthritis. Coronal proton-density (PD) FSE fat-suppressed image (**a**) and sagittal proton-density (PD) FSE image (**b**) show small cystic lesions (*arrows*) of the subchondral tibial and femoral bone in the medial compartment

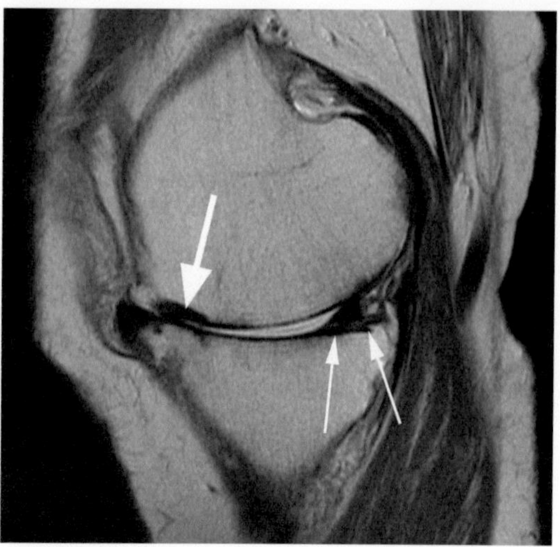

Fig. 6.9 Bone attrition. Sagittal proton-density (PD) FSE image shows depression of the bony surface on both, femoral condyle (*large arrow*) and posterior tibial plateau (*small arrows*). These changes are the result of subchondral microfractures and remodeling

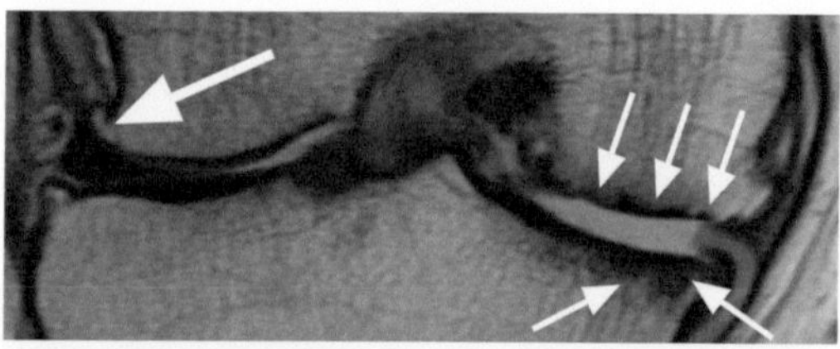

Fig. 6.10 Osteophytes and bone attrition. Coronal proton-density (PD) FSE image shows a lateral femoral osteophyte (*large arrow*) and complete denuded bone areas of the medial femoral condyle and medial tibial plateau with femoral and tibial bone attrition (*small arrows*)

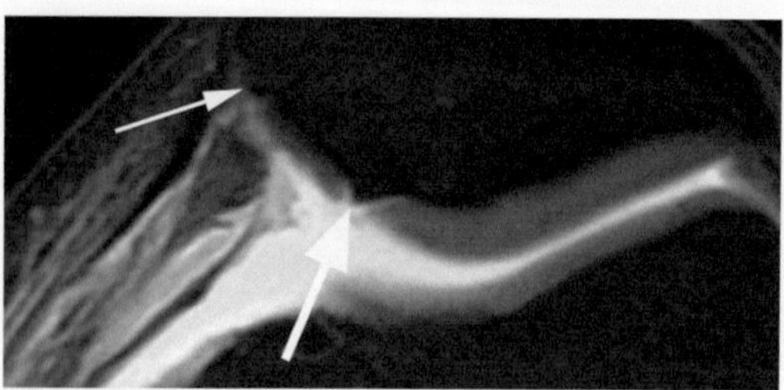

Fig. 6.11 Intracartilaginous osteophyte. Axial proton-density (PD) FSE fat-suppressed image shows an intracartilaginous osteophyte of the medial patellar facet which involves the entire thickness of the cartilage (*large arrow*). Note also the peripheral small osteophyte (*small arrow*)

6.2.2 Osteonecrosis of the Subchondral Bone

Spontaneous idiopathic osteonecrosis of the knee (SONK/Morbus Ahlback) affects middle-aged and elderly adults and is more frequently seen in women than in men with the medial side of the joint most commonly affected than the lateral side. The lesion usually results from circulatory impairment of the subchondral bone leading to ischemia. The etiology remains unclear, but the localized vascular insufficiency may explain subchondral osteonecrosis due to disruption of the nutrition supply to the cartilage above [33]. Spontaneous osteonecrosis of the knee has been also described as a complication after arthroscopic repair of the meniscal tears, and the lesion may be a late sequela of meniscal injury in association with cartilage defects and arthroscopic surgery [34].

Secondary osteonecrosis is caused by a number of well-recognized predisposing factors for osteonecrosis (e.g., systemic lupus erythematosus, steroid use, pancreatitis, alcoholism, HIV infection and renal transplants) or may be secondary to an old trauma [35].

MR imaging is the most accurate imaging technique for detecting osteonecrosis. The most specific MR imaging sign is the double-line sign at the periphery of osteonecrosis. The sign represents a reactive interface between necrotic bone and normal bone marrow and consists by an outer hypointense rim representing sclerotic bone and an inner rim and hyperintense on T2-weighted images, representing hypervascular granulation tissue (Fig. 6.12) [36]. This sign is more commonly seen in patients with secondary osteonecrosis compared to patients with idiopathic osteonecrosis in which the double-line sign can be absent (Fig. 6.13) [35]. However, there might be exceptions to this rule of thumb, and knowledge of the patient's history is necessary in these cases. Thus, whenever osteonecrosis is present, the patient's charts should be reviewed for predisposing factors. There is also a subcortical focal area of low-signal on both T1- and T2-weighted images representing the necrotic bone with

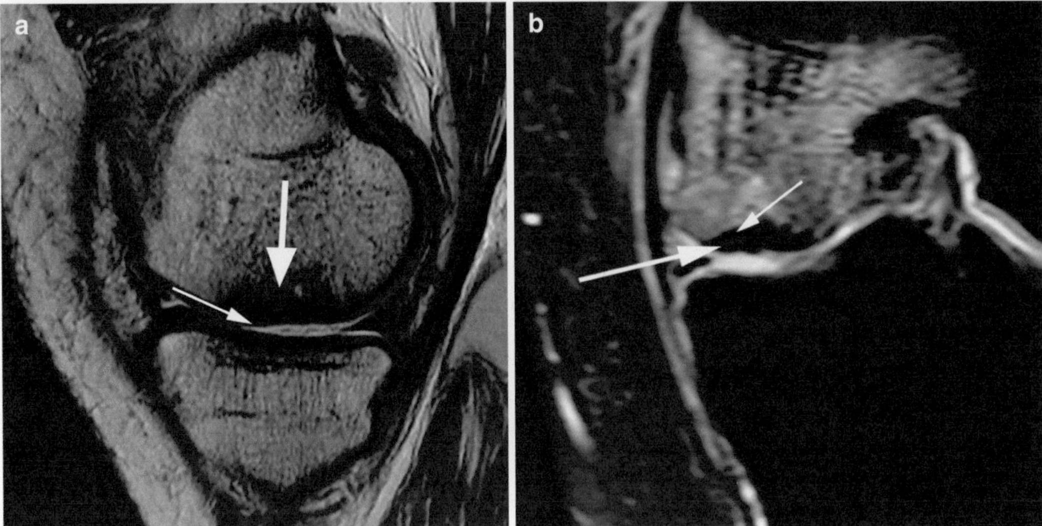

Fig. 6.12 Avascular osteonecrosis (SONK) of the medial femoral condyle in a 43 year old male (SONK). Sagittal proton-density (PD) FSE image (**a**) and coronal proton-density (PD) FSE fat-suppressed image (**b**) show a subcortical area of low signal intensity (*large arrow* in **a**) with depression of the subchondral bone. The cartilage thickness is almost normal (*small arrow* in **a**). The double-line sign at the periphery of osteonecrosis is demonstrated in the coronal plane (**b**): a hyperintense inner rim (*large arrow* in **b**) representing hypervascular granulation tissue and an outer hypointense rim representing sclerotic bone (*small arrow* in **b**)

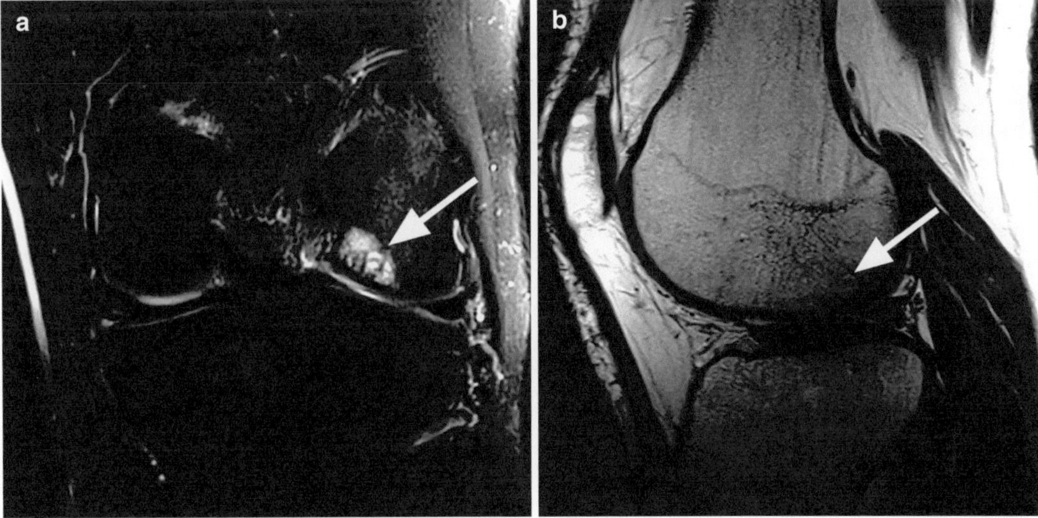

Fig. 6.13 Avascular osteonecrosis (SONK) of the lateral femoral condyle in a 50 year old female (SONK). Coronal proton-density (PD) FSE fat-suppressed image (**a**) and sagittal proton-density (PD) FSE image (**b**) show a subcortical area of high signal intensity (*arrow* in **a**, **b**) relatively well delineated. Note that the double-line sign is not present in this case

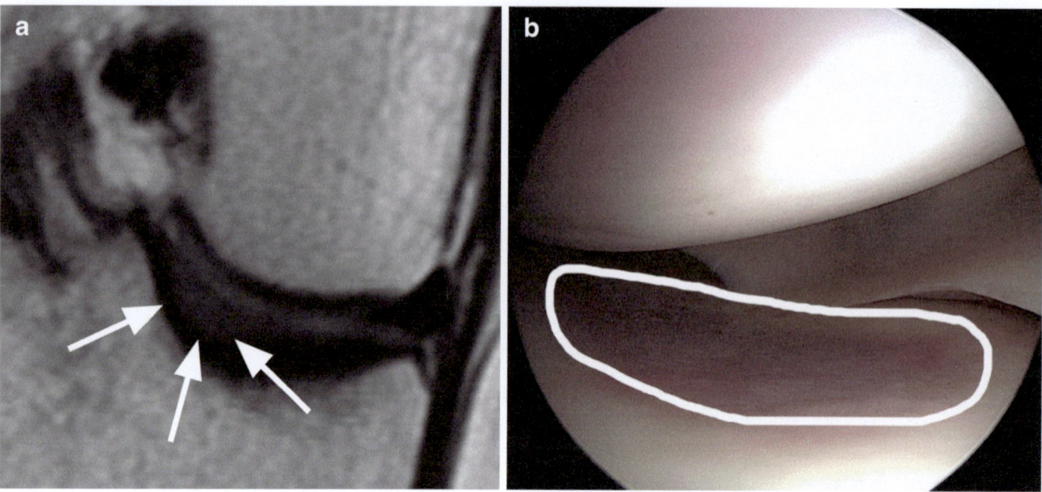

Fig. 6.14 Acute cartilage contusion (grade 1 lesion). Coronal proton-density (PD) FSE image (**a**) shows a focal hyperintense lesion involving the tibial cartilage (*arrows*). The lesion was confirmed at arthroscopy (**b**)

deformity and flattening of the articular surface (Fig. 6.12). Lesions may be surrounded by bone marrow edema.

6.2.3   Traumatic Osteochondral Lesions

Traumatic Cartilage Injuries

Cartilage contusions, cartilage fissures, and *cartilage fractures* may involve the cartilage superficial layer, the cartilage deep layers, or both without involving the subchondral bone (Figs. 6.13, 6.14, 6.15, 6.16, 6.17, and 6.18). Usually, the lesions are located at the weight-bearing surface, and avulsed and displaced fragments may be discovered in different location within the knee joint (intra-articular bodies). Pathologically, the cartilage lesions are classified into four grades of pathological changes (Table 6.3). On MR imaging, an acute cartilage lesion (contusion or fracture) is seen as a focal area of high signal intensity on T2-weighted images (Figs. 6.13, 6.14, 6.15, 6.16, and 6.17) or in the case of fractures as a cartilage defect filled with fluid with abrupt, well-delineated borders (Fig. 6.18). Subchondral edema may be seen in acute phase but it resolves in time. In chronic lesions, the margins are smoother due to healing

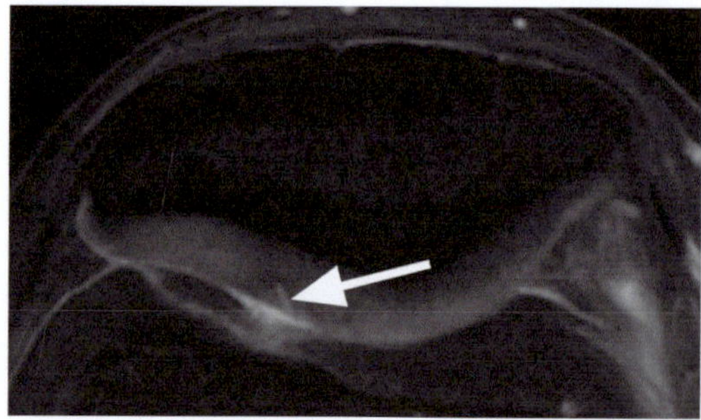

Fig. 6.15 Patellar cartilage fissure (grade 2 lesion). Axial proton-density (PD) FSE fat-suppressed image shows a small fissure of the cartilage (*arrow*) involving <50 % of the cartilage thickness

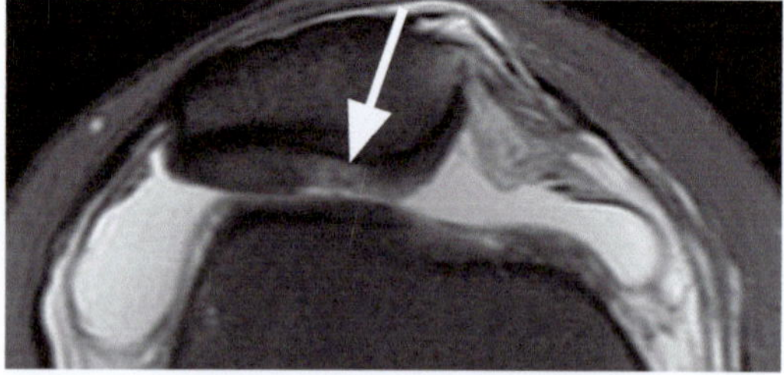

Fig. 6.16 Acute cartilage lesion (grade 3 lesion). Axial proton-density (PD) FSE fat-suppressed image shows a high-signal-intensity focal cartilage lesion (*arrow*) which is clearly delineated from the adjacent normal cartilage. The lesion involves >50 % of depth but not through subchondral bone

process, and over the time the defect may be replaced by fibrous tissue. MR arthrography can be used for a more accurate classification of the cartilage defect as well as for a better detection of intra-articular bodies. The MR report should include the location of the lesion, the size of the lesion, and the depth (<50 % of cartilage thickness, >50 % of cartilage thickness, full-thickness tear).

Cartilage delamination is the separation of the cartilage from the underlying bone at the deepest, calcified zone of the cartilage [38]. They result from shearing stress, and the delamination line

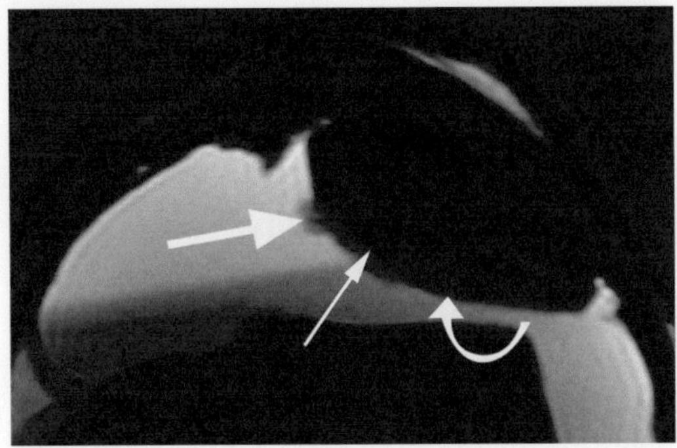

Fig. 6.17 Severe acute cartilage injury with different types of lesions. Axial proton-density (PD) FSE fat-suppressed image shows superficial fraying of the cartilage (*large arrow*), cartilage fissure (*small arrow*), and focal high-signal-intensity cartilage contusion (*curved arrow*). Note the presence of hemarthrosis in this patient with additional tibial fracture

runs parallel to the joint surface, but the overlying articular cartilage remains initially intact [39]. These lesions appear on MR imaging as linear increased signal intensity on T2-weighted images parallel to the cartilage surface at the junction of the articular cartilage and subchondral bone (Figs. 6.3 and 6.5) [39].

Osteochondritis Dissecans (Osteochondral Fracture)

Osteochondritis dissecans or osteochondral fracture is an acquired fracture in the subchondral bone extending through the articular cartilage having different grades of stability (Figs. 6.19, 6.20, and 6.21). The etiology seems to be multifactorial and related to an acute single event or to minor repetitive trauma that leads to subchondral fracture with possible necrosis in the deep area of the fragment margins [40]. Osteochondritis dissecans can be classified as stable (Fig. 6.19) or unstable according to partial or complete separation of the fragment (Table 6.4). The lesion may vary from few millimeters to several centimeters. On MR imaging, there is a curvilinear line that ends on both sides at the cartilage-bone junction (Fig. 6.20). The recommended MR sequences for diagnosis and classification are the T2-weighted, proton-density weighted, and 3-dimensional (3D) T1-weighted images in which the fracture line is best characterized. Usually, it appears as a

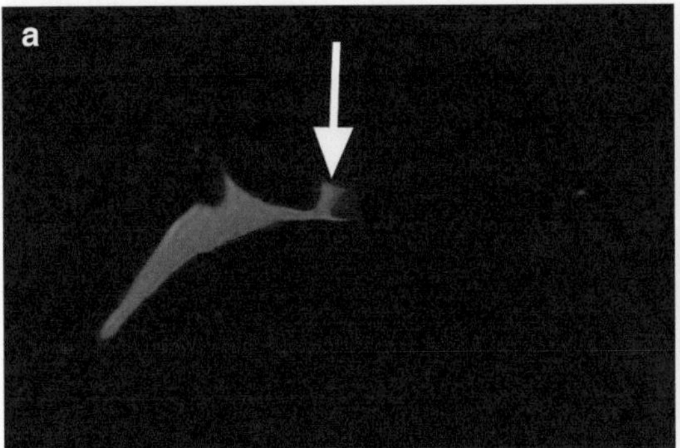

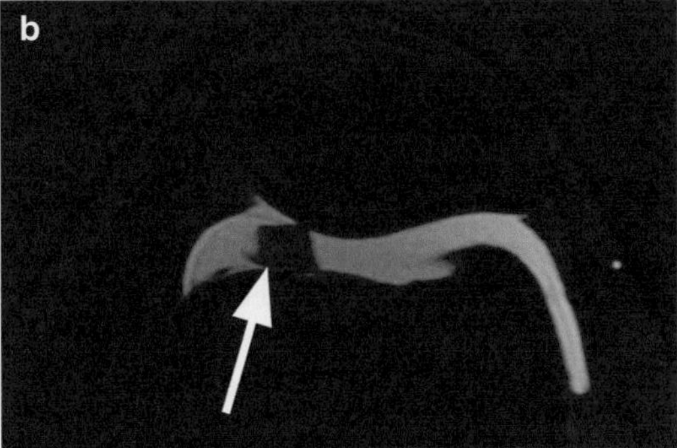

Fig. 6.18 Acute cartilage fracture with denudation of the subchondral bone (grade 4 lesion). Axial proton-density (PD) FSE fat-suppressed images (**a, b**) show a high-signal-intensity focal cartilage defect (*arrow* in **a**) with abrupt, well-delineated borders. The cartilage defect is filled with fluid. The missing cartilage fragment is displaced more cranially in the femoropatellar joint (*arrow* in **b**). Note that the dimension of the displaced fragment is similar to the dimension of the focal cartilage defect

Table. 6.3 Classification of cartilage injuries

	Pathologic change/arthroscopic findings	MRI findings
Grade 1 (Fig. 6.14)	Superficial lesion/chondral softening to probe	Normal appearance or increased focal or diffuse signal within the cartilage
Grade 2 (Fig. 6.15)	Lesion involving <50 % from the cartilage thickness/fissures involving <50 % thickness at arthroscopy	Irregularities of the cartilage surface or cartilage defect with increased signal intensity <50 % thickness
Grade 3 (Fig. 6.16)	Cartilage defect extending >50 % of depth but not through subchondral bone/fissures involving >50 % thickness at arthroscopy	Cartilage defect with increased signal intensity >50 % thickness
Grade 4 (Fig. 6.18)	Denudation/exposed subchondral bone at arthroscopy	Complete absence of the cartilage with fluidlike signal intensity in contact with the subchondral bone

Modified from International Cartilage Repair Society [37]

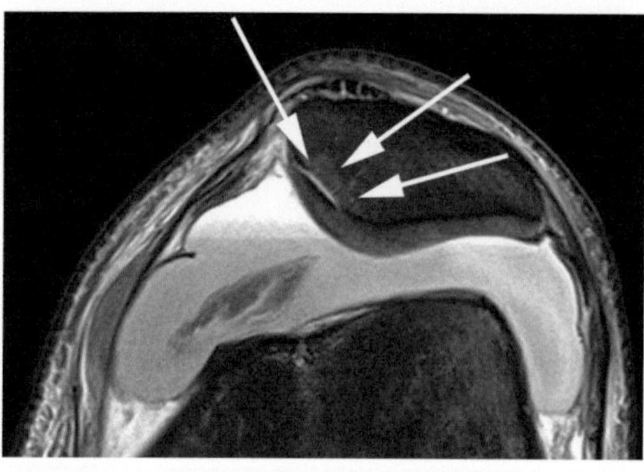

Fig. 6.19 Grade I (stable) osteochondritis dissecans or osteochondral fracture of the patella. Axial proton-density (PD) FSE fat-suppressed image shows a focal depressed fracture identified as a high-signal-intensity subchondral bone lesion without a clear delineation of the fragment (*arrows*). The lesion is stable

rim of high signal intensity. A confident diagnosis regarding the stability of the lesion is difficult even on MR arthrography. The presence of a fluidlike signal intensity rim on T2-weighted images may be an indicator of instability based on the fact that there should be a cartilage violation [42]. However, the high signal intensity around the lesion is not always the result of the presence of intra-articular fluid extending around the lesion. Similar hyperintense linear changes may appear in the presence of granulation tissue in stable lesions. The most accurate sign of instability is the identification of contrast material surrounding the lesion after intra-articular administration at direct MR arthrography. Bone marrow edema of the adjacent bone is present in most of the

cases. In the case of unstable lesions, the bone and cartilage fragment may detach and become a free intra-articular body (Fig. 6.21).

Bone Contusion (Trabecular Microfractures)

Bone contusions, bone bruises, or trabecular microfractures represent areas of hemorrhage, edema, or hyperemia secondary to trabecular traumatic injuries [43]. Different mechanisms of knee injury are responsible for bone contusions including the direct blow to the bone, compressive forces impacting adjacent bones, and shear and traction forces that occur during an avulsion injury [44]. These lesions can be isolated or are usually associated with other structures injuries of the knee. Although they alone may be a source of pain, they may also suggest a mechanism of injury to or a specific derangement of the knee joint (*see* Table 11.2). These types of occult bone lesions are not depicted by arthroscopy and can only be detected by MR imaging. Ill-defined areas with hyperintensity seen on T2-weighted images and hypointensity on T1-weighted images without the presence of a fracture line are commonly considered to represent bone marrow edema.

Subchondral Fractures

A subchondral fracture is defined as a fracture that does not extend through cortex and does not affect the overlying cartilage. The lesion remains subchondral and is surrounded by diffuse bone marrow edema. The subchondral fractures may be the result of insufficiency fractures of the

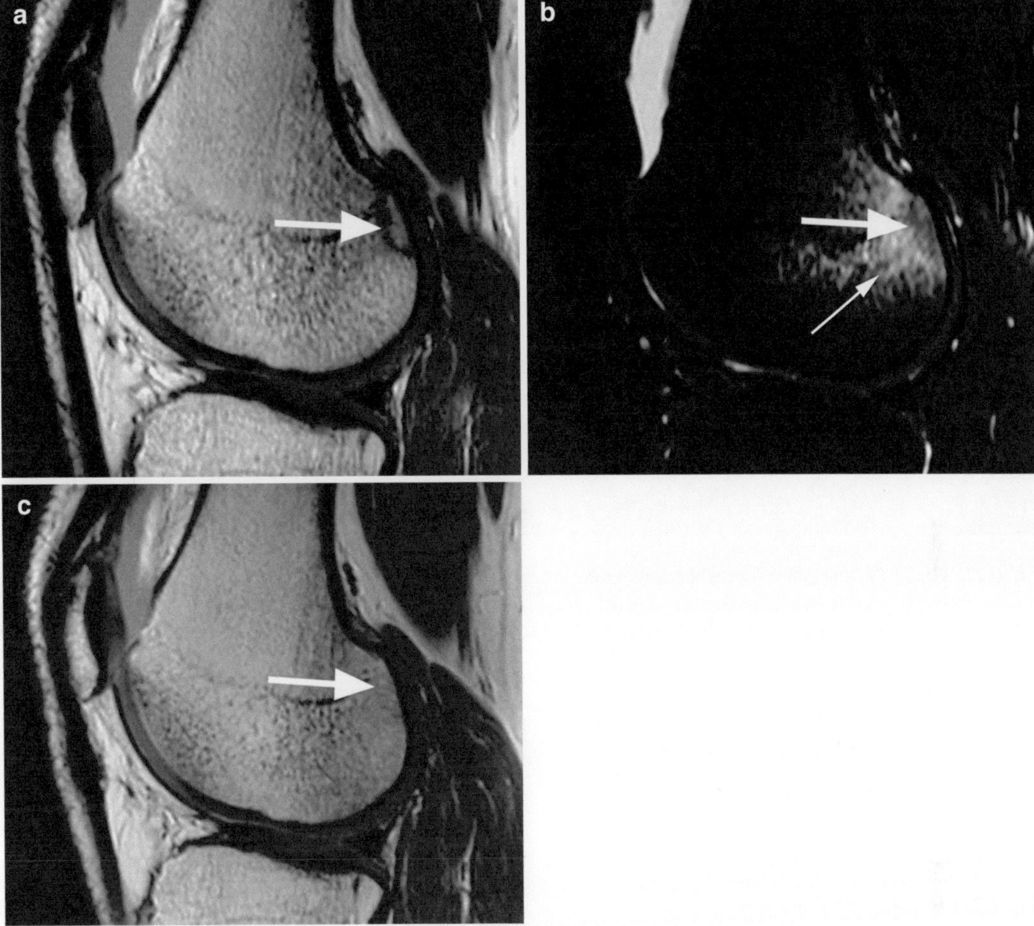

Fig. 6.20 Grade II (stable) osteochondritis dissecans or osteochondral fracture of posterior lateral femoral condyle in a 24 year old male. Sagittal proton-density (PD) FSE (**a**) and sagittal T2-weighted FSE fat-suppressed images (**b**) show a curvilinear line that ends on both sides at the cartilage-bone junction (*large arrow* in **a, b**). Note the diffuse bone marrow edema around the lesion (*small arrow* in **b**). Sagittal proton-density (PD) FSE (**c**) 18 months after the first examination shows a complete healing of the lesion (*arrow*)

subchondral bone (normal stress on abnormally bone) or of fatigue fractures (abnormal stress on normal bone). On MR imaging, the lesion appears as a discrete linear signal change situated in the subchondral area surrounded by diffuse edema without involving the articular cartilage.

6.3 MRI Postoperative Findings

The purpose of treatment of a cartilage defect is not only to repair or to replace the cartilage but also to prevent osteoarthritis. Cartilage lesions are not suitable for spontaneous repair due to the lack of vascularization. The indication of surgical intervention is based on different clinical and imaging algorithms such as the International Cartilage Repair Society score which is based on arthroscopic findings and the International Knee Documentation Committee functional score or the Hughston score [37, 45, 46]. Several surgical techniques are used currently in the cartilage repair, and they can be classified into marrow-stimulating techniques (abrasion, drilling, microfracturing) and regeneration techniques (autologous osteochondral transplants

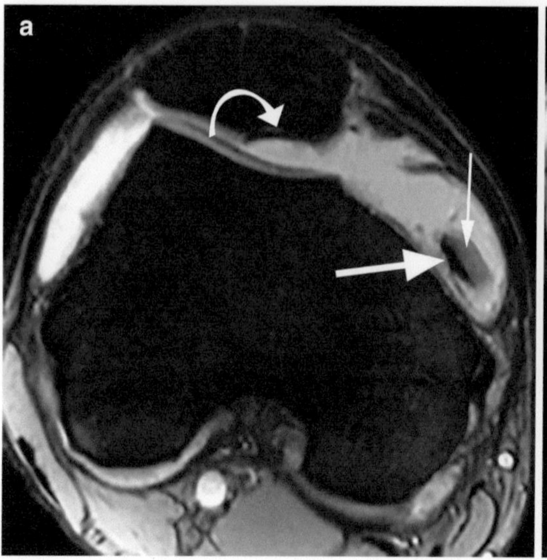 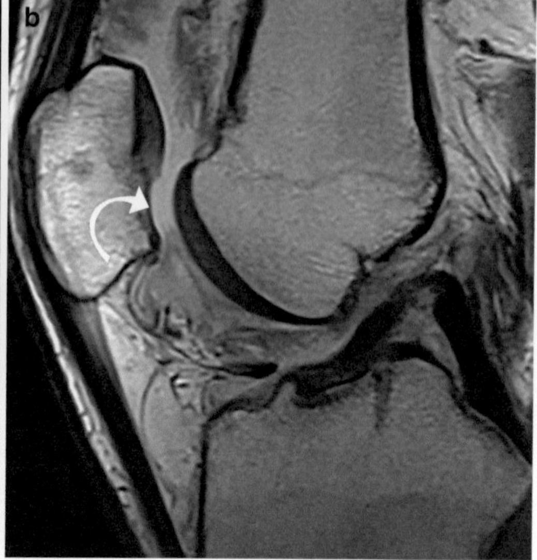

Fig. 6.21 Grade IV (unstable) osteochondritis dissecans or osteochondral fracture of patella. Axial image (**a**) shows a detached osteochondral fragment with a bony component (*large arrow*) covered by cartilage (*small arrow*). The frag-ment's origin is the medial facet of the patella (*curved arrow*). Sagittal proton-density (PD) FSE image (**b**) enables a better evaluation of the "donor" site (*curved arrow*)

Table 6.4 Grading of osteochondritis dissecans [41]

	Pathological description	Stability
Grade I (Fig. 6.19)	Depressed osteochondral fracture	Stable
Grade II (Fig. 6.20)	Osteochondral fragment attached by an osseous bridge	Stable
Grade III	Detached non-displaced fragment	Unstable
Grade IV (Fig. 6.21)	Displaced fragment	Unstable

and autologous chondrocyte implantation). MR imaging is the recommended noninvasive tool for evaluation of cartilage repair [47].

Regardless the treatment choice, the MR imaging assessment should include the relative signal intensity of the lesion after treatment, the presence or absence of delamination, the homogeneity of the structure including the presence or absence of fissures, the percentage fill of the lesion in two orthogonal planes, and the assessment of the subchondral bone [48–50]. In clinical routine MR examinations, all of these findings can be qualitatively evaluated on proton-density weighted, T2-weighted turbo-spin echo, and 3-dimensional (3D) T1 gradient-echo (GRE) sequences.

In marrow-stimulating techniques, the principle is to heal the cartilage defect with mesenchymal stem cells from subchondral bone by microfractures every 4–5 mm to a depth of maximum 6 mm into the vascularized subchondral bone [51]. The initial layer of fibrin within the cartilage defect reaches full thickness after 1–2 years [52]. The subchondral bone marrow edema may be persistent during this period. A normal MR appearance of the postoperative cartilage implies a complete filling of the defect without gaps between native cartilage and the repair tissue, a normal thickness of the repair tissue without cartilage irregularities [52, 53].

In autologous osteochondral transplants, there is a transfer of an osteochondral unit (usually from superomedial trochlea) to the cartilage defect the grafts (Figs. 6.22 and 6.23). The holes are typically 10–15 mm in length. Bone marrow signal appears as diffuse high signal intensity on T2-weighted images at the donor (usually femoral trochlea) and the recipient sites with regression of its intensity and during the first 6–9 months (Fig. 6.22). However, this signal may be discretely

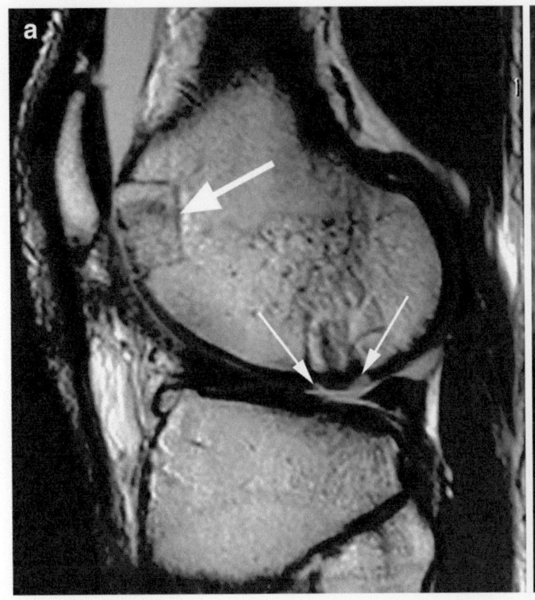
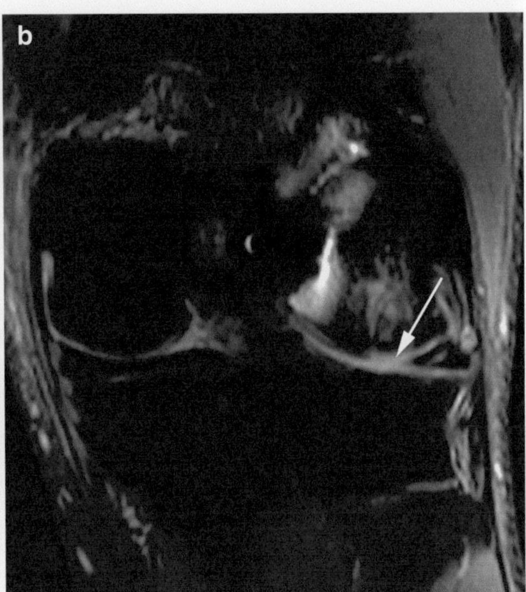

Fig. 6.22 Autologous osteochondral transplantation of the lateral femoral condyle 2 months after surgery in a 43 year old male. Sagittal proton-density (PD) FSE image (**a**) shows a step-off between surface of the implanted transplant relative and the surrounding native cartilage surface (*small arrows*) which may be an indicator of abnormality. Note the normal donor site appearance (lateral femoral trochlea) (*large arrow*). Coronal T2-weighted fat-suppressed image (**b**) shows a high-signal-intensity implanted cartilage (*arrow*) which can be another indicator of an abnormal postoperative evolution

present 12 months to 2 years after treatment [54]. After the transplant repair, the articular surface should be smoothly congruent on MR images in the region of repair (Fig. 6.23). Surface irregularities and the step-off between surface of the implanted transplant relative to the surrounding native cartilage surface are considered abnormal findings (Fig. 6.22) [54]. The transplanted cartilage should resemble the signal intensity of the normal cartilage, but postoperatively, the transplanted cartilage may be thinner and inhomogeneous signal intensity with discrete defects that will be filled in time by fibrinous clot and subsequent fibrocartilage (Fig. 6.23) [54]. Partial or complete loosing of the implanted transplant can be well appreciated on MR images and is usually not a diagnostic problem.

In autologous chondrocyte implantation, the chondrocytes are growing ex vivo and after that are injected into the cartilage defect under a patch of periosteum harvested from the tibia and sutured to the edge of the lesion [55]. There are three phases of healing after implantation. In the first 6 weeks, there is a proliferative phase, and the transplant tissue has a more homogeneous signal intensity due to the high content of chondrocytes without proteoglycans and collagen [54]. Normally, the defect should be filled with a smooth transition to the normal adjacent cartilage [56]. The proliferative phase is followed by remodeling and maturation phases (up to 9–18 months) [57, 58]. During maturation, MR imaging may show heterogeneity of the repair cartilage, and after the maturation phase, the cartilage implant should have the same signal intensity as the adjacent native cartilage. The pathological MR imaging findings include an incomplete filling, surface irregularities, and surface incongruity relative to the normal cartilage [56]. Delamination is a complication that may appear in the first 6 months after surgery [59, 60]. MR imaging shows a linear increased signal intensity on T2-weighted images parallel to the subchondral bone and represents the separation of the cartilage from the underlying bone. It may result from the failure of incorporation

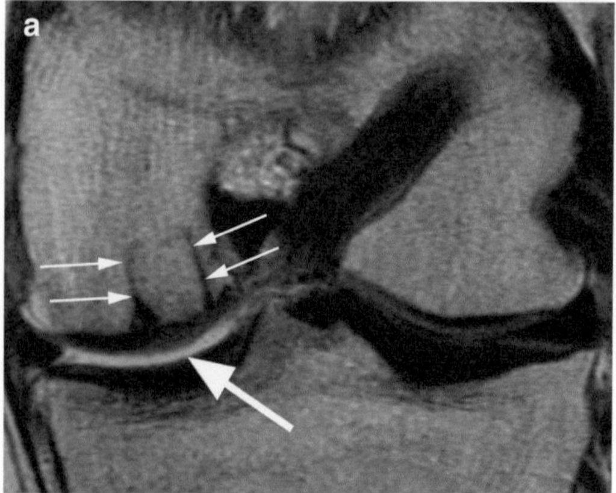

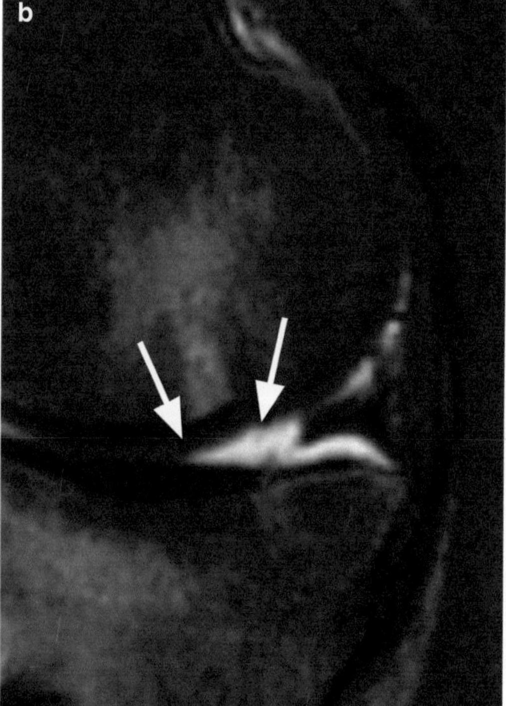

Fig. 6.23 Normal appearance of autologous osteochondral transplantation to the medial femoral condyle 4 months after surgery. Coronal proton-density (PD) FSE image (**a**) and sagittal T2-weighted fat-suppressed image (**b**) show a normal thickness of the implanted cartilage (*large arrow* in **a**). The small surface irregularities between surface of the implanted transplant relative to the surrounding native cartilage surface (*arrows* in **b**) will be filled in time by fibrinous clot and subsequent fibrocartilage. Note the osteochondral unit of 10–15 mm in length (*small arrows* in **a**)

into the subchondral bone or from shearing forces [56]. Another complication of the implantation is the fibrous overgrowth that can be seen on MR imaging as a protrusion of the cartilage surface due to hypertrophy of the periosteal flap. The bone marrow edema may be identified on MR images during the first year after implantation. The persistence of subchondral edema after 1 year is considered a pathological finding that may suggest a poor integration of the implant [61].

The compositional MR techniques are promising techniques in the quantitative assessment of cartilage repair and indeed often used in clinical research. The widely used compositional techniques in cartilage repair measurements are the diffusion-weighted imaging, the T2 mapping, and dGEMRIC. Currently, however, these techniques are not used for the clinical routine MR imaging after cartilage repair.

6.4 MRI Impression

6.4.1 Nonoperative Cartilage and Subchondral Bone

1. Cartilage thinning (location)
2. Cartilage defect with denudation of the bone (location and area of the lesion)
   - Without subchondral lesions
   - With subchondral changes: edema, attrition, osteophytes, cysts, and erosions
3. Subchondral osteonecrosis (location and dimension)
4. Acute cartilage contusion, fissure, and fracture with/without subchondral bone edema grades 1–4 (location, area of the lesion)
5. Cartilage fracture with detached loose intra-articular fragment (dimension and location of the fragment)
6. Cartilage delamination (location and dimension)
7. Osteochondritis dissecans or osteochondral fracture (grades I–IV)
8. Bone contusion without evidence of fracture lines (= subchondral edema, = subchondral trabecular microfractures)
9. Subchondral fracture (without involvement of cartilage)

6.4.2 Postoperative Osteochondral Findings

1. Normal postoperative MR imaging findings correlated to the interval time from the surgical intervention (bone edema may be normal during the first 2 years); no signs of complications at the site of repair or of the knee joint
2. Abnormal MR imaging findings
   - Incomplete defect filling
   - Irregularities and thin (compared to native cartilage) of the repair tissue/graft
   - Abnormal signal intensity of repair cartilage
   - Incongruence of articular surface
   - Delamination of repair cartilage
   - Protrusion of the cartilage surface suggesting fibrous overgrowth
   - Subchondral bone marrow edema after autologous chondrocyte implantation or autologous osteochondral transplants more than 1 year may suggest poor integration

References

1. Bhosale AM, Richardson JB. Articular cartilage: structure, injuries and review of management. Br Med Bull. 2008;87:77–95.
2. Bullough P, Goodfellow J. The significance of the fine structure of articular cartilage. J Bone Joint Surg Br. 1968;50(4):852–7.
3. Zhang L, Hu J, Athanasiou KA. The role of tissue engineering in articular cartilage repair and regeneration. Crit Rev Biomed Eng. 2009;37(1–2):1–57.
4. Imhof H, et al. Subchondral bone and cartilage disease: a rediscovered functional unit. Invest Radiol. 2000;35(10):581–8.
5. Shepherd DE, Seedhom BB. Thickness of human articular cartilage in joints of the lower limb. Ann Rheum Dis. 1999;58(1):27–34.
6. Kladny B, et al. Cartilage thickness measurement in magnetic resonance imaging. Osteoarthritis Cartilage. 1996;4(3):181–6.
7. Andreisek G, Weiger M. T2* mapping of articular cartilage: current status of research and first clinical applications. Invest Radiol. 2014;49(1):57–62.
8. Crema MD, et al. Articular cartilage in the knee: current MR imaging techniques and applications in clinical practice and research. Radiographics. 2011;31(1):37–61.
9. Andreisek G, et al. Delayed gadolinium-enhanced MR imaging of articular cartilage: three-dimensional T1 mapping with variable flip angles and B1 correction. Radiology. 2009;252(3):865–73.
10. Andreisek G, et al. Quantitative MR imaging evaluation of the cartilage thickness and subchondral bone area in patients with ACL-reconstructions 7 years after surgery. Osteoarthritis Cartilage. 2009;17(7):871–8.
11. Eckstein F, Guermazi A, Roemer FW. Quantitative MR imaging of cartilage and trabecular bone in osteoarthritis. Radiol Clin North Am. 2009;47(4):655–73.
12. Raya JG, et al. Diffusion-tensor imaging of human articular cartilage specimens with early signs of cartilage damage. Radiology. 2013;266(3):831–41.
13. Losch A, et al. A non-invasive technique for 3-dimensional assessment of articular cartilage thickness based on MRI. Part 1: development of a computational method. Magn Reson Imaging. 1997;15(7):795–804.
14. Trattnig S, et al. MR imaging of cartilage and its repair in the knee–a review. Eur Radiol. 2009;19(7):1582–94.
15. Andreisek G, et al. A systematic review of semiquantitative and qualitative radiologic criteria for the diagnosis of lumbar spinal stenosis. AJR Am J Roentgenol. 2013;201(5):W735–46.
16. Peterfy CG, et al. Whole-Organ Magnetic Resonance Imaging Score (WORMS) of the knee in osteoarthritis. Osteoarthritis Cartilage. 2004;12(3):177–90.
17. Kornaat PR, et al. MRI assessment of knee osteoarthritis: Knee Osteoarthritis Scoring System (KOSS)– inter-observer and intra-observer reproducibility of a compartment-based scoring system. Skeletal Radiol. 2005;34(2):95–102.
18. Hunter DJ, et al. The reliability of a new scoring system for knee osteoarthritis MRI and the validity of bone marrow lesion assessment: BLOKS (Boston Leeds Osteoarthritis Knee Score). Ann Rheum Dis. 2008;67(2):206–11.
19. Goodfellow J, Hungerford DS, Woods C. Patellofemoral joint mechanics and pathology. 2. Chondromalacia patellae. J Bone Joint Surg Br. 1976;58(3):291–9.
20. Rubenstein JD, et al. Image resolution and signal-to-noise ratio requirements for MR imaging of degenerative cartilage. AJR Am J Roentgenol. 1997;169(4):1089–96.
21. Cotofana S, et al. Relationship between knee pain and the presence, location, size and phenotype of femorotibial denuded areas of subchondral bone as visualized by MRI. Osteoarthritis Cartilage. 2013;21(9):1214–22.
22. Zanetti M, et al. Bone marrow edema pattern in osteoarthritic knees: correlation between MR imaging and histologic findings. Radiology. 2000;215(3):835–40.
23. Landells JW. The bone cysts of osteoarthritis. J Bone Joint Surg Br. 1953;35-B(4):643–9.
24. Rhaney K, Lamb DW. The cysts of osteoarthritis of the hip; a radiological and pathological study. J Bone Joint Surg Br. 1955;37-B(4):663–75.
25. Bancroft LW, Peterson JJ, Kransdorf MJ. Cysts, geodes, and erosions. Radiol Clin North Am. 2004;42(1):73–87.

26. McQueen FM. Bone marrow edema and osteitis in rheumatoid arthritis: the imaging perspective. Arthritis Res Ther. 2012;14(5):224.
27. Bullough PG, Bansal M. The differential diagnosis of geodes. Radiol Clin North Am. 1988;26(6):1165–84.
28. Tehranzadeh J, et al. MRI of large intraosseous lesions in patients with inflammatory arthritis. AJR Am J Roentgenol. 2004;183(5):1453–63.
29. Crema MD, et al. MR imaging of intra- and periarticular soft tissues and subchondral bone in knee osteoarthritis. Radiol Clin North Am. 2009;47(4):687–701.
30. Guermazi A, et al. MR findings in knee osteoarthritis. Eur Radiol. 2003;13(6):1370–86.
31. Waldschmidt JG, Braunstein EM, Buckwalter KA. Magnetic resonance imaging of osteoarthritis. Rheum Dis Clin North Am. 1999;25(2):451–65.
32. McCauley TR, Kornaat PR, Jee WH. Central osteophytes in the knee: prevalence and association with cartilage defects on MR imaging. AJR Am J Roentgenol. 2001;176(2):359–64.
33. Breer S, et al. Spontaneous osteonecrosis of the knee (SONK). Knee Surg Sports Traumatol Arthrosc. 2013;21(2):340–5.
34. Brahme SK, et al. Osteonecrosis of the knee after arthroscopic surgery: diagnosis with MR imaging. Radiology. 1991;178(3):851–3.
35. Narvaez J, et al. Osteonecrosis of the knee: differences among idiopathic and secondary types. Rheumatology (Oxford). 2000;39(9):982–9.
36. Mitchell DG, et al. Chemical-shift MR imaging of the femoral head: an in vitro study of normal hips and hips with avascular necrosis. AJR Am J Roentgenol. 1987;148(6):1159–64.
37. van den Borne MP, et al. International Cartilage Repair Society (ICRS) and Oswestry macroscopic cartilage evaluation scores validated for use in Autologous Chondrocyte Implantation (ACI) and microfracture. Osteoarthritis Cartilage. 2007;15(12): 1397–402.
38. Levy AS, et al. Chondral delamination of the knee in soccer players. Am J Sports Med. 1996;24(5):634–9.
39. Kendell SD, et al. MRI appearance of chondral delamination injuries of the knee. AJR Am J Roentgenol. 2005;184(5):1486–9.
40. Uozumi H, et al. Histologic findings and possible causes of osteochondritis dissecans of the knee. Am J Sports Med. 2009;37(10):2003–8.
41. Clanton TO, DeLee JC. Osteochondritis dissecans. History, pathophysiology and current treatment concepts. Clin Orthop Relat Res. 1982;167:50–64.
42. Mesgarzadeh M, et al. Osteochondritis dissecans: analysis of mechanical stability with radiography, scintigraphy, and MR imaging. Radiology. 1987;165(3): 775–80.
43. Steiner RM, et al. Magnetic resonance imaging of diffuse bone marrow disease. Radiol Clin North Am. 1993;31(2):383–409.
44. Lynch TC, et al. Bone abnormalities of the knee: prevalence and significance at MR imaging. Radiology. 1989;171(3):761–6.
45. Hooper DM, et al. Validation of the Hughston Clinic subjective knee questionnaire using gait analysis. Med Sci Sports Exerc. 2001;33(9):1456–62.
46. Irrgang JJ, et al. Development and validation of the international knee documentation committee subjective knee form. Am J Sports Med. 2001;29(5): 600–13.
47. Versier G, Dubrana F, Society French Arthroscopy. Treatment of knee cartilage defect in 2010. Orthop Traumatol Surg Res. 2011;97(8 Suppl):S140–53.
48. Brown WE, et al. Magnetic resonance imaging appearance of cartilage repair in the knee. Clin Orthop Relat Res. 2004;422:214–23.
49. Marlovits S, et al. Magnetic resonance observation of cartilage repair tissue (MOCART) for the evaluation of autologous chondrocyte transplantation: determination of interobserver variability and correlation to clinical outcome after 2 years. Eur J Radiol. 2006; 57(1):16–23.
50. Trattnig S, et al. MR imaging of osteochondral grafts and autologous chondrocyte implantation. Eur Radiol. 2007;17(1):103–18.
51. Steadman JR, et al. The microfracture technique in the treatment of full-thickness chondral lesions of the knee in National Football League players. J Knee Surg. 2003;16(2):83–6.
52. Gnannt R, et al. MR imaging of the postoperative knee. J Magn Reson Imaging. 2011;34(5):1007–21.
53. Alparslan L, et al. Postoperative magnetic resonance imaging of articular cartilage repair. Semin Musculoskelet Radiol. 2001;5(4):345–63.
54. Polster J, Recht M. Postoperative MR evaluation of chondral repair in the knee. Eur J Radiol. 2005; 54(2):206–13.
55. Brittberg M, et al. Treatment of deep cartilage defects in the knee with autologous chondrocyte transplantation. N Engl J Med. 1994;331(14):889–95.
56. Nehrer S, et al. Chondrocyte-seeded collagen matrices implanted in a chondral defect in a canine model. Biomaterials. 1998;19(24):2313–28.
57. Richardson JB, et al. Repair of human articular cartilage after implantation of autologous chondrocytes. J Bone Joint Surg Br. 1999;81(6):1064–8.
58. Minas T, Chiu R. Autologous chondrocyte implantation. Am J Knee Surg. 2000;13(1):41–50.
59. Minas T, Peterson L. Advanced techniques in autologous chondrocyte transplantation. Clin Sports Med. 1999;18(1):13–44, v–vi.
60. Peterson L, et al. Two- to 9-year outcome after autologous chondrocyte transplantation of the knee. Clin Orthop Relat Res. 2000;374:212–34.
61. Recht MP, Kramer J. MR imaging of the postoperative knee: a pictorial essay. Radiographics. 2002;22(4): 765–74.

Patella, Femoropatellar Joint, and Infrapatellar Fat Pad

Nicolae Bolog, Gustav Andreisek,
and Erika Ulbrich

7.1 Anatomy and Normal MRI Appearance

7.1.1 Patella and Patellar Retinaculum

The patella is the largest sesamoid bone in the body and is part of the extensor mechanism of the knee together with the quadriceps muscle and tendon, patellar tendon, and patellar retinaculum [1]. The bone has two surfaces, three borders, a base, and an apex. The vastus intermedius and the rectus femoris tendons attach to the base (syn. proximal pole) of the patella and the vastus medialis and vastus lateralis to the medial and, respectively, lateral border. The quadriceps muscle is the active stabilizer of the patella. The apex (syn. distal pole) of the patella is extra-articular and is the site of the attachment of the patellar tendon. The patellar tendon, the major passive stabilizer of the patella, inserts distally to the tibial tuberosity and has a length of approximately 4–6 cm. The thickness of the tendon is 5–6 mm and the width is 3 cm at the patellar insertion and 2.5 cm at the tibial insertion [2]. Normal tendons have uniformly low signal intensity on all MRI sequences and display distinct margins [3]. The quadriceps muscle and tendon, patellar tendon, patella, and patellar retinaculum represent the extensor mechanism of the knee [1].

The patellar anterior surface is related to the quadriceps tendon and to the prepatellar bursa that is not apparent on MR images in the absence of bursitis. The patellar posterior surface is divided into a superior intra-articular surface and a lower extra-articular portion. The mean patellar height varies between approximately 4 and 5 cm from which a height of 2.4–3.7 cm represents the intra-articular segment [4]. The intra-articular surface is divided into seven facets [5]. Three medial and three lateral facets are in contact with the medial and lateral femoral condyles, and the odd facet on the medial border of the patella articulates with the medial femoral condyle only in deep knee flexion [5].

The medial and lateral retinacula are passive stabilizers of the patella. The medial patellar retinaculum is part of the anterior third of the medial joint capsule and is formed by the superficial layer of MCL and the deep crural fascia [6]. It extends from the proximal aspect of the medial border of the patella to the medial femoral epicondyle and represents, together with the medial femoropatellar ligament (MPFL), the most important patellar ligamentous stabilizers. The medial femoropatellar ligament inserts to the medial femoral epicondyle, and its fibers fan out to the patella where they insert to the most prominent medial edge of the patella [7]. The ligament is adherent to the vastus medialis obliquus, and its fibers may be hidden to a variable extent by the overlying muscle and tendon [8]. The ligament is 55 mm long and 3–30 mm wide and is the primary passive restraint to patellar lateral displacement [7]. On MR imaging, the medial retinaculum and the medial femoropatellar ligament

N.V. Bolog et al., *MRI of the Knee: A Guide to Evaluation and Reporting*,
DOI 10.1007/978-3-319-08165-6_7, © Springer International Publishing Switzerland 2015

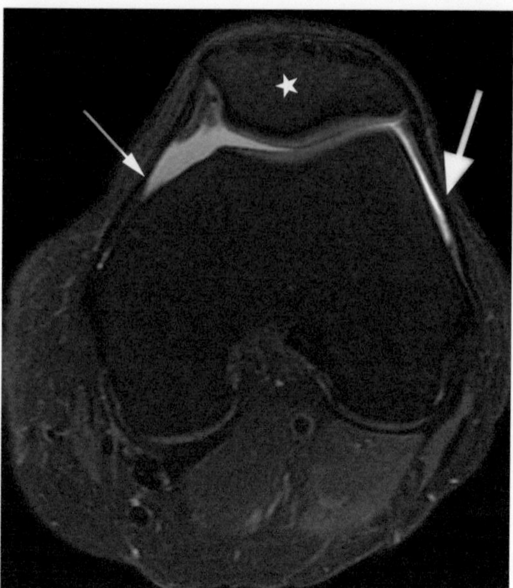

Fig. 7.1 Normal medial and lateral retinaculum in a 34 year old female. Axial proton-density (PD) FSE fat-suppressed image shows the medial (*small arrow*) and lateral retinacula (*large arrow*) as well-defined low-signal-intensity bands connecting the patella (*star*) with the femoral condyles

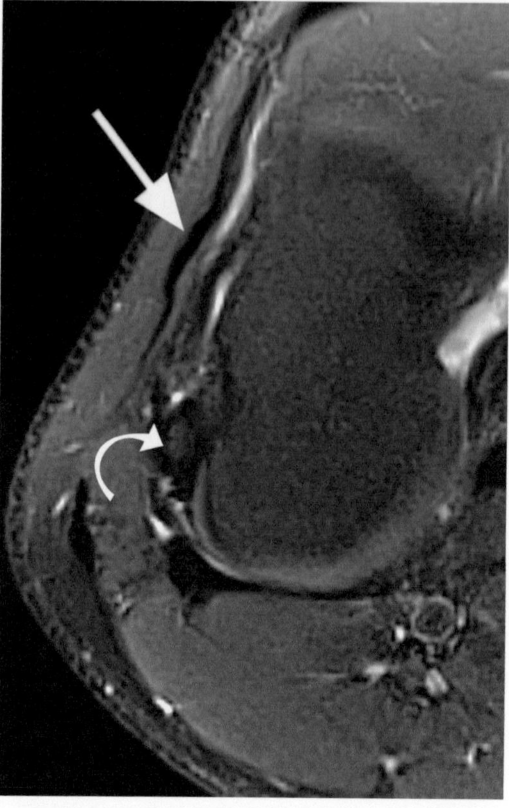

Fig. 7.2 The intermediate layer of the lateral retinaculum in a 17 year old male. Axial proton-density (PD) FSE fat-suppressed image shows the anterior longitudinal expansion of the iliotibial tract (*large arrow*). Note that there is no direct connection to the femur or to the lateral collateral ligament (*curved arrow*)

are seen as well-defined low-signal-intensity bands but are often difficult to be distinguished from each other (Fig. 7.1) [9].

The lateral retinaculum has a more complex anatomy with three layers difficult to delineate both macroscopically and on MR imaging, because of converging and interdigitating structures (Fig. 7.1) [10]. The superficial layer is represented by the deep fascia that is not adherent to the patella. Deep to it, there is the anterior longitudinal expansion of the iliotibial tract that merges with the anterior quadriceps aponeurosis and attaches to the patella (syn. intermediate layer) [11]. The intermediate layer is the most substantial layer of the lateral retinaculum [10]. Although these fibers are often called the lateral femoropatellar band, there is no attachment to the femur, except indirectly via proximal and distal attachment of the iliotibial band (Fig. 7.2) [12]. The deepest layer of the lateral retinaculum is part of the joint capsule and is referred to as the lateral femoropatellar ligament reinforced by an epicondylopatellar and a patellotibial band that are less substantial [10].

7.1.2 Femoropatellar Joint

The femoropatellar joint is formed by the posterior intra-articular surface of the patella and its counterpart represented by the femur trochlea. The articular congruence between femoral and patellar surfaces enables the static stability of the patella. However, there are anatomical variants of the patellar facet sizes by comparing the configuration of the medial and lateral bony facets [13]. In Wiberg type I patella (prevalence of 10 %), the medial and lateral facets are concave and are almost equal in size (Fig. 7.3). In Wiberg type II patella (prevalence of 65 %), the medial facet is flat and is smaller than the lateral facet (Fig. 7.4). In Wiberg type III patella (prevalence of 25 %), the medial facet is also smaller than the lateral

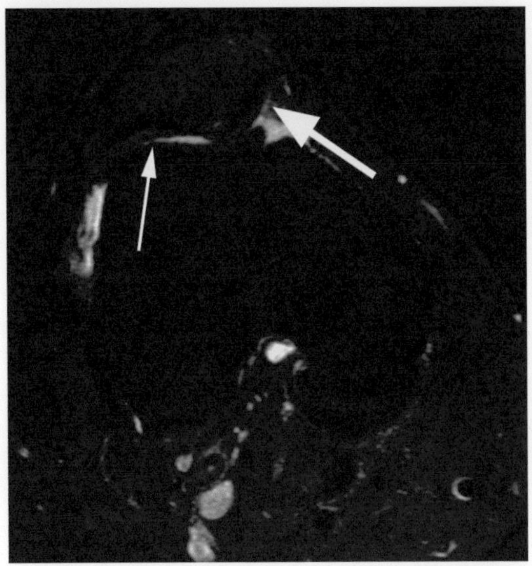

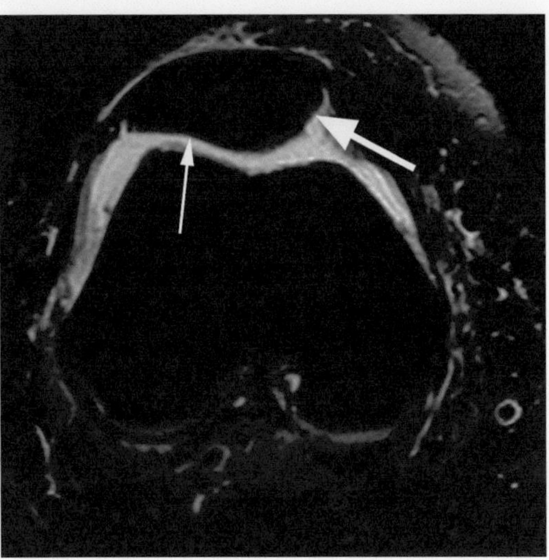

Fig. 7.5 Wiberg type III patella in a 50 year old female. Axial proton-density (PD) FSE fat-suppressed image shows that the medial facet (*large arrow*) is much smaller than the lateral facet (*small arrow*) and has a convex shape

Fig. 7.3 Wiberg type I patella in a 45 year old female. Axial proton-density (PD) FSE fat-suppressed image shows that the medial (*large arrow*) and lateral (*small arrow*) facets are concave and are almost equal in size

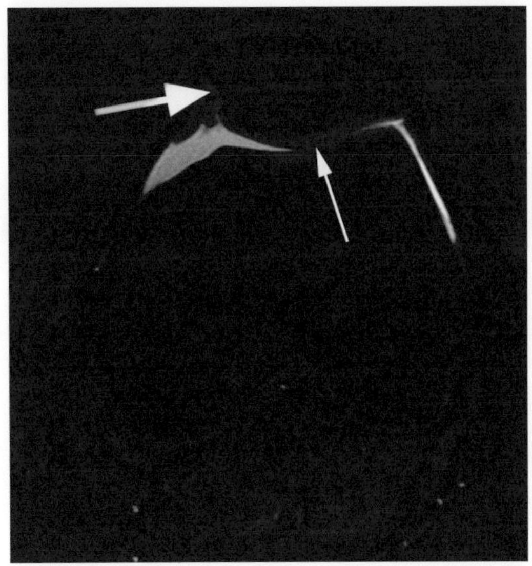

Fig. 7.4 Wiberg type II patella in a 34 year old female. Axial proton-density (PD) FSE fat-suppressed image shows that the medial facet (*large arrow*) is much smaller than the lateral facet (*small arrow*) and is flat or even concave

facet but has a convex shape (Fig. 7.5). The femoral trochlea consists of the medial and lateral facets of the femoral sulcus or femoral groove. On axial MR imaging, the lateral facet of the trochlea is more elevated and larger than the medial facet. The sulcus angle of the trochlea is normally less than 144° [14].

Both surfaces, patellar facets and femoral trochlea, are covered by articular cartilage, but there are significant differences between the subchondral bone geometry and the articular cartilage surface geometry [15]. This means that the measurements on plain radiographs or on computed tomography (CT) may not represent the real articular femoropatellar congruence and all measurements, which are based on these imaging modalities, should be used with caution. MRI is the only imaging method that is able to reveal the real articular congruence due to visualization of the articular cartilage and the subchondral bone at the same time. This especially applies to cases with normal morphology of trochlea or in a low-grade dysplasia.

Whenever quantitative or semiquantitative measures of the patellar position are required or asked for, we suggest determining the position of the articular patellar cartilage in relation to the trochlear cartilage [16]. This relation can be quantitatively assessed on sagittal MR images by using the patellotrochlear index measured with the knee fully extended (Fig. 7.6) [17].

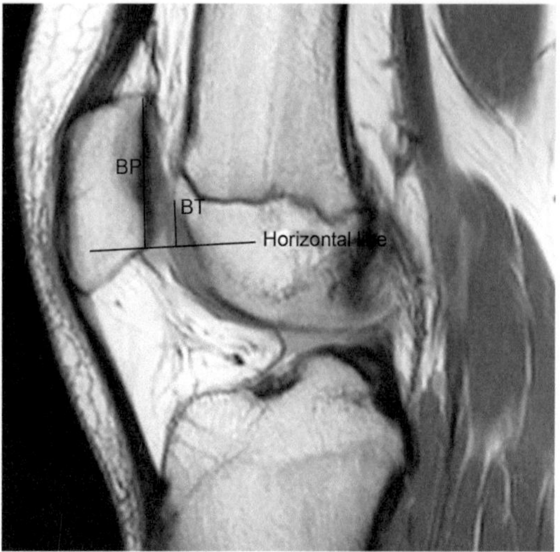

Fig. 7.6 The patellotrochlear index in a 16 year old female. Sagittal proton-density (PD) FSE image enables the calculation of the patellotrochlear index. The baseline trochlea (*BT*) is measured as the distance from the most proximal trochlear cartilage margin to an horizontal line which is drawn at the inferior margin of the patellar cartilage (*horizontal line*). The baseline patella represents the length of the patellar cartilage measured from the most proximal margin of the patellar cartilage to the most distal margin of the cartilage (*BP*). The patellotrochlear index is calculated using the formula: BT/BP × 100. An index value of more than 50 % documents patella baja and an index value less than 12.5 % documents patella alta. These values are not valid in the cases of patients with patellar dislocation

7.1.3 Infrapatellar Fat Pad and Suprapatellar Fat Pad

The infrapatellar fat pad, also referred as Hoffa's fat pad, is intracapsular and extrasynovial and is bordered by the patellar tendon and joint capsule anteriorly, proximal tibia and deep infrapatellar bursa inferiorly, synovia posteriorly, and the inferior pole of the patella superiorly. On MR images, it appears as a relatively homogeneous triangular shape fatty tissue on sagittal plane. Some vessels might be seen within the fat pad (Fig. 7.7). An infrapatellar synovial plica may be present, extending from the distal pole of the patellar to the intercondylar notch close to the anterior cruciate ligament (Fig. 7.8).

The suprapatellar fat pad is also intracapsular and extrasynovial and is divided into an anterior suprapatellar fat pad (quadriceps fat pad) and a posterior suprapatellar fat pad (prefemoral fat pad). Both fat pads are often separated by the suprapatellar bursa (Fig. 7.7).

7.1.4 Patellar Calcar

Patellar calcar is a constant and normal anatomical finding of the patella represented by a dense bone lying as a ridge within the subchondral

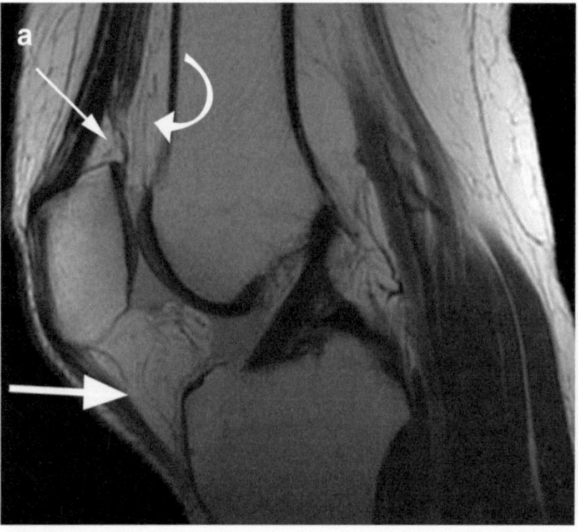
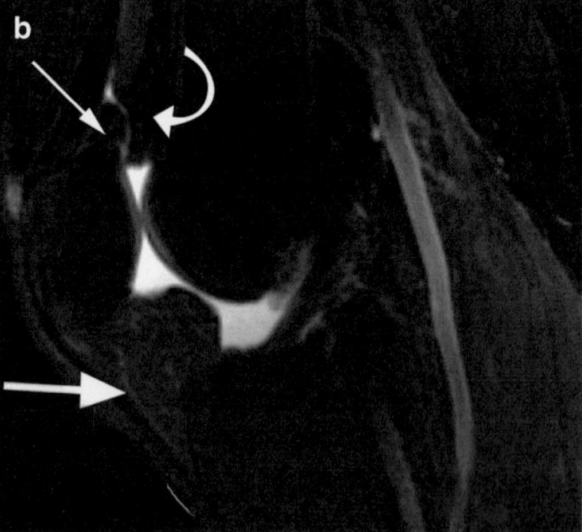

Fig. 7.7 The infrapatellar fat pad (Hoffa's fat pad) and the suprapatellar fat pad in a 34 year old female. Sagittal proton-density (PD) FSE image (**a**) and sagittal T2-weighted FSE fat-suppressed image (**b**) show the infrapatellar fat pad as a triangular shape fatty tissue between the patella and proximal tibia (*large arrows* in **a**, **b**). Note the presence of small vessels within the fat pad. The suprapatellar fat pad is divided into an anterior suprapatellar fat pad (*small arrows* in **a**, **b**) and a posterior suprapatellar fat pad (*curved arrows* in **a**, **b**)

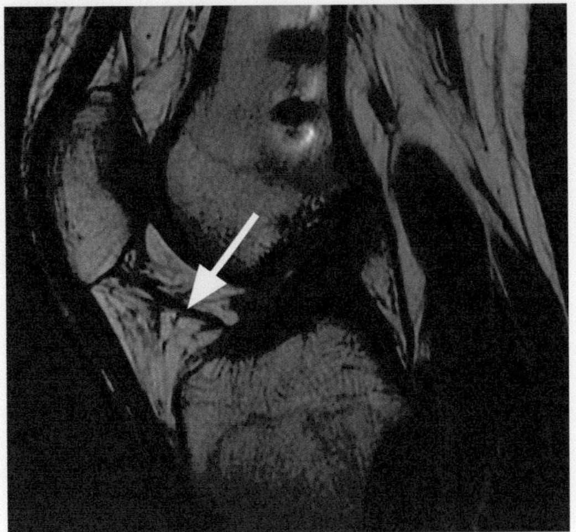

Fig. 7.8 Infrapatellar synovial plica in a 22 year old male. Sagittal proton-density (PD) FSE image shows a linear hypointense structure extending from the distal pole of the patellar to the intercondylar notch (*arrow*)

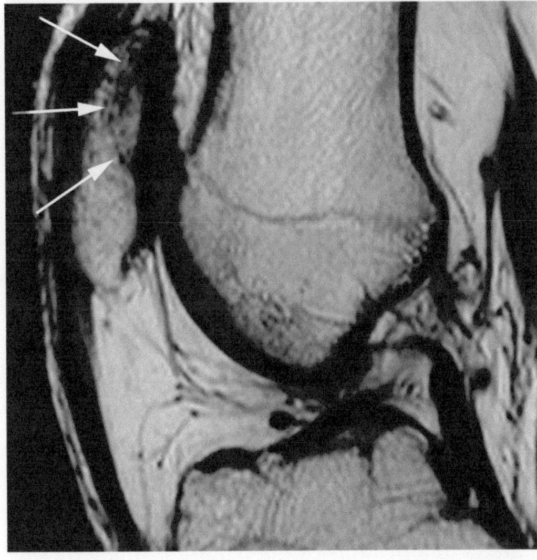

Fig. 7.9 Patellar calcar in a 27 year old male. Sagittal proton-density (PD) FSE image shows a linear low-signal intensity line within the subchondral area of the lateral facet of the patella (*arrows*) which represents a normal bone condensation

patellar bone. The patellar calcar is always present on the lateral facet of the patella and is better seen on sagittal images as a linear low-intensity-signal change or the subchondral patellar bone (Fig. 7.9) [18]. Although the presence of this normal bone condensation is not correlated with any clinical symptoms, recognizing the imaging appearance is important in order to exclude a misinterpretation of a normal finding as osteochondritis dissecans or patellar fracture [18].

7.2   MRI Pathological Findings

Abnormalities of the patella, femoropatellar joint, and infrapatellar fat pad are often associated with anterior knee pain which is one of the most frequent complaints in orthopedics and sports medicine practice. However, there is a long list of possible differential diagnoses of anterior knee pain that implies bone and/or soft tissue pathology (Table 7.1) [19].

7.2.1   Patellar Dysplasia

The patella is cartilaginous at birth and ossifies from one or several centers after the age of three years. The most common patellar dysplasias are hypoplasia, aplasia, patella bipartite or multipartite, duplication, and fragmentation. Congenital hypoplasia and aplasia are very rare diseases and are the result of the phenotype and gene defects including the nail patella syndrome or hereditary osteo-onychodysplasia (HOOD disease), small patella syndrome, isolated patella aplasia or hypoplasia, Meier-Gorlin syndrome, RAPADILINO syndrome, and genitopatellar syndrome [20].

Patellar duplication or double-layered patella may be seen in multiple epiphyseal dysplasia and is identified on axial and sagittal MR images as two separate anterior and posterior layers [21]. The fragmentation of the patella may involve the superior or the inferior pole. It may be seen in patients with cerebral palsy. The excessive tension in the quadriceps tendon, usually in the presence of a flexion contracture, appears to cause the lesion [22].

Patella bipartite is a developmental dysplasia in which the ossification centers fail to fuse and may be a cause of anterior knee pain. Usually, the bipartite fragment is situated at the superolateral quadrant of the patella at the insertion of the vastus lateralis muscle (type III patella bipartite).

Table 7.1 Possible causes of anterior knee pain

Anatomical structure	Pathology
Patella	Patella bipartite
	Unstable synchondrosis
	Pseudoarthrosis
	Patellar alta/patella baja
	Patellar dislocation/subluxation
	Patellar/femoral fractures/contusions
Subchondral bone and cartilage (patella/femur)	Cartilage injuries – osteoarthritis/arthritis
	Subchondral edema
	Subchondral cysts
	Osteochondritis dissecans
	Bone tumors
Meniscus	Meniscal tear
	Meniscal cyst
	Meniscal extrusion
Muscles and tendons	Tendinosis – quadricipital tendon/patellar tendon
	Tendon tear – quadricipital tendon/patellar tendon
	Osgood-Schlatter disease
	Sinding-Larsen-Johansson disease
	Muscle tumors
Synovia	Inflammatory synovitis
	Pigmented villonodular synovitis (PVNS)
	Prepatellar/infrapatellar bursitis
	Medial plica syndrome
	Infrapatellar plica syndrome
	Synovial osteochondromatosis
	Synovial sarcoma
Infrapatellar fat pad	Hoffa disease
	Intra-articular chondroma
	Postoperative fibrosis (including cyclops lesion)

Patella bipartite occurs usually bilaterally. Very rarely the fragment is located at the medial border (type II patella bipartite) or at the inferior pole (type I patella bipartite) [23]. The bone fragments are connected through a synchondrosis, and the associated patellar articular cartilage remains intact in most of the cases. However, due to overuse or acute injury, synchondrosis may be disrupted allowing friction and abnormal motion that can lead finally to pseudoarthrosis [24]. In clinical practice, patella bipartite is repeatedly misdiagnosed as patellar fracture. The continuity

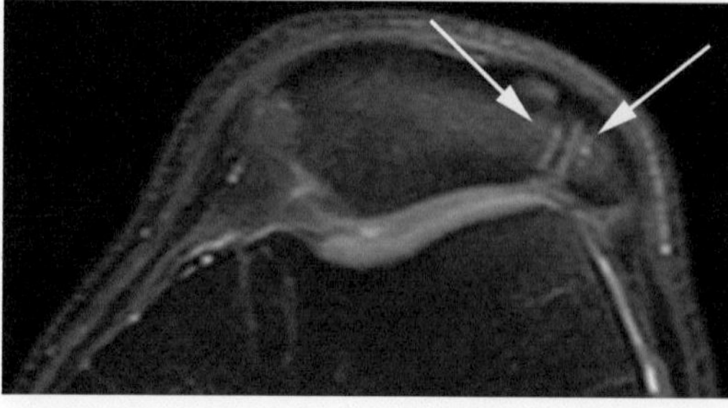

Fig. 7.10 Patella bipartite in a 21 year old male with intermittent anterior knee pain. Axial proton-density (PD) FSE fat-suppressed image shows normal synchondrosis (presence of the cartilage) between patellar fragments with subchondral bone marrow edema along the margins of synchondrosis (*arrows*)

of the articular cartilage, the presence of the cartilage between the fragments (normal synchondrosis), and the absence of abnormal signal intensity within the fragments are normal MRI findings in uncomplicated patella bipartite.

MR imaging is also the method of choice for differentiation between symptomatic and asymptomatic patients with patella bipartite by demonstrating the presence of bone edema within the patellar fragment and along the margins of synchondrosis that is the result of impaction and trabecular injuries of the bone (Fig. 7.10). The presence of fluid signal between the patellar body and the bipartite fragment represents a suggestive MRI finding for pseudoarthrosis (Fig. 7.11) [23].

7.2.2 Patella Alta and Patella Baja

Patella alta or high-riding patella is a patella that is situated too high above the femoral trochlea. Although patella alta is considered a normal anatomical variant secondary to a long patellar tendon, the high position of the patella leads to reduced contact area with the femoral trochlea and may cause pain due to instability. In conjunction with other factors, this increases the risk of patellar lateral dislocation [25, 26]. Patella baja is the result of the shortening of the patellar tendon and may occur following trauma or surgery (harvesting of a patellar tendon autograft) [27].

Numerous methods are used to determine the patellar height, but there is a high frequency of

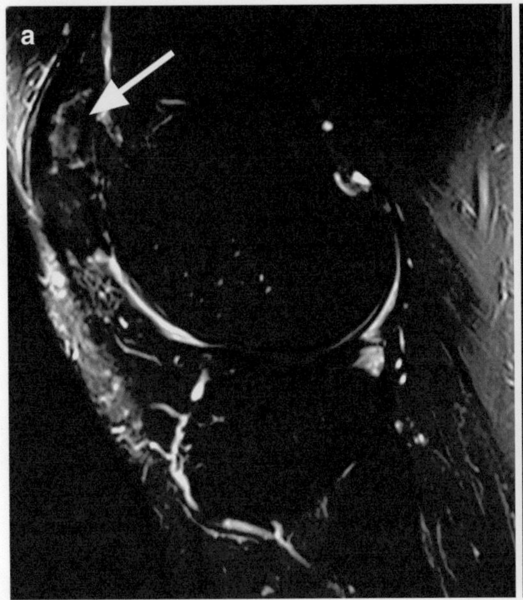

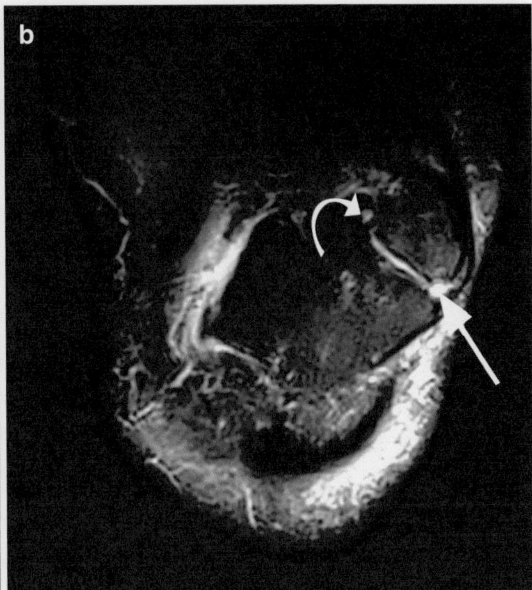

Fig. 7.11 Complicated patella bipartite in a 57 year old male. Sagittal T2-weighted fat-suppressed image (**a**) shows an irregular bipartite fragment (*arrow*). Coronal proton-density (PD) FSE fat-suppressed image (**b**) shows the presence of fluid signal between the patellar body and the bipartite fragment (*arrow*) and even a small subchondral cyst (*curved arrow*). Both signs are suggestive for pseudoarthrosis

differing results in determination of patellar position [28]. This finding has led many clinicians to question the utility of commonly used ratios for accurate assessment of patellar position [28]. Nevertheless, some of these measures are still used and requested.

The first method described was the Insall-Salvati ratio that is calculated as the ratio between the length of the patellar tendon and the length of the patella on lateral radiographs. It is ideally measured with the knee in 30° flexion [29]. As on radiographs, the Insall-Salvati ratio can be reliably assessed on sagittal MR images independent on the degree of knee flexion (Fig. 7.12), and a ratio greater than 1.3 is suggestive for patella alta, while a ratio smaller than 0.8 is suggestive for patella baja [5, 30].

Several studies have demonstrated that the Insall-Salvati ratio and modified Insall-Salvati ratios do not correlate with femoropatellar cartilage congruence [28, 31]. Moreover, this ratio may be influenced by form variations of the patella and variations of the patellar tendon (Sinding-Larsen or Osgood-Schlatter diseases, surgical interventions) [17]. Biedert and Albrecht [17] have thus proposed another measure,

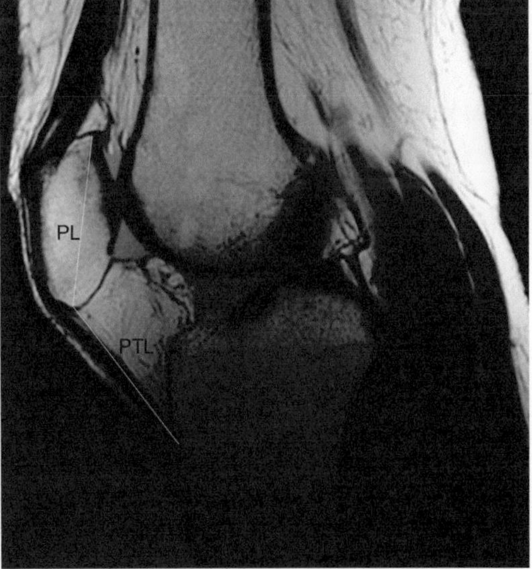

Fig. 7.12 Insall-Salvati ratio in a 34 year old female. Insall-Salvati ratio is calculated as the ratio between the length of the patellar tendon (*PTL*) and the length of the patella (*PL*). A ratio greater than 1.3 is suggestive for patella alta, while a ratio smaller than 0.8 is suggestive for patella baja

namely, the patellotrochlear index. It is thought to provide a more reliable measurement of the patellar height because the most important factor

Table 7.2 Factors that influence patellar stability [33–35]

Structure	Role in patellar stability
Femoropatellar bone and cartilage congruence	*Static stability:* restraint to lateral patellar displacement at flexion angles more than 30°
Quadriceps muscle	*Active stability:* quadriceps contraction pulls the patella proximally, posteriorly, and slightly laterally; the force of quadriceps is resisted by patellar tendon tension
Retinacula	*Passive stability:* medial femoropatellar ligament is the most important passive restraint to lateral patellar displacement in early flexion (0–30°)

in patellar position evaluation is the position of the articular cartilage in relation to the trochlear cartilage [16]. The patellotrochlear index is calculated as the ratio between the baseline trochlea, measured as the vertical length of the femoral trochlea that is engaged with the patella, and the baseline patella, calculated as the vertical length of the patellar articular surface (Fig. 7.6). An index value of more than 50 % documents patella baja, and an index value less than 12.5 % documents patella alta [17].

7.2.3   Patellar Instability

The stability of the patella is maintained by a complex interaction between bone and soft tissue structures (Table 7.2). Morphological variations of the bone anatomy of the femoropatellar joint and ligamentous insufficiencies can disturb this interaction resulting in patellar instability [32]. Patellar instability is one of the most frequent clinical syndromes and is defined as an abnormal lateral course of the patella during knee flexion with or without dislocation. Chronic instability of the femoropatellar joint and recurrent dislocation may lead to progressive cartilage damage and severe arthritis if not treated adequately [9]. In patients without any history of knee dislocation, the diagnosis is difficult because anterior knee pain is often nonspecific and the clinical examination of the knee may be normal. The

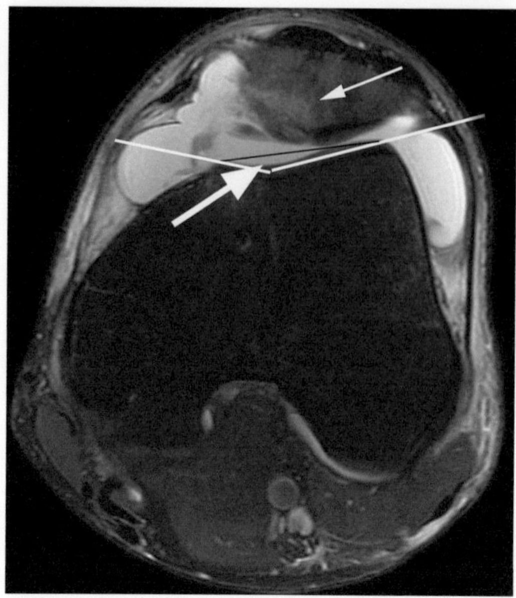

Fig. 7.13 Trochlear dysplasia in a 32 year old male. Axial proton-density (PD) FSE fat-suppressed image 3 cm above femorotibial joint level shows that the trochlear depth is less than 3 mm (*large arrow*). Note the osteochondral fracture of the medial patellar facet (*small arrow*) resulting from lateral patellar dislocation

most important predisposing factors for instability are trochlear dysplasia, patella alta, and the lateralization of the tibial tuberosity.

Trochlear dysplasia is believed to be a developmental morphological abnormality, often present bilaterally, defined by the flattening of the femoral trochlea that can result in lateral patellar dislocation with flexion [36]. There are several quantitative and qualitative MRI criteria for the diagnosis of trochlear dysplasia. The mean trochlear depth in normal knees 3 cm above femorotibial joint level including the cartilaginous surface is 5.2 mm (Fig. 7.13) [19]. On axial MR images at this level, a trochlear depth less than 3 mm has a sensitivity of 100 % and a specificity of 96 % for trochlear dysplasia [19].

The lateral trochlear inclination and trochlear facets asymmetry are other quantitative MR findings that can be measured on axial images. The lateral trochlea inclination enables evaluation for the presence of dysplasia at the proximal portion of trochlea and is measured on the first craniocaudal image that demonstrates cartilaginous

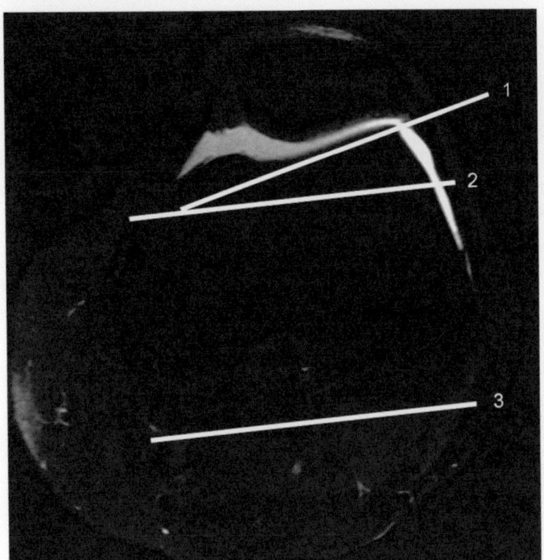

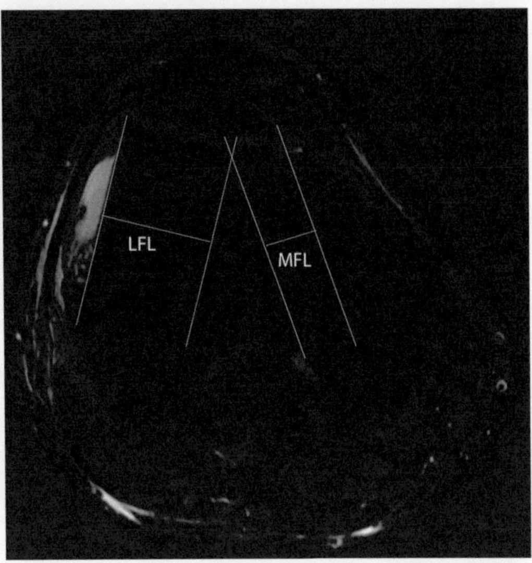

Fig. 7.14 The lateral trochlear inclination in a 34 year old female. The first craniocaudal axial proton-density (PD) FSE fat-suppressed image that demonstrates cartilaginous trochlea enables the measurement of the lateral trochlear inclination. An inclination angle smaller than 11° is suggestive for trochlear dysplasia. The angle is measured between the cartilaginous femoral trochlea (*line 1*) and a parallel line (*line 2*) with the posterior plane of the femoral condyles (*line 3*)

Fig. 7.15 Measurement of the trochlear facet asymmetry in a 43 year old male on axial proton-density (PD) FSE fat-suppressed image 3 cm above femorotibial joint level. The trochlear facet asymmetry is measured by lateral facet length (*LFL*) to medial facet length (*MFL*) ratio (LFL/MFL × 100). A value of 40 % or less shows a decrease of the lateral facet length having a sensitivity of 100 % and a specificity of 96 % for diagnosis of trochlear dysplasia

trochlea by means of a line tangential to the subchondral bone of the posterior aspect of the two femoral condyles crossed with a line tangential to the subchondral bone of the lateral trochlear facet (Fig. 7.14) [37]. A horizontal lateral facet with an inclination angle smaller than 11° is suggestive for diagnosis [37]. Trochlear facet asymmetry 3 cm above the femorotibial joint level is measured by lateral facet length (LFL) to medial facet length (MFL) ratio (LFL/MFL × 100) (Fig. 7.15) [19]. A value of 40 % or less shows a decrease of the lateral facet length having a sensitivity of 100 % and a specificity of 96 % for diagnosis [19].

The presence of a nipplelike anterior prominence at the superior border of the trochlea on midsagittal MR images can be used as semi-quantitative criteria for trochlea dysplasia with a 91 % specificity when the nipplelike prominence is larger than 2 mm (Fig. 7.16) [19]. However, the sign is reliable only in patients without degenerative changes of the femoropatellar joint.

The lateralization of the tibial tuberosity and the lateralization of the patella are other quantitative findings that can be used in the evaluation of patellar

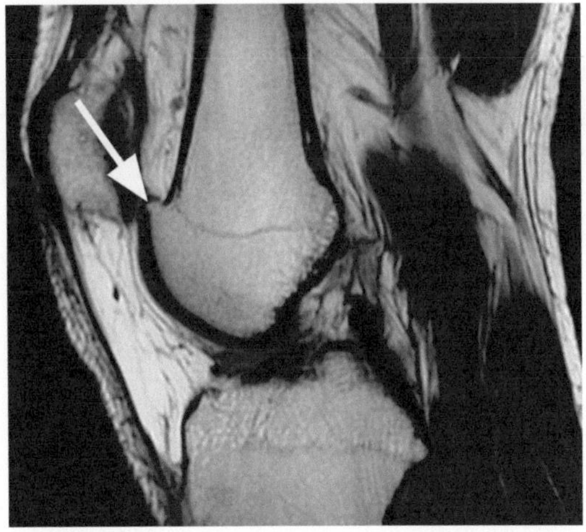

Fig. 7.16 Semi-quantitative criteria for trochlea dysplasia: nipplelike anterior prominence at the superior border of the trochlea in a 43 year old male. Midsagittal proton-density (PD) FSE image shows a prominence larger than 2 mm in a patient with trochlear dysplasia (*arrow*)

instability. The lateralization of the tibial tuberosity results in lateral displacement of the patella during flexion. On axial MR images, the lateralization of the tibial tuberosity can be measured by using the

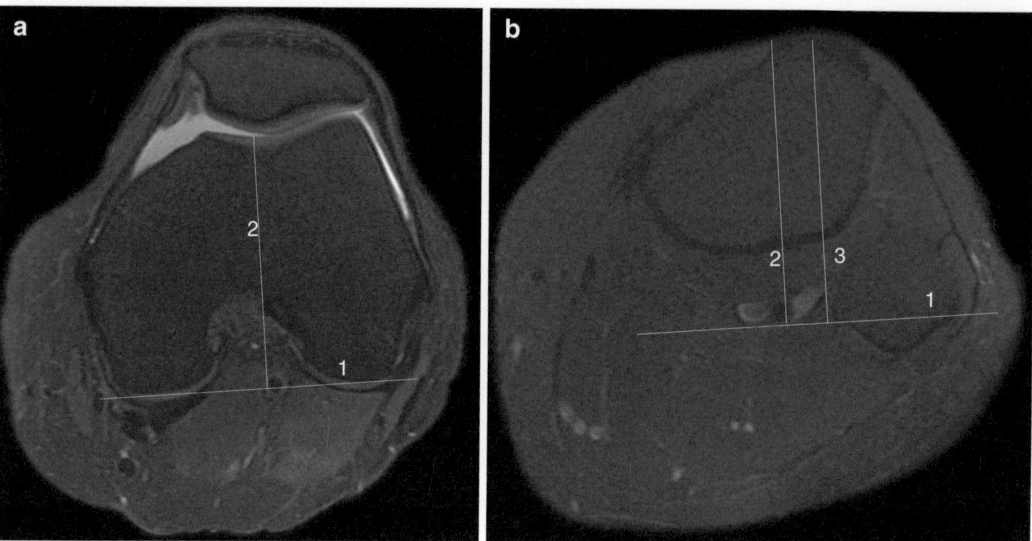

Fig. 7.17 Tibial tuberosity-trochlear groove distance (TTTG) in a 34 year old male. On axial MR images, the lateralization of the tibial tuberosity can be measured by using the tibial tuberosity-trochlear groove distance by superimposing axial images through the tibial tuberosity and the apex of the intercondylar groove. First, a line through the posterior femoral condyle is drawn (*line 1* in **a**). The line is superimposed on an axial image through the tibial apex (*line 1* in **b**). A perpendicular line through the deepest point of the trochlea is drawn (*line 2* in **a**) and after that is superimposed on the axial image through the tibial apex (*line 2* in **b**). On the axial image through the tibial apex, a parallel line is drawn through the most anterior part of the tibial tuberosity (*line 3* in **b**). The tibial tuberosity-trochlear groove distance (TTTG) is measured at this level as the distance between line 2 and line 3. A distance greater than 2 cm is suggestive for patellar instability

tibial tuberosity-trochlear groove distance by superimposing axial images through the tibial tuberosity and the apex of the intercondylar groove (Fig. 7.17) [9, 38]. A distance greater than 2 cm is usually associated with patellar instability [9].

Measuring the distance between the most lateral point of the patella and the line paralleling the lateral surface of the femoral condyle (Fig. 7.18) enables information regarding the lateralization of the patella [19]. Patellar lateralization of more than 6 mm has a sensitivity of 75 % and a specificity of 83 % for trochlear dysplasia [19]. As in the evaluation of the anterior nipple-like prominence, the articular degenerative changes with the presence of lateral patellar osteophytes may influence the measurements.

7.2.4   Patellar Dislocation

Patellar dislocation is defined as the loss of contact between the femoropatellar joint surfaces [9]. The incidence of patellar dislocation

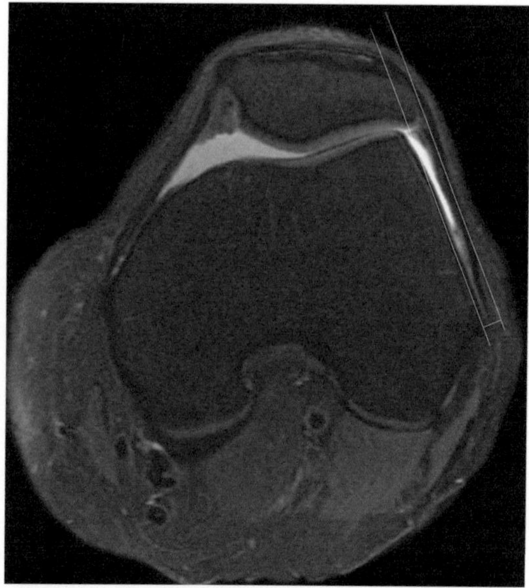

Fig. 7.18 Lateralization of patella in a 34 year old male on axial proton-density (PD) FSE fat-suppressed image. Two parallel lines are drawn through the most lateral point of the patella and through the lateral surface of the femoral condyle. Patellar lateralization of more than 6 mm has a sensitivity of 75 % and a specificity of 83 % for trochlear dysplasia

represents 2–3 % of all knee injuries. The dislocation is usually lateral and seen in young and active individuals. Interestingly, patients are often unaware of the dislocation, and in 50–75 % of the cases, the diagnosis is missed at the time of the initial clinical evaluation [39, 40]. Lateral patellar dislocation may be atraumatic or traumatic, transient or persistent, and complete or incomplete. A high correlation between trochlear dysplasia and recurrent patellar dislocation with atraumatic onset has been reported [41]. MR imaging has replaced diagnostic arthroscopy and is recognized as a standard procedure for the primary diagnostic modality [9]. The pattern seen on MR imaging may reflect the mechanism of injury by evaluating ligamentous and bone injuries associated with patellar dislocation. A crucial injury that occurs in patellar dislocation is the disruption of the medial femoropatellar ligament, and, because of its extrasynovial location, these injuries were not always visible in the past when arthroscopy was used as a standard diagnostic tool [42].

Soft tissue injuries in patellar dislocations are represented by lesions of the capsule, medial retinaculum, and medial femoropatellar ligament. Although on MR imaging the medial femoropatellar ligament is not distinguishable from the medial retinaculum, injuries of the medial retinaculum complex are easily recognized on axial images. Periligamentous edema is present in sprains with intact fibers of the retinaculum (Fig. 7.19). In partial or incomplete tears, MRI findings include intrasubstance retinaculum edema and thickening (Fig. 7.20). Discontinuity of the structure with wavy or retracted fibers is characteristic of complete tears of the medial retinaculum (Fig. 7.21) [36]. The MR report should include the site of the tear: patellar insertion (anterior third), midsubstance, or femoral attachment (posterior third) [36]. The medial femoropatellar ligament injuries usually occur at the femoral insertion, and these injuries may be accompanied by avulsion fracture of the medial femoral condyle [38, 43]. In chronic patellar instability with recurrent patellar dislocations, subtle scarring of the medial retinaculum or residual bone changes at the medial patellar border may be seen on MR imaging [19]. Often the tendon or the

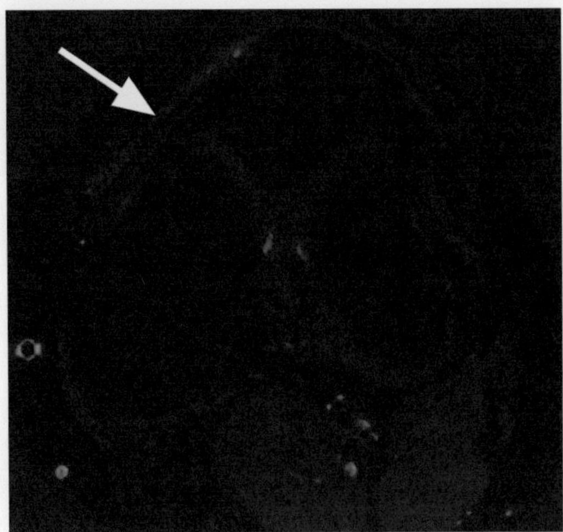

Fig. 7.19 Sprain of the medial retinaculum in an 18 year old female. Axial proton-density (PD) FSE fat-suppressed image shows intact fibers of the retinaculum with periligamentous edema (*arrow*)

musculotendinous junction of the vastus medialis muscle is involved, and diffuse areas of high signal intensity on T2-weighted MR images can be seen (Fig. 7.22).

Resultant impaction of the medial patellar facet on the lateral femoral condyle causes fractures or contusions (trabecular microfractures) that are seen on MRI as areas of high signal intensity on T2-weighted images and low signal intensity on T1-weighted images (Fig. 7.23) [36]. These lesions are also referred as "kissing contusions" [39].

Osteochondral injuries with or without cartilaginous or osseous loose bodies may appear and the most frequent donor site at the inferomedial aspect of the medial border of the patella (Fig. 7.24) [44, 45]. Any sharp-margined cartilage lesion, i.e., in younger patients, should raise the attention of an acute traumatic cartilage injury, and frequently the dislocated cartilage fragment can be found within the joint space. The size of the loose body should fit to the size of the articular cartilage donor site.

Joint effusion is usually present in acute patellar dislocation and may extend through the medial retinaculum in complete tears (Fig. 7.24) [36]. In case of hemarthrosis or associated fractures with lipohemarthrosis, fluid-fluid levels are seen on axial and sagittal MR images (Fig. 7.25).

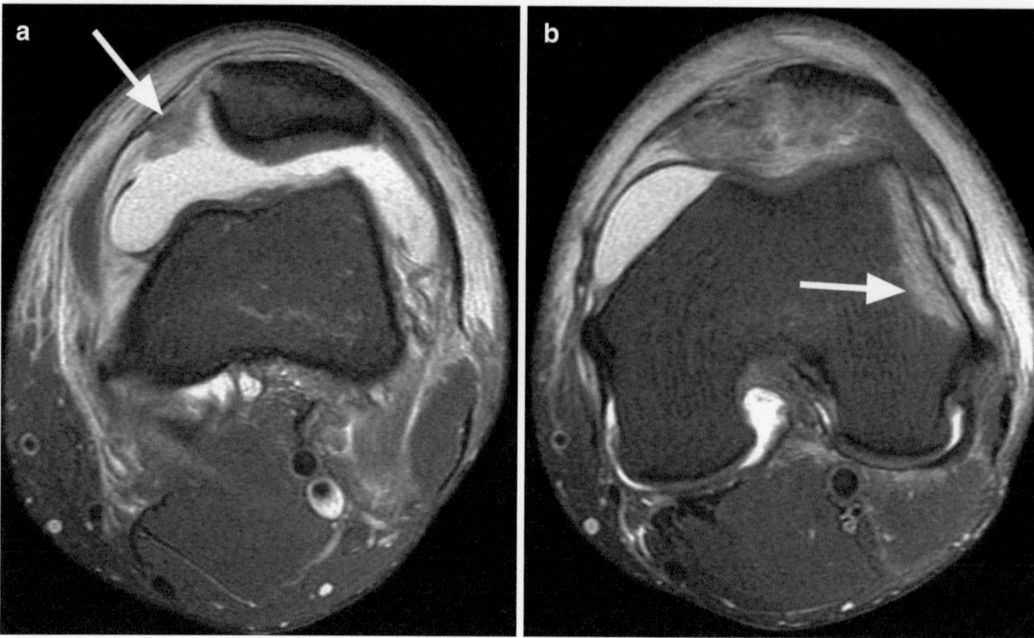

Fig. 7.20 Partial or incomplete tear of the medial retinaculum in a 28 year old male with patellar dislocation. Axial proton-density (PD) FSE fat-suppressed image (**a**) shows intrasubstance hemorrhage and thickening of the anterior third of the retinaculum (*arrow*). Axial proton-density (PD) FSE fat-suppressed image obtained more caudally (**b**) shows the bone contusion of the lateral femoral condyle (*arrow*) resulting from the impaction of the medial patellar facet on the lateral femoral condyle during dislocation

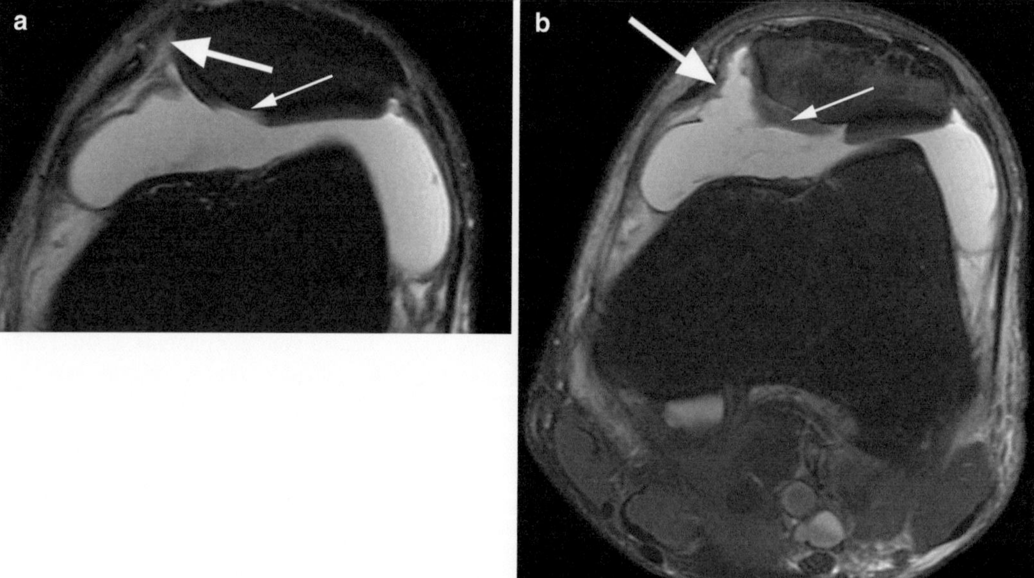

Fig. 7.21 Complete tear of the medial femoropatellar ligament in a 32 year old male with patellar dislocation. Two consecutive axial proton-density (PD) FSE fat-suppressed images (**a**, **b**) show the complete discontinuity of the ligament (*large arrow* in **a**) and a wavy contour of the fibers (*large arrow* in **b**). Note the patellar cartilage defect after as a result of impaction with the femoral condyle during dislocation (*small arrow* in **a**). The detached cartilage is seen distally (*small arrow* in **b**)

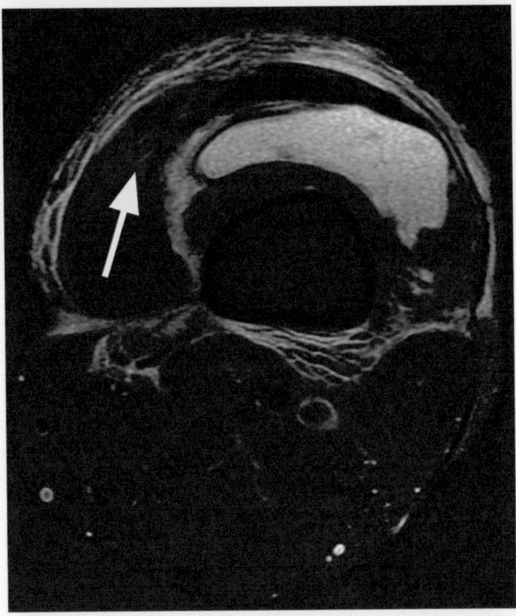

Fig. 7.22 Musculotendinous junction lesion of vastus medialis muscle in a 28 year old male with chronic patellar dislocation. Axial proton-density (PD) FSE fat-suppressed image shows a diffuse area of high signal intensity (*arrow*) indicating the involvement of musculotendinous junction of the vastus medialis

7.2.5 Pathological Findings of the Patellar Tendon

Patellar Tendinosis and Patellar Tendon Tears

Activities that include running, jumping, and kicking may affect the patellar tendon due to sudden extension of the knee or repetitive peak strain to the tendon [3]. Pathologically, it has been shown that microtears, mucoid degeneration, fibrinoid necrosis, and inflammation due to repair process are characteristic changes in patellar tendinosis [46]. A different terminology can be also used to define these findings including patellar tendinitis, patellar tendinopathy, or "jumper's knee" in cases that are located at the proximal insertion of the tendon [3, 46, 47]. The clinical symptoms range from pain inferior to the patella only after sports activity to persistent and severe pain during and after activities [47, 48]. On MR images, the tendon may show segmental thickening especially at the proximal portion where the anterior-posterior diameter of more than 7 mm is suggestive for tendinosis (Fig. 7.26) [3].

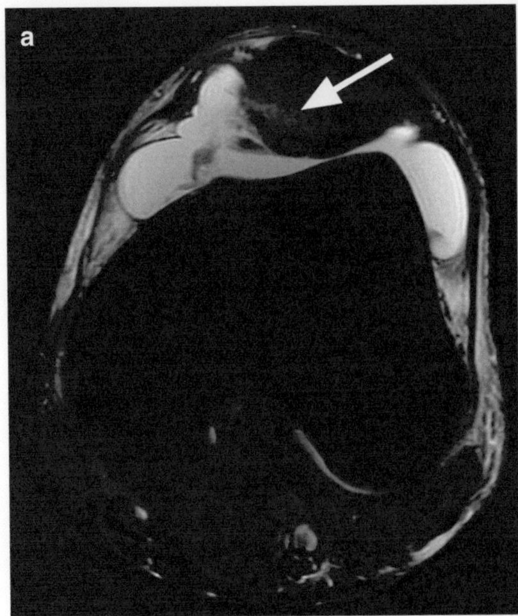

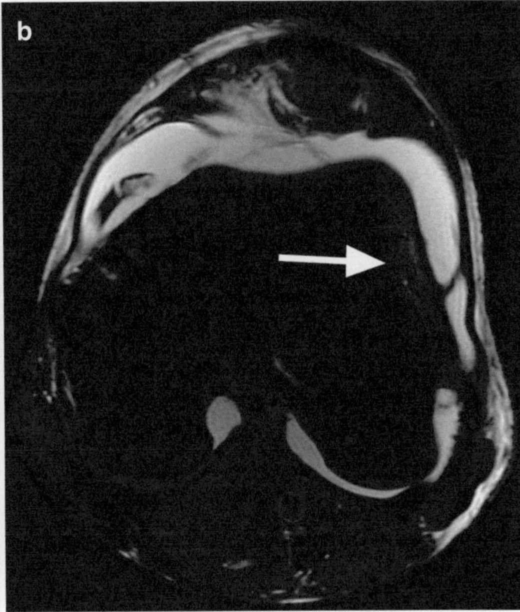

Fig. 7.23 "Kissing contusions" in a 32 year old male with acute patellar dislocation. Axial proton-density (PD) FSE fat-suppressed images (**a, b**) show areas of high signal intensity of the medial patellar facet (*arrow* in **a**) and of the lateral femoral condyle (*arrow* in **b**) resulting from impaction of patella on the femoral condyle during dislocation

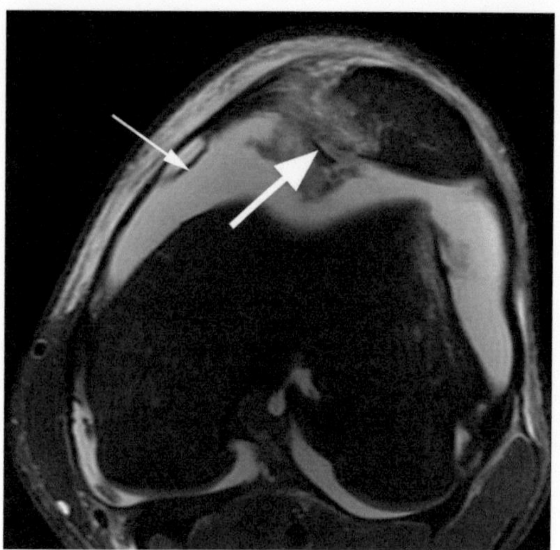

Fig. 7.24 Free osteochondral fragment in a 31 year old male with patellar dislocation and complete tear of the medial retinaculum. Axial proton-density (PD) FSE fat-suppressed image shows a small osteochondral fragment (*large arrow*) completely detached from the medial patellar facet. The bone component of the fragment is low signal intensity on this fat-suppressed image. Note the large joint effusion (*small arrow*)

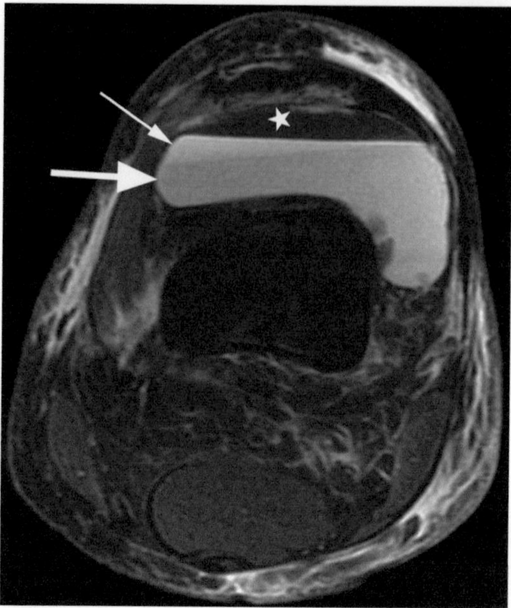

Fig. 7.25 Lipohemarthrosis in a 48 year old female with patellar dislocation and associated fracture. Axial proton-density (PD) FSE fat-suppressed image shows the typical three-layer appearance: the superior layer with fat signal intensity because of the fat suppression (*star*), the intermediate layer as a normal joint fluid representing the blood serum (*small arrow*), and the inferior layer of cellular debris as intermediate signal intensity (*large arrow*)

The tendon also shows an increased intrasubstance signal intensity on T1- and T2-weighted images with indistinct posterior margins of the tendon especially posterior to the thickened segment (Fig. 7.26) [3]. In chronic cases, quadriceps muscle atrophy may be seen.

Partial or complete tendon tears usually appear in association with underlying tendinosis. High-grade forces on normal tendon or lesser forces on a weakened tendon due to systemic diseases (diabetes, chronic renal failure, collagen diseases, or chronic systemic inflammatory diseases) may also result in tears at different locations along the tendon. MR imaging shows focal incomplete discontinuity or complete discontinuity of the tendon with wavy contour (Figs. 7.27 and 7.28). The tendon tears are usually in the proximal portion of the tendon and may include osseous avulsion fragment from the inferior pole of the patella.

Osgood-Schlatter Syndrome

Osgood-Schlatter syndrome represents an avulsion injury of the tibial tuberosity by the patellar tendon. The injury is bilateral in up to 50 % of cases, and MR imaging is an additional tool that confirms the clinical and radiological diagnosis and provides additional information [49]. Sagittal MR images show cortical irregularities of the tibial tuberosity with possible one or more small bone fragments detached accompanied by high bone marrow signal intensity on T2-weighted images (Fig. 7.29). Other MRI findings include distal patellar tendon enlargement and inhomogeneity, thickened cartilage anterior to tibial tuberosity, deep infrapatellar bursitis, and surrounding soft tissue edema.

Sinding-Larsen-Johansson Syndrome

Sinding-Larsen-Johansson syndrome refers to a spectrum of pathological entities that involves the proximal patellar tendon and the inferior pole of the patella including "the jumper's knee" and the patellar sleeve avulsion [49]. The MR imaging findings are best seen on sagittal images and are represented by thickening and signal

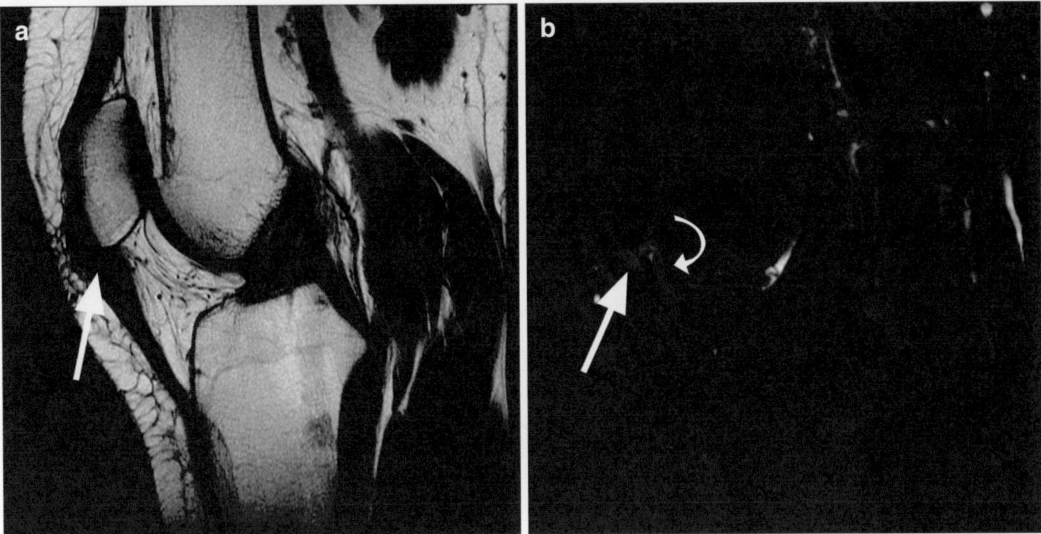

Fig. 7.26 Proximal patellar tendinopathy or "jumper's knee" in a 41 year old male. Sagittal proton-density (PD) FSE image (**a**) and sagittal T2-weighted fat-suppressed image (**b**) show proximal thickening and increased intrasubstance signal intensity of the patellar tendon (*large arrows* in **a**, **b**). Note the indistinct posterior margin of the tendon (*curved arrow* in **b**)

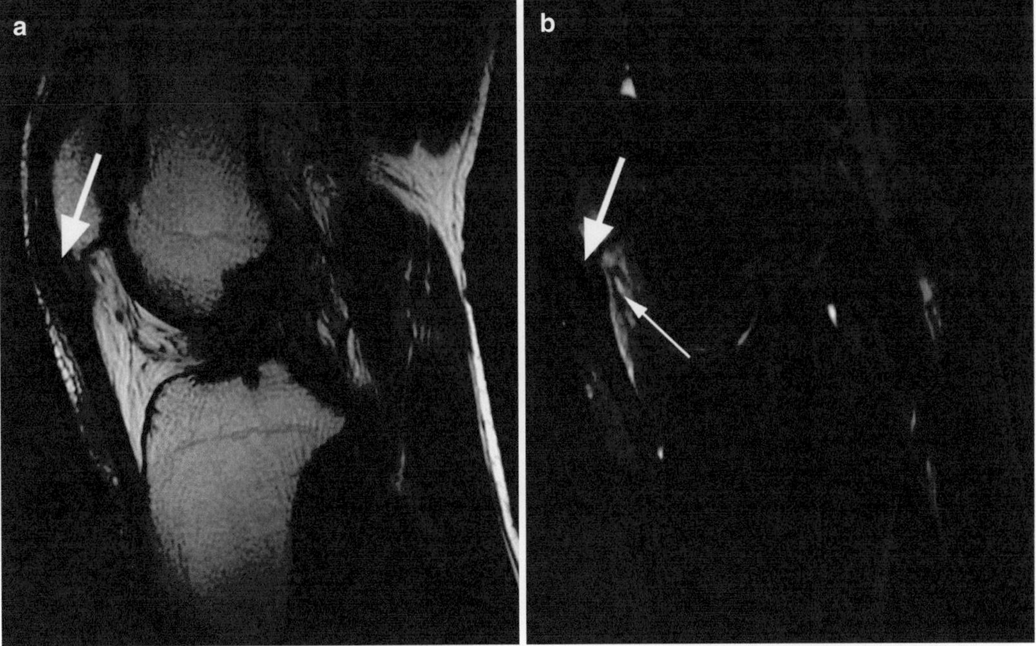

Fig. 7.27 Partial tear of the patellar tendon in a 28 year old male with "jumper's knee." Sagittal proton-density (PD) FSE image (**a**) and sagittal T2-weighted fat-suppressed image (**b**) show a longitudinal linear increased intrasubstance signal intensity within the proximal tendon (*large arrows* in **a**, **b**). Note the diffuse edema of the adjacent fat pad which is also suggestive for "jumper's knee" appearance (*small arrow* in **b**)

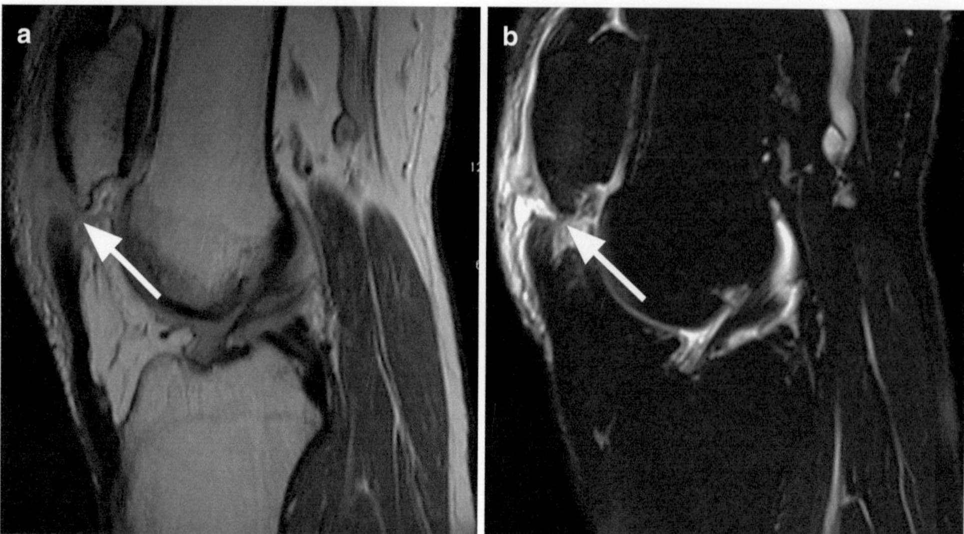

Fig. 7.28 Complete tear of the patellar tendon in a 43 year old male. Sagittal proton-density (PD) FSE image (**a**) and sagittal T2-weighted fat-suppressed image (**b**) show complete discontinuity of the tendon from its proximal insertion with hemorrhage between the tendon and patella (*arrows* in **a, b**)

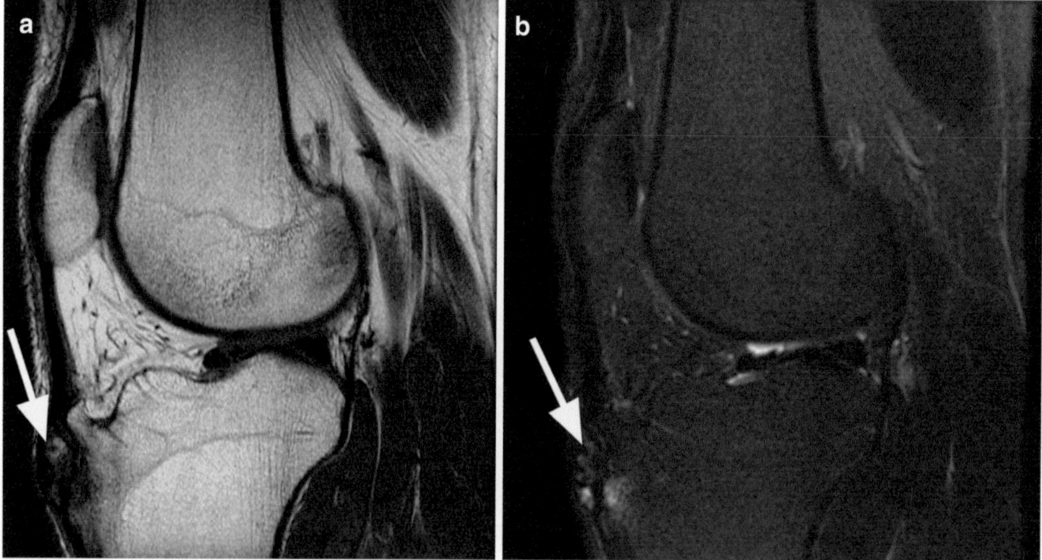

Fig. 7.29 Osgood-Schlatter syndrome in a 51 year old male. Sagittal proton-density (PD) FSE image (**a**) and sagittal T2-weighted fat-suppressed image (**b**) show a small fragment detached from the tibial tuberosity (*arrows*). Note the bone marrow at the insertion

changes of the proximal tendon, irregularities or erosions at the tendon insertion, and possible small bone fragment detached from the inferior pole of the patella. Some authors consider Sinding-Larsen-Johansson syndrome and patellar sleeve avulsion as two different entities [50]. Although the mechanism of injury is similar in both cases (e.g., forceful contraction of the

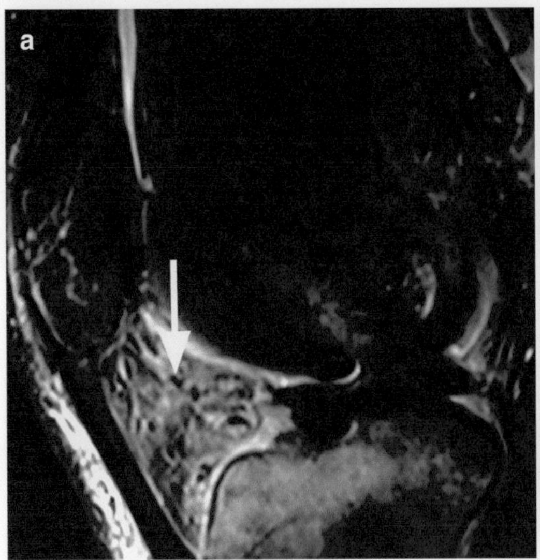
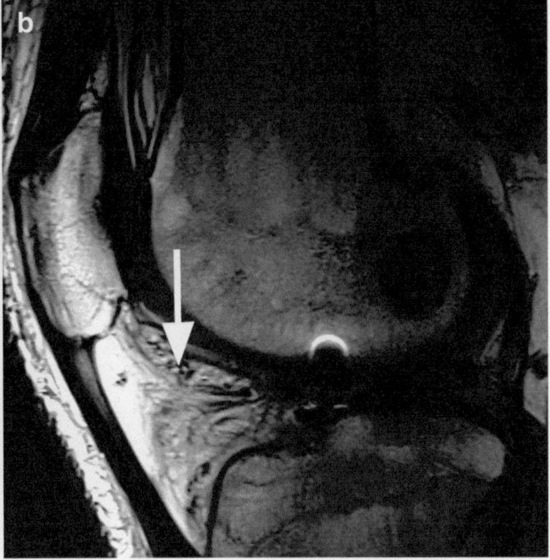

Fig. 7.30 Hoffa disease in a 34 year old male. Sagittal T2-weighted fat-suppressed image (**a**) and sagittal proton-density (PD) FSE image (**b**) show diffuse high-signal changes within the infrapatellar fat pad due to inflammation and hemorrhage. The result is an impingement of the anterior femorotibial space

quadriceps tendon against resistance), the authors consider that only a bone avulsion is present in Sinding-Larsen-Johansson syndrome, while in patellar sleeve avulsion, extensive cartilaginous injury is present, and the differentiation should be made because the two entities are managed differently [49, 50].

7.2.6   Pathological Findings of the Infrapatellar Fat Pad

The infrapatellar fat pad is an intracapsular structure that can be the site of different pathological entities including inflammation (Hoffa disease), synovial diseases such as intracapsular chondroma and nodular synovitis, shear injuries, lipoma arborescens, and postoperative localized or diffuse fibrosis [51].

The Hoffa disease (syn. Hoffa syndrome) represents an impingement of the fat pad resulting in scar tissue formation. The etiology can be traumatic or atraumatic. In traumatic disease, acute or repetitive chronic trauma leads to inflammation and hemorrhage within the fat pad that becomes hypertrophic and predisposes to impingement between the tibia and femur. In acute Hoffa disease, diffuse high-signal-intensity changes are seen on T2-weighted MR images (Fig. 7.30). The patellar tendon may be displaced anteriorly and small joint effusion may be present [51]. In chronic disease, the main pathological finding is fibrosis that is identified on MR imaging as diffuse areas of low signal intensity on T1- and T2-weighted images. In cases in which small foci of metaplastic bone or cartilage are suspected on MR imaging, correlation with radiography is essential to differentiate fibrosis from ossification [51].

Intracapsular chondroma is an intra-articular benign soft tissue mass that involves most often the knee compared to other joints and commonly arises in the infrapatellar fat pad. Intracapsular chondroma results from extrasynovial capsule metaplasia and, histologically, has a chondroid structure with punctate calcifications. Erosions of the adjacent bone may be present [51]. MR imaging shows a mass with inhomogeneous signal intensity on T1- and T2-weighted images which obliterates the infrapatellar fat pad. It shows small foci of low signal intensity representing calcifications (Fig. 7.31).

Intra-articular nodular synovitis is a localized synovial proliferation within the knee and is

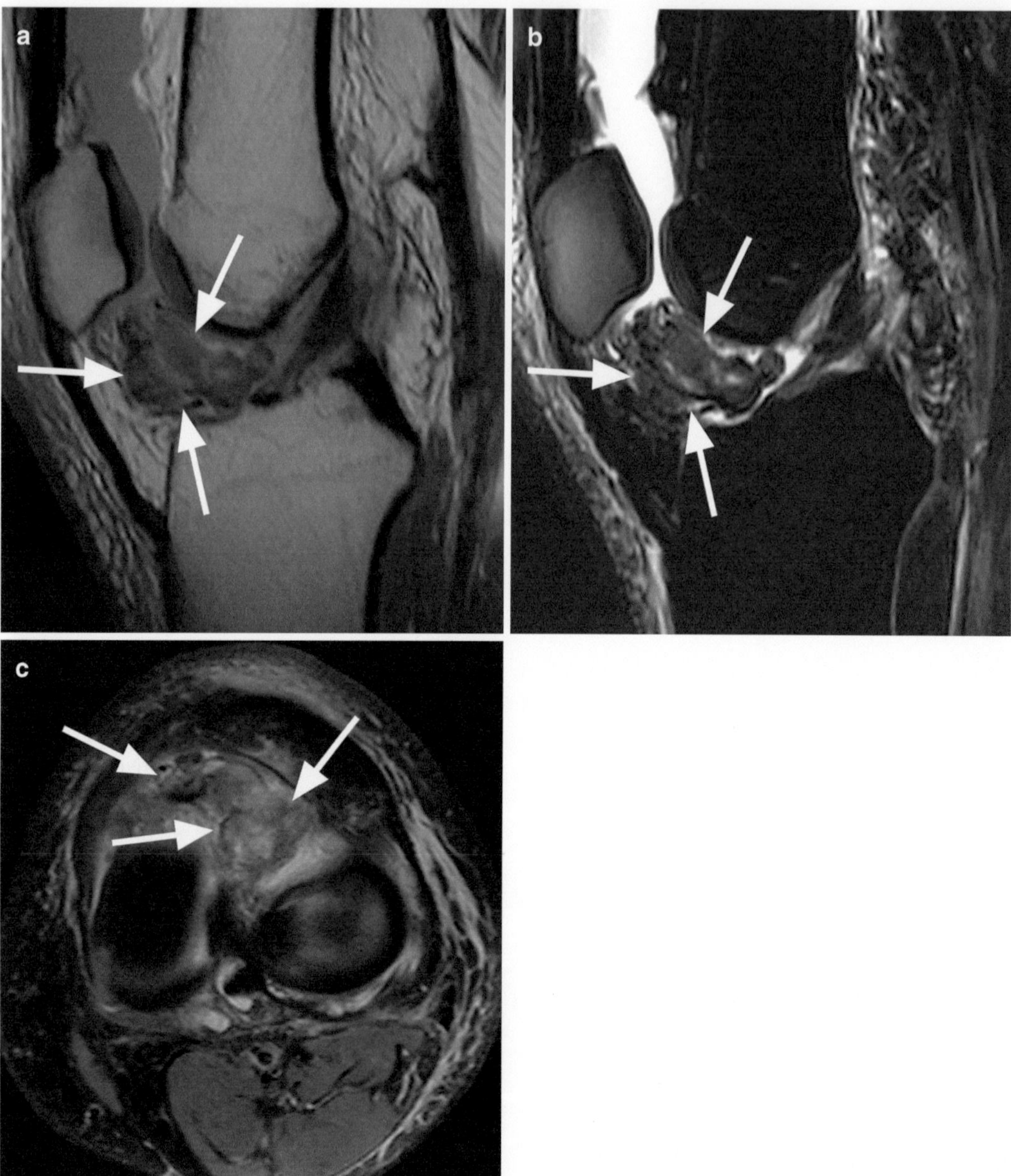

Fig. 7.31 Intracapsular chondroma in a 33 year old male. Sagittal proton-density (PD) FSE image (**a**), sagittal T2-weighted fat-suppressed image (**b**), and axial proton-density (PD) FSE fat-suppressed image (**c**) show a polilobulated mass within the infrapatellar fat pad (*arrows*). The chondroid origin of the lesion is demonstrated by the fact that the lesion and the articular cartilage have similar signal intensities on all sequences

considered by some authors the localized form of the pigmented villonodular synovitis (PVNS) [52, 53]. MR imaging demonstrates nodules of intermediate to low signal intensity on T1-weighted images and inhomogeneous high signal intensity on T2-weighted images with variable foci of low signal intensity representing hemosiderin (Fig. 7.32).

The shear injury of the infrapatellar fat pad usually appears as a secondary finding of anterior

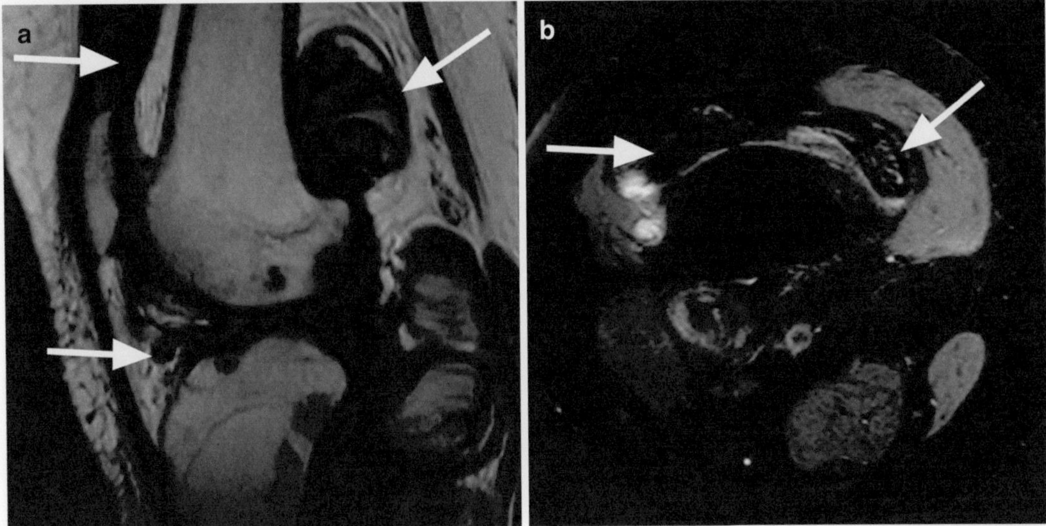

Fig. 7.32 Intra-articular nodular synovitis in a 40 year old male. Sagittal proton-density (PD) FSE image (**a**) shows multiple nodules of various dimensions located within the infrapatellar fat pad, suprapattelar fat pad and posteriorly (*arrows*). The nodules are heterogeneous intermediate to low signal intensity with variable foci of low signal intensity representing hemosiderin. Axial proton-density (PD) FSE fat-suppressed image (**b**) through the suprapatellar fat pad also shows heterogeneous hypointensity foci within the lesion indicating the hemosiderin (*arrows*)

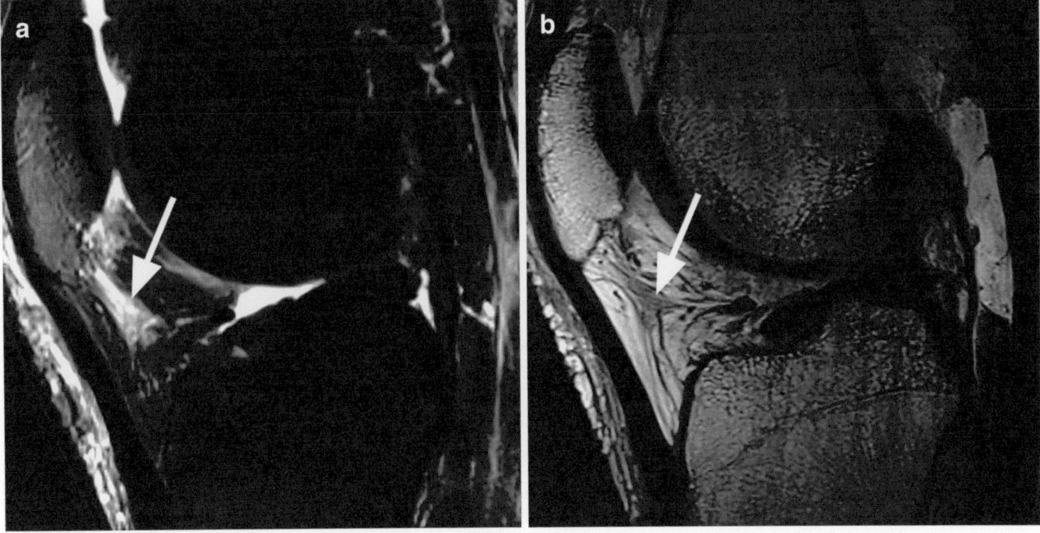

Fig. 7.33 Shear injury of the infrapatellar fat pad in a 38 year old male with partial anterior cruciate ligament tear. Sagittal T2-weighted fat-suppressed image (**a**) and sagittal proton-density (PD) FSE image (**b**) show linear fluid collection within the fat pad (*arrow*)

cruciate ligament injuries and is identified on T2-weighted images as a linear fluid collection within the fat pad at the level of the menisci (Fig. 7.33) [54].

Lipoma arborescens appears as a reaction to chronic inflammatory irritation of the synovia and can be bilateral and multifocal. The lesion is commonly located within the suprapatellar fat pad and

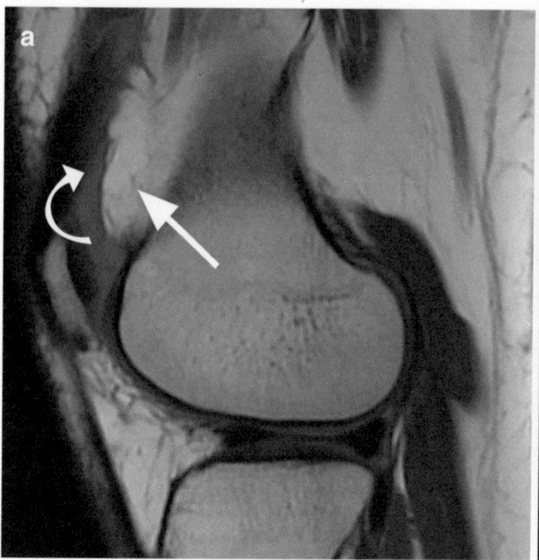

Fig. 7.34 Lipoma arborescens in a 53 year old male. Sagittal proton-density (PD) FSE image (**a**) and coronal proton-density (PD) FSE fat-suppressed image (**b**) show a lobulated mass with similar signal intensity to the subcutaneous fat (*large arrows* in **a, b**). Note the fluid collection in the suprapatellar bursa (*curved arrows* in **a, b**)

less often in the infrapatellar fat pad. The lesion is lobulated and has similar signal intensity to the subcutaneous fat on MR imaging (Fig. 7.34).

Postoperative fibrosis or arthrofibrosis appears after arthroscopy and may be classified into diffuse or focal fibrosis. Diffuse arthrofibrosis appears on MR imaging as linear strands or as diffuse areas of fibrosis of low signal intensity within the fat pad (Fig. 7.35). The focal form of arthrofibrosis is better known by its synonym "cyclops lesion" which is a focal mass that is situated anterior in the midline of the joint space. It is a finding which is usually seen after ACL or PCL reconstructions (Fig. 7.36).

7.3   MRI Postoperative Findings

A great number of surgical options are available to treat patients with lesions of the extensor structures of the knee that refers to patellar instability and dislocation, patellar tendon tear, or patella bipartite.

The treatment of patellar dislocation requires a profound understanding of predisposing factors and injury pattern and should be based on the individual's risk of recurrent dislocation, pain, and disability [42, 55]. In primary acute dislocation without severe structural damages, the

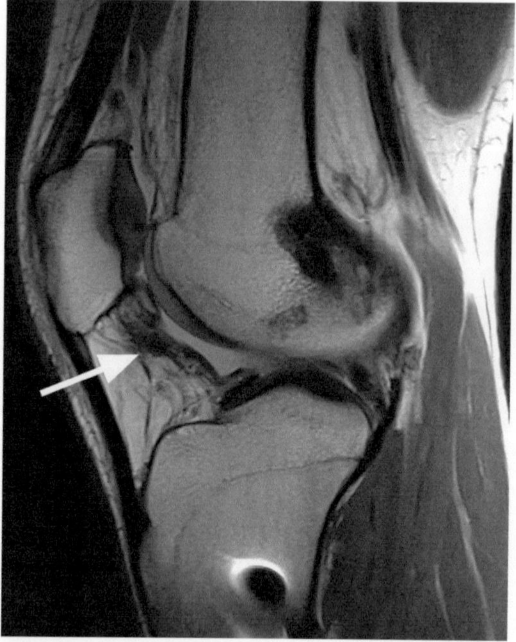

Fig. 7.35 Diffuse arthrofibrosis in a 25 year old female after arthroscopy. Sagittal proton-density (PD) FSE image shows linear strands of fibrosis of low signal intensity within the fat pad (*arrow*)

therapy of choice is the conservative treatment (e.g., physical therapy, behavioral education, bracing). However, the surgical intervention is

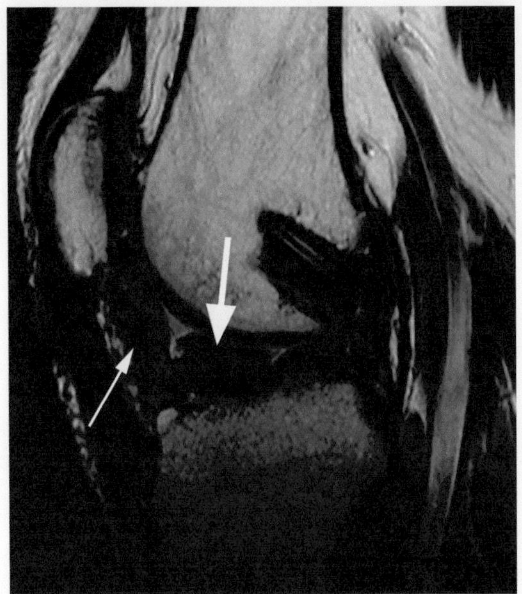

Fig. 7.36 Complex fibrotic changes of the Hoffa's fat pad in a 30 year old male after anterior cruciate ligament (ACL) reconstruction. Sagittal proton-density (PD) FSE image shows the focal form of arthrofibrosis or the "cyclops lesion" (*large arrow*) as well as the diffuse arthrofibrosis as diffuse areas of fibrosis of low signal intensity within the fat pad (*small arrow*)

recommended in primary acute traumatic dislocation that includes severe trochlear dysplasia, the presence of unstable or free osteochondral fragments, extensive cartilage damage, or a relevant disruption of the medial ligamentous stabilizers [56]. The surgical interventions may be classified as procedures that involve the soft tissue stabilizers (medial ligamentous repair and lateral release) and procedures that involve the bone (trochleoplasty and tibial tuberosity transfer).

The medial femoropatellar ligament reconstruction restores the restraining function of the medial stabilizers by using different anchoring techniques and graft materials (e.g., gracilis tendon, semimembranosus tendon) [9]. The ligament is extracapsular, and, therefore, the femoral disruption might not be reliably diagnosed by standard arthroscopy [42].

The role of the preoperative MR imaging is crucial since the determination of the site of the injury is the first factor that may influence a satisfactory result. Some authors reported that the positioning of the femoral tunnel during surgery

is important for the patellar stability. The anatomic location of the normal femoral tunnel is just anterior to the intersection of the posterior femoral cortical line and Blumensaat's line [57]. A too proximally placed tunnel would lead to an increased stress on the non-isometric ligament and failure of the reconstruction [58, 59] as well as increase stress and contact pressure on the medial facet cartilage [57]. However, it seems that regardless of the tunnel position, a key factor in medial femoropatellar ligament reconstruction is to set the correct graft length or tension [57].

The role of MR imaging after surgery is to exclude the general surgical complications (septic arthritis), to evaluate the femoral tunnel position and ligament length in cases with insufficient outcome, and to follow up the outcome of the intervention regarding the normal patellar position.

The lateral retinaculum release and the lateral retinaculum lengthening were widely used as primary intervention for patellar dislocation when combined with medial capsular plication [60]. However, this technique is rarely used nowadays and, if used, usually only in patients with lateral hypercompression syndrome or in patients with positive patellar tilt test [61]. MR imaging after lateral interventions may identify extensive scar formation at the site of intervention that can cause additional compression and tilting of the lateral femoropatellar joint [9].

The trochleoplasty is a very demanding technique that implies an osteotomy with femoral sulcus deepening and showed improved physical activities of the patients. The role of postoperative MR imaging is to assess the resulting femoral groove depth and the lateral femoral inclination. However, 10–30 % of patients may suffer increased pain after intervention, and MR images may show progression of degenerative changes in the femoropatellar joint [62].

The *tibial tubercle transfer technique* involves medial transfer of the tibial attachment of the patellar tendon. It is usually performed when the tibial tuberosity-trochlear groove distance is more than 2 cm, measured on axial images. Although redislocation is rare after tibial tuberosity transfer, it seems that this procedure cannot prevent the progress of femoropatellar joint degeneration.

7.4 MRI Impression

7.4.1 Nonoperative Findings

1. Normal femoropatellar joint with normally positioned patella; Wiberg patella type I, II, or III
2. Patella alta/patella baja – based on Biedert index
3. Patella bipartite/multipartite
   - Uncomplicated
   - MRI suggestive for complicated patella bipartite: subchondral edema or pseudoarthrosis (fluid between fragments)
4. The MRI findings suggestive for trochlear dysplasia with/without findings of dislocation
   - Trochlear depth less than 3 mm
   - Horizontal lateral facet inclination angle smaller than 11°
   - Trochlear facet asymmetry 3 cm above the femorotibial joint level of 40 % or less
   - Nipplelike anterior prominence at the superior border of the trochlea larger than 2 mm
   - Tibial tuberosity-trochlear groove distance greater than 2 cm
5. MRI findings suggestive for acute patellar dislocation
   - Lesions of the medial patellar retinaculum (sprain, partial tear, complete tear)
   - "Kissing contusions" (trabecular microfractures of the medial patellar facet and the lateral femoral condyle)
   - With/without avulsion fracture of the medial femoral epicondyle
   - With/without involvement of the musculotendinous junction of the vastus medialis muscle
   - With/without patellar or femoral fractures
   - With/without osteochondral injuries with or without cartilaginous or osseous loose bodies (including location of the loose bodies and their origin)
6. MR findings suggestive of patellar tendon pathology
   - Tendinosis or tendinopathy
   - Partial tear
   - Complete tear
7. Osgood-Schlatter syndrome
8. Sinding-Larsen-Johansson syndrome
9. Infrapatellar fat pad abnormalities
   - MRI findings of Hoffa disease
   - Soft tissue mass (suggestive for intracapsular chondroma, intra-articular nodular synovitis or lipoma arborescens)
   - Fibrosis (diffuse or focal)
   - MRI findings that suggest a shear injury

7.4.2 Postoperative Findings (Intervention for Instability and Dislocation)

1. Normal postoperative MR imaging findings including patellar position and trochlear qualitative and quantitative assessment
2. Without signs of recurrent dislocation
3. Abnormal MR imaging findings:
   - Fibrosis of the lateral or medial retinaculum
   - Incorrect positioning of the femoral tunnel after medial femoropatellar ligament repair
   - Insufficient depth of the femoral groove after trochleoplasty
   - Incorrect positioning of the patella after tibial tubercle translation
   - Femoropatellar degenerative changes

References

1. Sonin AH, et al. MR imaging appearance of the extensor mechanism of the knee: functional anatomy and injury patterns. Radiographics. 1995;15(2):367–82.
2. Reider B, et al. The anterior aspect of the knee joint. J Bone Joint Surg Am. 1981;63(3):351–6.
3. el-Khoury GY, et al. MR imaging of patellar tendinitis. Radiology. 1992;184(3):849–54.
4. Grelsamer RP, Proctor CS, Bazos AN. Evaluation of patellar shape in the sagittal plane. A clinical analysis. Am J Sports Med. 1994;22(1):61–6.
5. Tecklenburg K, et al. Bony and cartilaginous anatomy of the patellofemoral joint. Knee Surg Sports Traumatol Arthrosc. 2006;14(3):235–40.
6. Ruiz ME, Erickson SJ. Medial and lateral supporting structures of the knee. Normal MR imaging anatomy and pathologic findings. Magn Reson Imaging Clin N Am. 1994;2(3):381–99.
7. Amis AA, et al. Anatomy and biomechanics of the medial patellofemoral ligament. Knee. 2003;10(3):215–20.

8. Bicos J, Fulkerson JP, Amis A. Current concepts review: the medial patellofemoral ligament. Am J Sports Med. 2007;35(3):484–92.

9. Diederichs G, Issever AS, Scheffler S. MR imaging of patellar instability: injury patterns and assessment of risk factors. Radiographics. 2010;30(4):961–81.

10. Merican AM, Amis AA. Anatomy of the lateral retinaculum of the knee. J Bone Joint Surg Br. 2008; 90(4):527–34.

11. Fulkerson JP, Gossling HR. Anatomy of the knee joint lateral retinaculum. Clin Orthop Relat Res. 1980; 153:183–8.

12. Terry GC, Hughston JC, Norwood LA. The anatomy of the iliopatellar band and iliotibial tract. Am J Sports Med. 1986;14(1):39–45.

13. Wiberg G. Roentgenographic and anatomic studies on the femoro-patellar joint. Acta Orthop Scand. 1941; 15(1):39–46.

14. Dejour D, Le Coultre B. Osteotomies in patellofemoral instabilities. Sports Med Arthrosc. 2007; 15(1):39–46.

15. Staeubli HU, et al. Magnetic resonance imaging for articular cartilage: cartilage-bone mismatch. Clin Sports Med. 2002;21(3):417–33, viii–ix.

16. Seil R, et al. Reliability and interobserver variability in radiological patellar height ratios. Knee Surg Sports Traumatol Arthrosc. 2000;8(4):231–6.

17. Biedert RM, Albrecht S. The patellotrochlear index: a new index for assessing patellar height. Knee Surg Sports Traumatol Arthrosc. 2006;14(8):707–12.

18. Collins MS, Tiegs-Heiden CA, Stuart MJ. Patellar calcar: MRI appearance of a previously undescribed anatomical entity. Skeletal Radiol. 2014;43(2): 219–25.

19. Pfirrmann CW, et al. Femoral trochlear dysplasia: MR findings. Radiology. 2000;216(3):858–64.

20. Bongers EM, et al. Human syndromes with congenital patellar anomalies and the underlying gene defects. Clin Genet. 2005;68(4):302–19.

21. Sheffield EG. Double-layered patella in multiple epiphyseal dysplasia: a valuable clue in the diagnosis. J Pediatr Orthop. 1998;18(1):123–8.

22. Rosenthal RK, Levine DB. Fragmentation of the distal pole of the patella in spastic cerebral palsy. J Bone Joint Surg Am. 1977;59(7):934–9.

23. Saupe E. Primare knochenmarkseiterung der kniescheibe. Deutsche Z Chir. 1943;258:386–92.

24. Kavanagh EC, et al. MRI findings in bipartite patella. Skeletal Radiol. 2007;36(3):209–14.

25. Neyret P, et al. Patellar tendon length–the factor in patellar instability? Knee. 2002;9(1):3–6.

26. Shabshin N, et al. MRI criteria for patella alta and baja. Skeletal Radiol. 2004;33(8):445–50.

27. Dejour D, et al. The introduction of a new MRI index to evaluate sagittal patellofemoral engagement. Orthop Traumatol Surg Res. 2013;99(8 Suppl):S391–8.

28. Ali SA, Helmer R, Terk MR. Patella alta: lack of correlation between patellotrochlear cartilage congruence and commonly used patellar height ratios. AJR Am J Roentgenol. 2009;193(5):1361–6.

29. Insall J, Salvati E. Patella position in the normal knee joint. Radiology. 1971;101(1):101–4.

30. Miller TT, Staron RB, Feldman F. Patellar height on sagittal MR imaging of the knee. AJR Am J Roentgenol. 1996;167(2):339–41.

31. Endo Y, et al. MRI quantitative morphologic analysis of patellofemoral region: lack of correlation with chondromalacia patellae at surgery. AJR Am J Roentgenol. 2007;189(5):1165–8.

32. Weber-Spickschen TS, et al. The relationship between trochlear dysplasia and medial patellofemoral ligament rupture location after patellar dislocation: an MRI evaluation. Knee. 2011;18(3):185–8.

33. Farahmand F, Senavongse W, Amis AA. Quantitative study of the quadriceps muscles and trochlear groove geometry related to instability of the patellofemoral joint. J Orthop Res. 1998;16(1):136–43.

34. Ahmed AM, Duncan NA. Correlation of patellar tracking pattern with trochlear and retropatellar surface topographies. J Biomech Eng. 2000;122(6): 652–60.

35. Amis AA, Senavongse W, Darcy P. Biomechanics of patellofemoral joint prostheses. Clin Orthop Relat Res. 2005;436:20–9.

36. Earhart C, et al. Transient lateral patellar dislocation: review of imaging findings, patellofemoral anatomy, and treatment options. Emerg Radiol. 2013;20(1): 11–23.

37. Carrillon Y, et al. Patellar instability: assessment on MR images by measuring the lateral trochlear inclination-initial experience. Radiology. 2000; 216(2):582–5.

38. Elias DA, White LM. Imaging of patellofemoral disorders. Clin Radiol. 2004;59(7):543–57.

39. Kirsch MD, et al. Transient lateral patellar dislocation: diagnosis with MR imaging. AJR Am J Roentgenol. 1993;161(1):109–13.

40. Zaidi A, et al. MRI of traumatic patellar dislocation in children. Pediatr Radiol. 2006;36(11):1163–70.

41. Dejour H, et al. Factors of patellar instability: an anatomic radiographic study. Knee Surg Sports Traumatol Arthrosc. 1994;2(1):19–26.

42. Balcarek P, et al. MRI but not arthroscopy accurately diagnoses femoral MPFL injury in first-time patellar dislocations. Knee Surg Sports Traumatol Arthrosc. 2012;20(8):1575–80.

43. Spritzer CE, et al. Medial retinacular complex injury in acute patellar dislocation: MR findings and surgical implications. AJR Am J Roentgenol. 1997;168(1):117–22.

44. Vellet AD, et al. Occult posttraumatic osteochondral lesions of the knee: prevalence, classification, and short-term sequelae evaluated with MR imaging. Radiology. 1991;178(1):271–6.

45. Elias DA, White LM, Fithian DC. Acute lateral patellar dislocation at MR imaging: injury patterns of medial patellar soft-tissue restraints and osteochondral injuries of the inferomedial patella. Radiology. 2002;225(3):736–43.

46. Roels J, et al. Patellar tendinitis (jumper's knee). Am J Sports Med. 1978;6(6):362–8.

47. Martens M, et al. Patellar tendinitis: pathology and results of treatment. Acta Orthop Scand. 1982;53(3):445–50.
48. Blazina ME, et al. Jumper's knee. Orthop Clin North Am. 1973;4(3):665–78.
49. Gottsegen CJ, et al. Avulsion fractures of the knee: imaging findings and clinical significance. Radiographics. 2008;28(6):1755–70.
50. Bates DG, Hresko MT, Jaramillo D. Patellar sleeve fracture: demonstration with MR imaging. Radiology. 1994;193(3):825–7.
51. Jacobson JA, et al. MR imaging of the infrapatellar fat pad of Hoffa. Radiographics. 1997;17(3):675–91.
52. Cavanagh RC, Schwamm HA. RPC of the month from the AFIP. Radiology. 1971;100(2):409–14.
53. Jelinek JS, et al. Imaging of pigmented villonodular synovitis with emphasis on MR imaging. AJR Am J Roentgenol. 1989;152(2):337–42.
54. Robertson PL, et al. Anterior cruciate ligament tears: evaluation of multiple signs with MR imaging. Radiology. 1994;193(3):829–34.
55. Fithian DC, Paxton EW, Cohen AB. Indications in the treatment of patellar instability. J Knee Surg. 2004; 17(1):47–56.
56. Stefancin JJ, Parker RD. First-time traumatic patellar dislocation: a systematic review. Clin Orthop Relat Res. 2007;455:93–101.
57. McCarthy M, et al. Femoral tunnel placement in medial patellofemoral ligament reconstruction. Iowa Orthop J. 2013;33:58–63.
58. Elias JJ, Cosgarea AJ. Technical errors during medial patellofemoral ligament reconstruction could overload medial patellofemoral cartilage: a computational analysis. Am J Sports Med. 2006;34(9):1478–85.
59. Bollier M, et al. Technical failure of medial patellofemoral ligament reconstruction. Arthroscopy. 2011;27(8):1153–9.
60. Haspl M, et al. Fully arthroscopic stabilization of the patella. Arthroscopy. 2002;18(1):E2.
61. Arendt EA, Fithian DC, Cohen E. Current concepts of lateral patella dislocation. Clin Sports Med. 2002; 21(3):499–519.
62. Fucentese SF, et al. Classification of trochlear dysplasia as predictor of clinical outcome after trochleoplasty. Knee Surg Sports Traumatol Arthrosc. 2011; 19(10):1655–61.

Synovium and Capsule

8

Nicolae Bolog, Gustav Andreisek, and Erika Ulbrich

8.1 Anatomy and Normal MRI Appearance

8.1.1 Capsule and Synovial Compartments

The articular capsule of the knee consists of a thick outer layer, the fibrous capsule, and a thinner inner layer, the synovial membrane (synovium).

The synovium is a mesenchymal tissue composed of two to three layers of specialized cells (synoviocytes) and a supporting connective tissue that includes a well-developed vascular network and relatively abundant adipose tissue [1]. This hypervascular membrane is responsible for the secretion of the synovial fluid, which lubricates and nourishes the joint [2]. The synoviocytes also have a role in removing intra-articular particles including cartilaginous debris [2].

The knee joint can be seen as common joint space that is subdivided by synovial membranes into several interconnected compartments. Anteriorly, at the central femoropatellar compartment, the synovial membrane attaches to the patellar borders and extends circumferentially beneath vastus lateralis and vastus medialis muscles to the anterior femoral shaft. It covers also the anterior aspects of the cruciate ligaments. The medial and lateral femorotibial compartments of the synovial membrane are represented by the lateral and medial extensions of the central portion [2]. These compartments are separated by the infrapatellar synovial fold anteriorly and by a reflection of the synovium that extends from the sides of the posterior cruciate ligament onto the fibrous capsule, posteriorly [2]. The anterior and posterior cruciate ligaments, menisci, and the infrapatellar fat pad are located "extrasynovially" which means that they are located outside the abovementioned synovial compartments.

8.1.2 Synovial Bursae and Synovial Recesses

Synovial bursae or synovial recesses are extensions of the synovial membrane between different anatomical structures, and their role is to reduce the friction during the motion of these structures. The knee bursae are numerous and, in the absence of pathological changes, rarely apparent on MR imaging [3]. The knowledge of the locations of synovial bursae is important since in pathological conditions, they may become apparent and a cause for misdiagnosis or diagnostic uncertainty [2]. The classification of the bursae is made on their anatomic location (Table 8.1). Readers of MR images should look for anterior and posterior bursae on sagittal planes and for medial and lateral bursae on axial planes. However, they should have in mind that normal bursae are generally not visible on MR imaging.

N.V. Bolog et al., *MRI of the Knee: A Guide to Evaluation and Reporting*,
DOI 10.1007/978-3-319-08165-6_8, © Springer International Publishing Switzerland 2015

Table 8.1 Anatomy and pathology of synovial bursae and recesses around the knee [2, 3, 5–10]

Compartment	Bursa/recess	Anatomy
Anterior	Suprapatellar bursa (Fig. 8.2)	Located between the quadriceps tendon and femur
	Prepatellar bursa (Fig. 8.3)	Superficially located between the patella and subcutaneous tissue
	Superficial infrapatellar or pretibial bursa	Superficially located between the tibial tubercle and subcutaneous tissue
	Deep infrapatellar bursa (Fig. 8.4)	Located posterior to the distal part of the patellar tendon between the tendon and anterior tibia
	Suprahoffatic recess (Fig. 8.5)	Located close to the inferior border of the patella
	Infrahoffatic recess (Fig. 8.5)	Located anterior to the inferior portion of the infrapatellar plica (also called ligamentum mucosum)
	Central synovial recess (Fig. 8.6)	Located anterior to the anterior cruciate ligament
Posterior	Medial posterior femoral recess or medial gastrocnemius bursa (Fig. 8.7)	Located between the posterior horn of the medial meniscus and the knee capsule and the medial head of the gastrocnemius muscle; may communicate with the articular cavity
	Lateral posterior femoral recess or lateral gastrocnemius bursa (Fig. 8.7)	Located between the posterior horn of the lateral meniscus and the knee capsule and lateral head of the gastrocnemius muscle; may communicate with the articular cavity
	Gastrocnemius-semimembranosus bursa (Fig. 8.8)	Double-bursa located between the semimembranosus and the medial head of the gastrocnemius muscle
	Subpopliteus bursa (Fig. 8.9)	Located between the posterior horn of the lateral meniscus and the popliteus tendon; communicates with the superior tibiofibular joint in 10 % of adults
	Posterior capsular recess (Fig. 8.10)	Located in the midline behind the posterior cruciate ligament; is an extension of the medial femorotibial compartment
Lateral	Iliotibial bursa	Located between the distal portion of the iliotibial band and the adjacent tibia
	Lateral collateral ligament-biceps femoris bursa (Fig. 8.11)	Located at the fibular insertion, the lateral collateral ligament and the biceps tendon form a conjoined tendon. Between the two structures, the lateral collateral ligament-biceps femoris bursa is constantly described
	Parameniscal recesses (Fig. 8.12)	Located superior and inferior to the level of the lateral meniscus in contact with the lateral femoral and tibial condyle
Medial	Medial collateral bursa	Located between the superficial and deep layer of medial collateral ligament
	Pes anserinus bursa	Located between the pes anserinus (tendons of sartorius, gracilis, and semitendinosus muscles) and the medial collateral ligament; does not typically communicate with the joint
	Medial collateral ligament-semimembranosus bursa	Located between the semimembranosus tendon and the medial collateral ligament

8.1.3   Synovial Plicae

Synovial plicae are normal anatomical structures representing embryologic remnants of the synovial membrane and are defined as thin, vascularized synovial folds without a known function [2, 4]. The plicae are usually asymptomatic, and they can be found at MR imaging within the knee joints as low-signal-intensity thin bands (Fig. 8.1). The most encountered plicae of the knee are the suprapatellar plica, the infrapatellar plica, the lateral patellar plica, and the mediopatellar plica (Table 8.2).

8.2   MRI Pathological Findings

8.2.1   Joint Effusions

Synovial Fluid

The synovial fluid is a viscid fluid secreted by the synovium. The knee synovial fluid is commonly depicted on MR imaging, but a definitive criterion that enables to define the quantity of the effusion as normal or pathological has not been clearly established. Clinically, knee effusions of less than 6–8 mL cannot be appreciated. However, on MR imaging, a volume of 1 mL of effusion may be visible adjacent to the femoral condyles [13]. Some authors demonstrated that a volume of 4 mL of fluid is depicted on plain radiography and, on midline sagittal MR images, leads to an anteroposterior diameter of the midline suprapatellar recess of 4 mm [13, 14]. This volume of

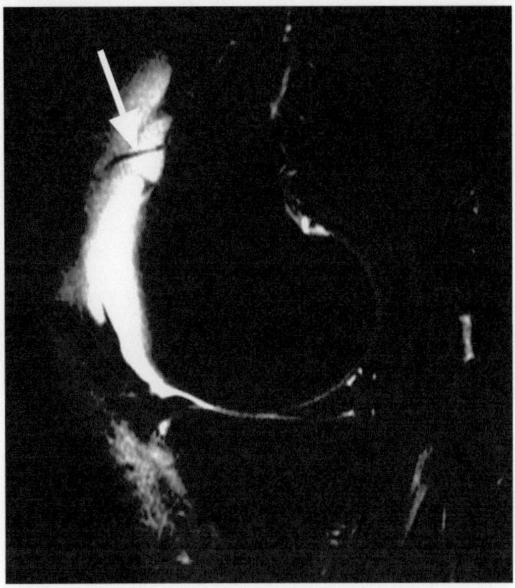

Fig. 8.1 Suprapatellar plica in a 28 year old female. Sagittal T2-weighted fat-suppressed image shows the synovial plica as a low-signal-intensity thin band (*arrow*)

Table 8.2 Synovial plicae of the knee [4, 11, 12]

	Anatomy	MR imaging appearance
Suprapatellar plica (Fig. 8.13)	Located between the suprapatellar bursa and the knee joint cavity; runs from the posterior aspect of quadriceps tendon, above the patella upward to the anterior aspect of the femur	Low-signal-intensity linear band posterior to the patella
Infrapatellar plica or ligamentum mucosum (Fig. 8.14)	The most commonly plica in the knee; runs from the femoral origin anterior to the intercondylar notch downward to the inferior pole of the patella	Low-signal-intensity band of various dimensions anterior and parallel to the anterior cruciate ligament, often within the infrapatellar fat pad
Mediopatellar plica (Fig. 8.15)	Runs from the medial capsule of the knee obliquely downward to the synovium of the infrapatellar fat pad	Low-signal-intensity linear band that may be connected to the suprapatellar plica; can extend between the medial facet of the patella and medial face of the trochlea
Lateral patellar plica (Fig. 8.16)	The least common plica of the knee; runs from the popliteus hiatus and attaches to the infrapatellar fat pad	Low-signal-intensity linear longitudinal band 1–2 cm lateral to the patella

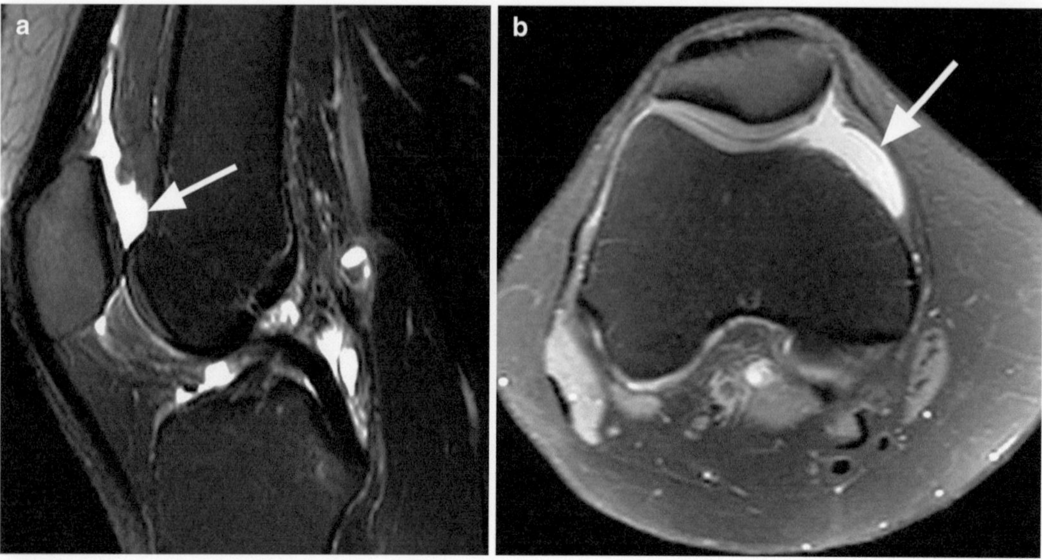

Fig. 8.2 Suprapatellar bursa in a 40 year old female. Sagittal T2-weighted fat-suppressed image (**a**) and axial proton-density (PD) fat-suppressed image (**b**) show the fluid in the suprapatellar bursa (*arrow*)

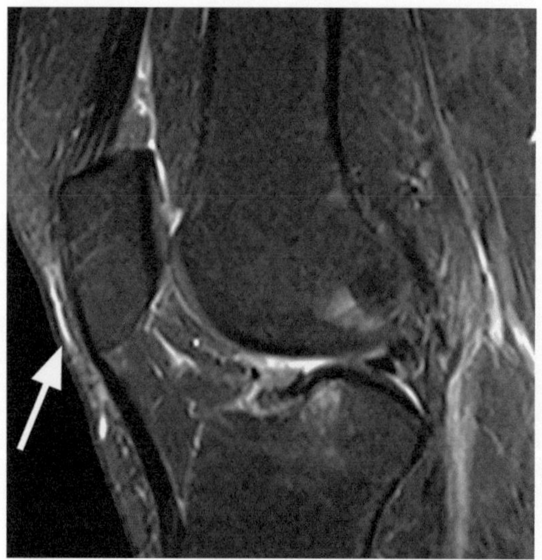

Fig. 8.3 Prepatellar bursa in a 55 year old male. Sagittal T2-weighted fat-suppressed image shows a small amount of fluid in the prepatellar bursa (*arrow*)

effusion was considered to be clinically important [15]. With increasing volumes of effusion, the fluid first collects in the suprapatellar bursa and subsequently in the posterior recesses and popliteal tendon sheath [13].

Although the knee effusion may be the only finding on MR imaging, most commonly the

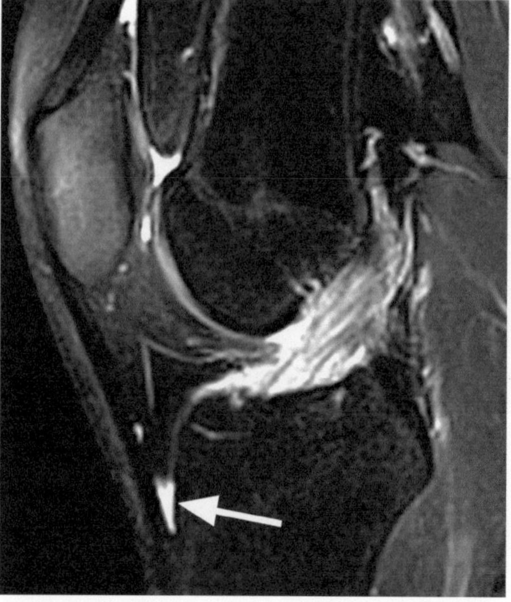

Fig. 8.4 Deep infrapatellar bursa in a 22 year old female. Sagittal T2-weighted fat-suppressed image shows the deep infrapatellar bursa posterior to the distal part of the patellar tendon between the tendon and anterior tibia (*arrow*)

synovial fluid is the result of a different underlying pathology (e.g., inflammatory diseases, trauma, degenerative changes, tumors). On MR imaging, the joint fluid appears homogeneously

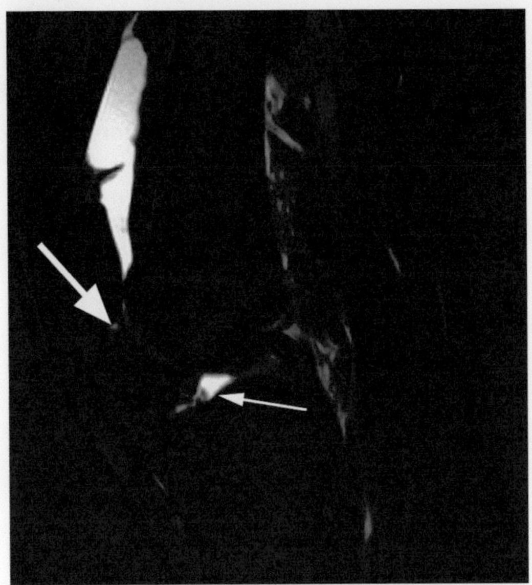

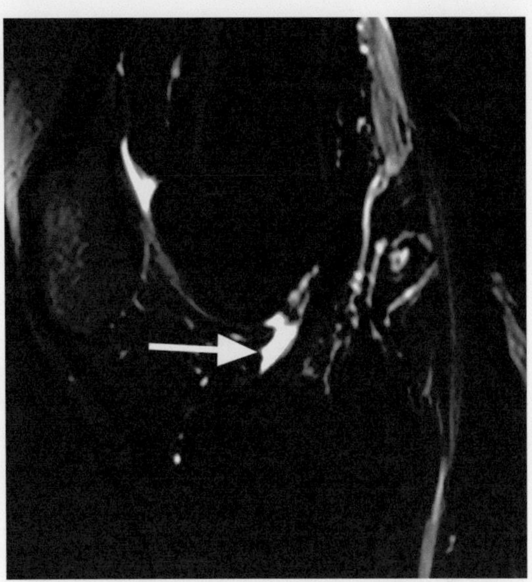

Fig. 8.5 Suprahoffatic and infrahoffatic recesses in a 19 year old female. Sagittal T2-weighted fat-suppressed image shows the suprahoffatic recess (*large arrow*) close to the inferior border of the patella and the infrahoffatic recess (*small arrow*)

Fig. 8.6 Central synovial recess in a 30 year old female. Sagittal T2-weighted fat-suppressed image shows the recess located anterior to the anterior cruciate ligament (*arrow*)

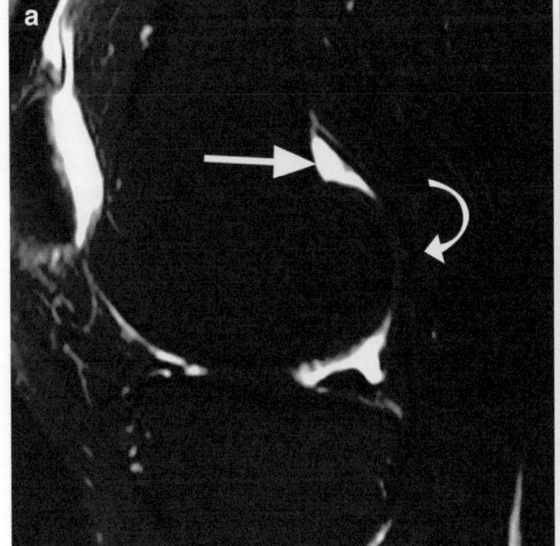

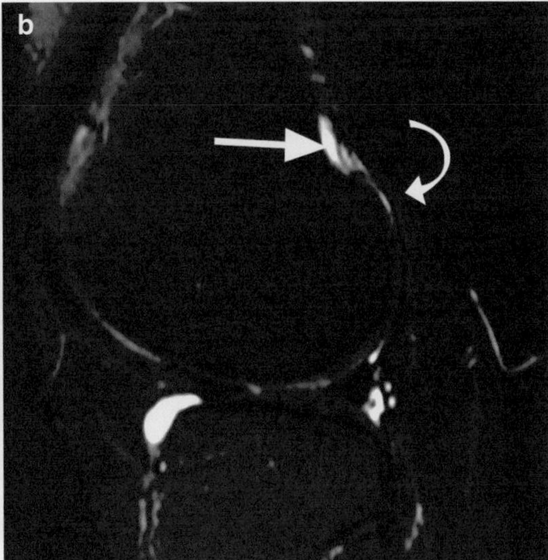

Fig. 8.7 Medial posterior femoral recess (medial gastrocnemius bursa) and lateral posterior femoral recess (lateral gastrocnemius bursa) in a 40 year old female. Sagittal T2-weighted fat-suppressed images through the medial compartment (**a**) and lateral compartment (**b**) show the medial gastrocnemius bursa (*arrow* in **a**) between the knee capsule and the medial head of the gastrocnemius muscle (*curved arrow* in **a**) and the lateral gastrocnemius bursa (*arrow* in **b**) between the knee capsule and the lateral head of the gastrocnemius muscle (*curved arrow* in **b**)

hypointense or of intermediate signal intensity on T1-weighted images and hyperintense on T2-weighted images.

Hemarthrosis and Lipohemarthrosis

Hemarthrosis is the result of the hemorrhage within the joint due to ligamentous injury, bone fracture, patellar dislocation, or other diseases including pigmented villonodular synovitis, hemophilia, articular tumors, neuroarthropathy, gout, and anticoagulant therapy [12, 16,

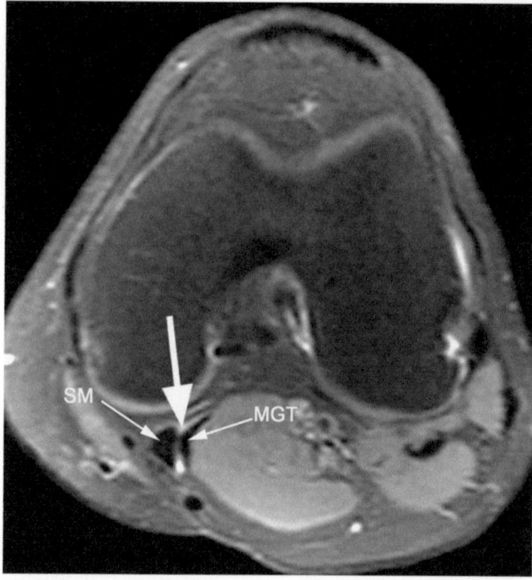

Fig. 8.8 Gastrocnemius-semimembranosus bursa (popliteal cyst or Baker's cyst) in a 36 year old male. Axial proton-density (PD) fat-suppressed image shows a small amount of fluid in the popliteal bursa (*arrow*) which is located between the semimembranosus (*SM*) and the medial head of the gastrocnemius muscle (*MGT*)

17]. The MRI appearance of hemarthrosis depends on the stage of the hemorrhage. In the early stage, the hemorrhage has a double-layer fluid level appearance with a superior layer of blood serum floating on an inferior layer of cellular debris of intermediate signal intensity on T1- and T2-weighted images. Gradient-echo images are especially useful for the identification of blood products due to the "blooming" effect.

Lipohemarthrosis, the presence of blood and fat within the joint, is a very strong indicator for intraarticular fracture. Most commonly, lipohemarthrosis is seen on MR imaging as a three-layer fluid level that appears approximately 3 h after trauma (Fig. 8.17) [18]. The superior layer with fat signal intensity (hyperintense on T1- and T2-weighted images and hypointense on fat-suppressed images) represents the floating fat. The intermediate or the central layer appears as a normal joint fluid and represents the blood serum, and the inferior layer of cellular debris is seen as intermediate signal intensity on T1- and T2-weighted images. In the very early stage, lipohemarthrosis may show a double-layer appearance with entrapment of globules of fat [18].

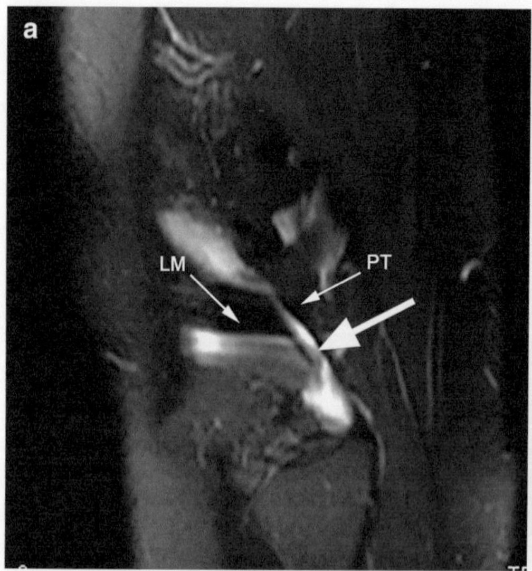

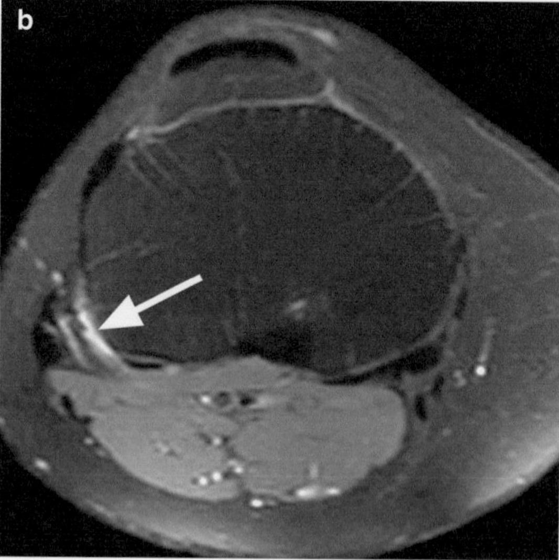

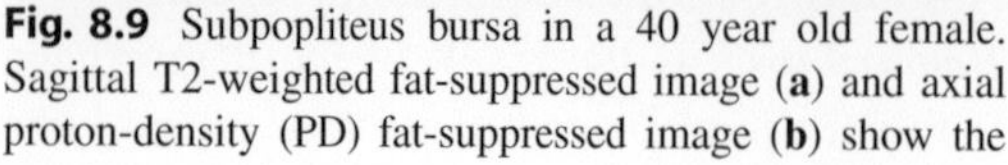

Fig. 8.9 Subpopliteus bursa in a 40 year old female. Sagittal T2-weighted fat-suppressed image (**a**) and axial proton-density (PD) fat-suppressed image (**b**) show the subpopliteal bursa (*large arrow* in **a**, **b**) located between the posterior horn of the lateral meniscus (*LM*) and the popliteus tendon (*PT*)

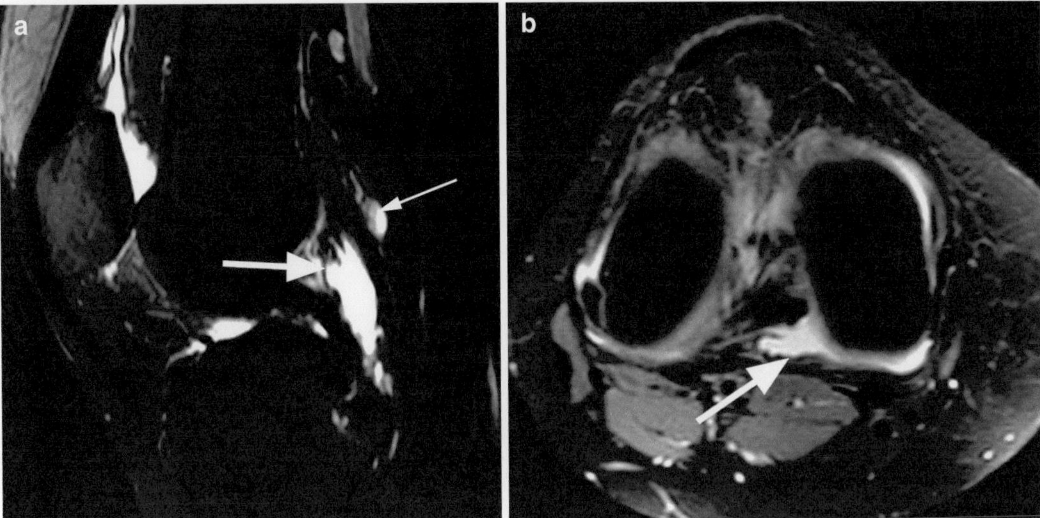

Fig. 8.10 Posterior capsular recess in a 40 year old female. Sagittal T2-weighted fat-suppressed image (**a**) and axial proton-density (PD) fat-suppressed image (**b**) show the posterior capsular recess (*large arrow* in **a**, **b**) located in the midline behind the posterior cruciate ligament. In cases of posterior capsule lesions, the fluid from this recess may be identified posteriorly to the capsule (*small arrow* in **a**)

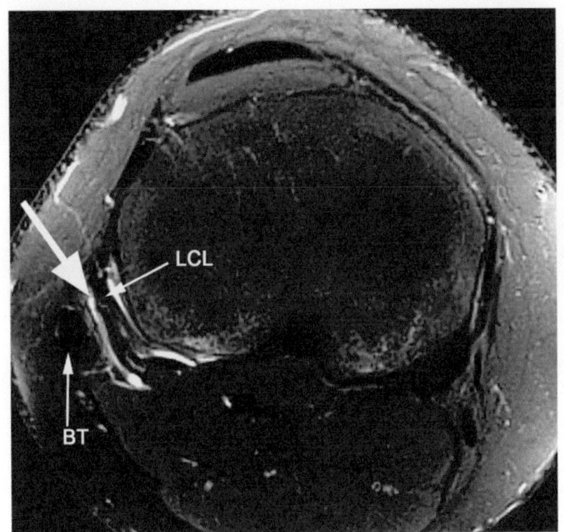

Fig. 8.11 Lateral collateral ligament-biceps femoris bursa in a 25 year old male. Axial proton-density (PD) fat-suppressed image shows a small amount of fluid in the lateral collateral ligament-biceps femoris bursa (*large arrow*) which is located between the lateral collateral ligament (*LCL*) and the biceps femoris tendon (*BT*)

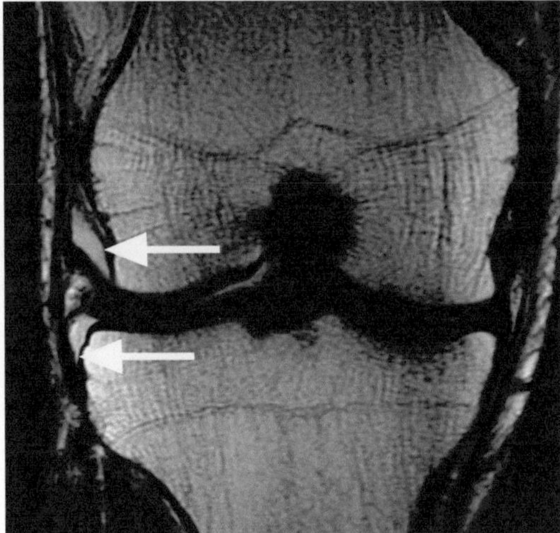

Fig. 8.12 Parameniscal recesses in a 41 year old male. Coronal proton-density (PD) image shows the parameniscal recesses (*arrows*) in contact with the lateral femoral and lateral tibial condyle

8.2.2   Intra-articular Bodies

Intra-articular bodies are best depicted on MR imaging in the presence of joint effusion as they are nicely outlined by the surrounding joint fluid. They appear as filling defects within the fluid (Figs. 8.18, 8.19, 8.20, and 8.21). The best technique to visualize intra-articular bodies is direct MR arthrography where the contrast agent is administered directly into the joint space increasing the amount of the intra-articular joint fluid. However, in the knee, intra-artic-

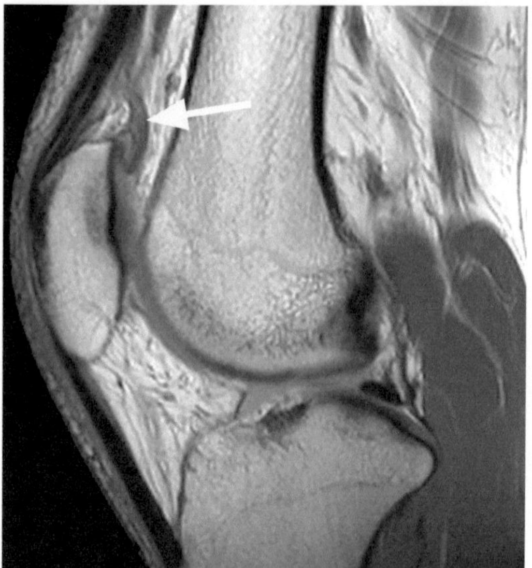

Fig. 8.13 Suprapatellar plica in a 33 year old male. Sagittal proton-density (PD) image shows the suprapatellar plica within the suprapatellar fat pad (*arrow*). The plica appears thickened indicating a suprapatellar plica syndrome

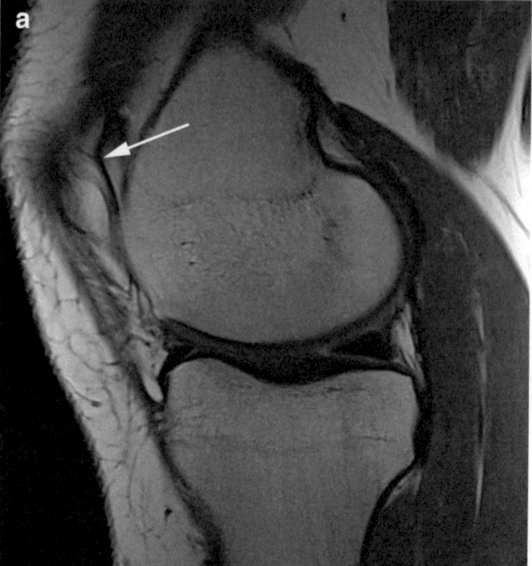

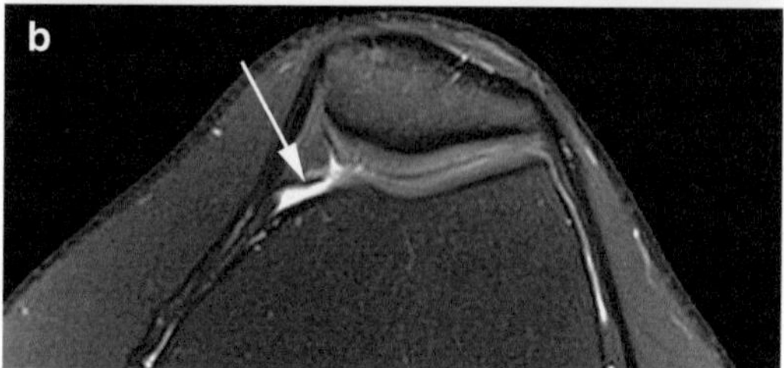

Fig. 8.15 Mediopatellar plica in a 26 year old male. Sagittal proton-density (PD) image (**a**) and axial proton-density (PD) fat-suppressed image (**b**) show a normal mediopatellar plica (*arrow* in **a**, **b**) as a thin low-signal-intensity band in the medial suprapatellar fat pad

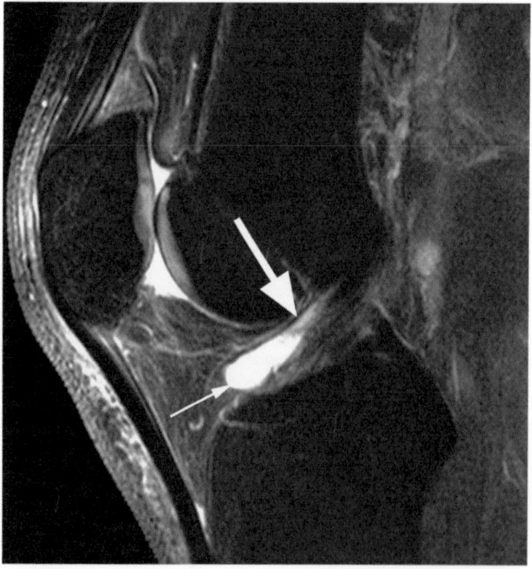

Fig. 8.14 Infrapatellar plica or ligamentum mucosum in a 43 year old male. Sagittal T2-weighted fat-suppressed image shows the ligamentum as low-signal-intensity thin band (*large arrow*) anterior and parallel to the anterior cruciate ligament. Note the fluid in the central synovial recess (*small arrow*)

ular bodies are often large, and usually there is enough joint fluid present. Thus, MR arthrography in the knee for the detection of intra-articular bodies is not recommended as a standard procedure, but can be helpful in cases where intra-articular bodies are suspected but cannot be otherwise detected.

Intra-articular bodies may have different etiologies, and the MRI signal appearance depends on the structure and origin of the bodies (Table 8.3). In the knee, intra-articular bodies are usually found beneath the medial collateral ligament, within the intercondylar notch, and in the tendon sheath of the popliteus tendon, or they can migrate into Baker's cysts [12]. It needs to be noted that intra-articular bodies are difficult to detect during arthroscopy, i.e., when they are located in recesses or compartments, which are hardly or even non-accessible by the arthroscope.

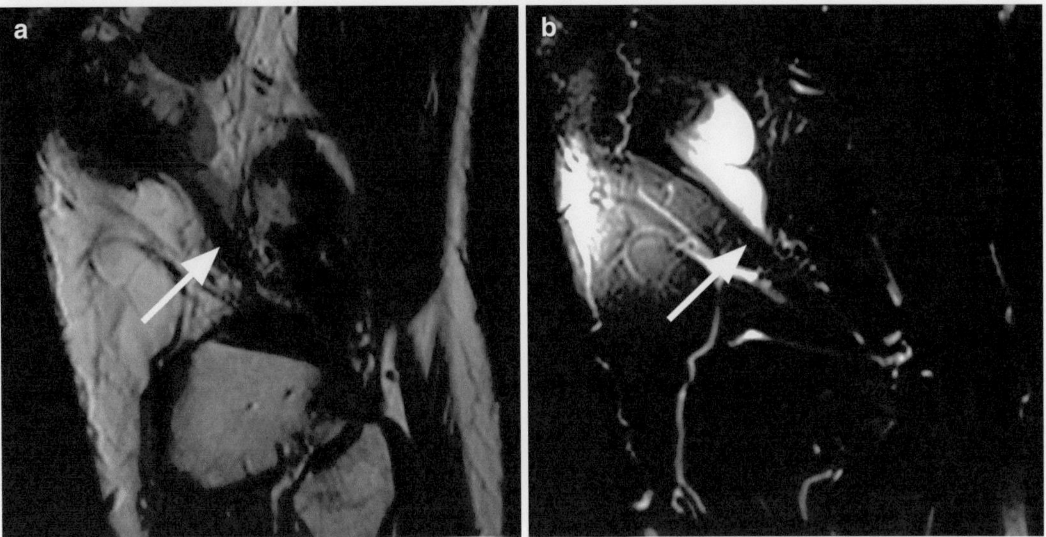

Fig. 8.16 Lateral patellar plica in a 38 year old male. Sagittal proton-density (PD) image (**a**) and sagittal T2-weighted fat-suppressed image (**b**) show the lateral patellar plica (*arrow* in **a**, **b**) extending from the popliteus hiatus to the patella

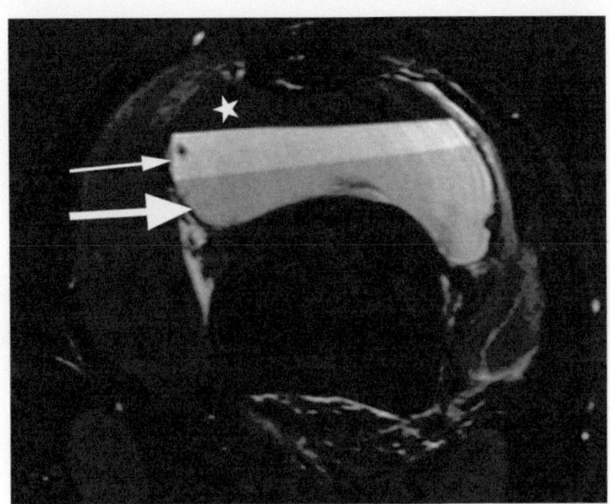

Fig. 8.17 Lipohemarthrosis in a 16 year old female. Axial proton-density (PD) fat-suppressed image shows the superior layer of floating fat which appears hypointense on fat-suppressed sequences (*star*), the intermediate or the central layer which appears as a normal joint fluid and represents the blood serum (*small arrow*), and the inferior layer of cellular debris which is seen as intermediate signal intensity (*large arrow*)

8.2.3 Synovitis

Synovitis, the inflammation of the synovial membrane, can be the result of several disorders including inflammatory arthritis, osteoarthritis, infection, pigmented villonodular synovitis, chronic intra-articular hemorrhage, metabolic

diseases, tumors, and trauma. The MR imaging diagnosis of synovitis is based on the evaluation of the synovium thickness and the presence of synovial effusion. The synovial hypertrophy may involve the entire knee synovium or may be focal and is seen on T2-weighted and on gradient-weighted images as hyperintense synovial membrane having a thickness of more than 2–3 mm (Fig. 8.22) [19]. A better appreciation of synovitis is obtained on postcontrast T1-weighted MR images that enable a superior delineation of the hypertrophied synovial membrane from the joint effusion (Fig. 8.23). Due to hyperemia of the inflamed synovium, there is an increased synovial enhancement on postcontrast T1-weighted images that can be also used to differentiate between acute and chronic inflammation.

Signal alterations in Hoffa's fat pad are a finding that can be seen in a multitude of diseases and can be used as a surrogate for knee synovitis [20–22].

Inflammatory Synovitis in Rheumatological Disorders

In rheumatological disorders (rheumatoid arthritis, psoriatic arthritis, and ankylosing spondylitis), the synovium is affected first, followed by involvement of the cartilage and bones. MR imaging

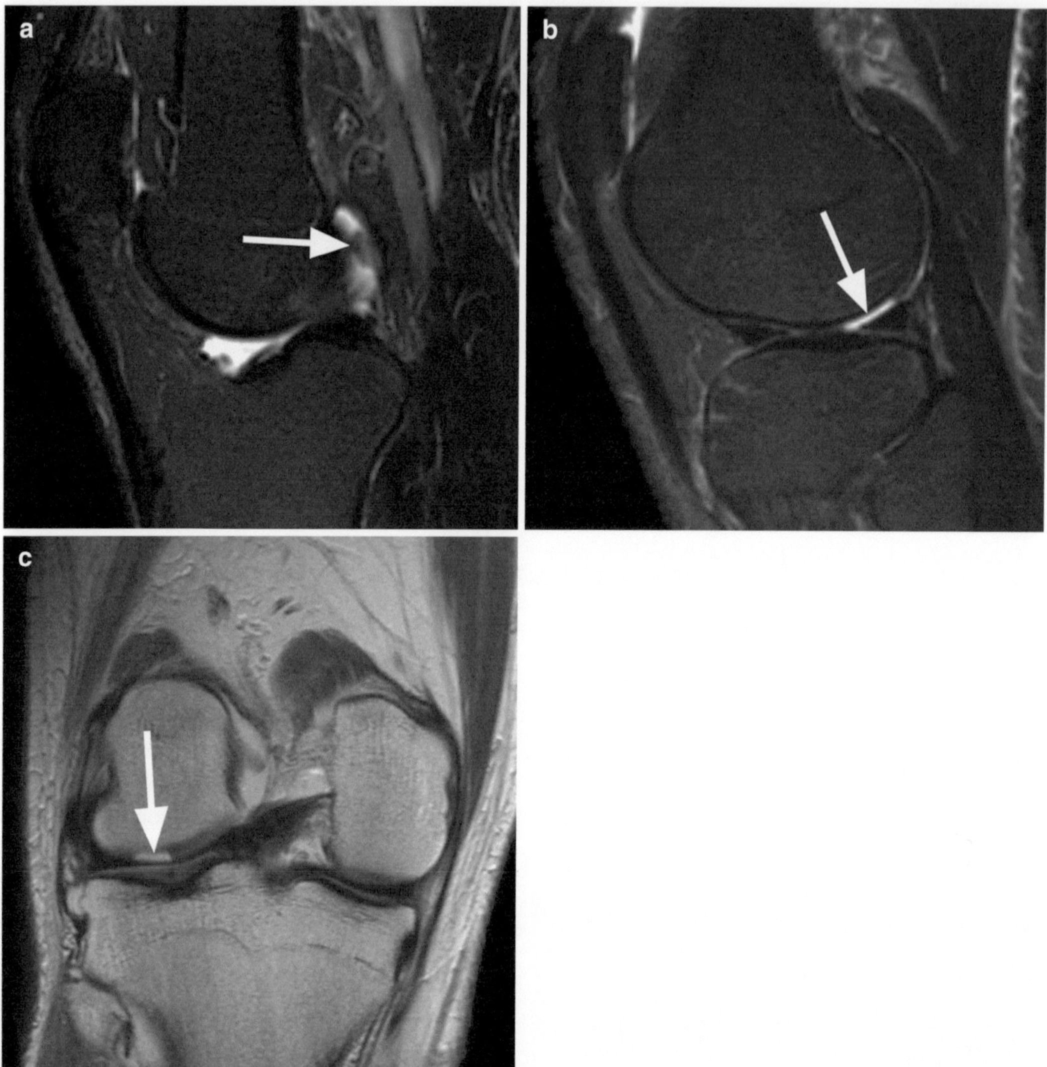

Fig. 8.18 Intra-articular free cartilage fragment in a 43 year old male. Sagittal T2-weighted fat-suppressed image (**a**) shows a small fragment of cartilage surrounded by joint fluid (*arrow*). Sagittal T2-weighted fat-suppressed image (**b**) and coronal proton-density (PD) image (**c**) demonstrate the lateral femoral condyle as the donor site (*arrows* in **b, c**)

enables the diagnosis of all intra-articular pathological changes including synovitis and joint effusion, bone marrow edema, and subchondral erosions (Fig. 8.20). There are different MRI techniques used in the evaluation of the synovial proliferation that are used either for qualitative or quantitative evaluation. Synovitis is best identified on T2-weighted images and postcontrast T1-weighted images as uniform or irregular thickening of the synovial membrane. Different quantitative evaluations of synovitis have been described

including the synovial volume measurement and the rate of contrast enhancement. Dynamic contrast-enhanced T1-weighted sequences may differentiate between active and chronic phases of the disease with a rapid synovial enhancement (30–60 s) after contrast administration in active or acute phases [23, 24]. Nevertheless, synovial volume or enhancement rate measurements require post-processing work, which is time consuming in clinical practice and thus rarely used [12]. Apart from demonstrating the synovial proliferation,

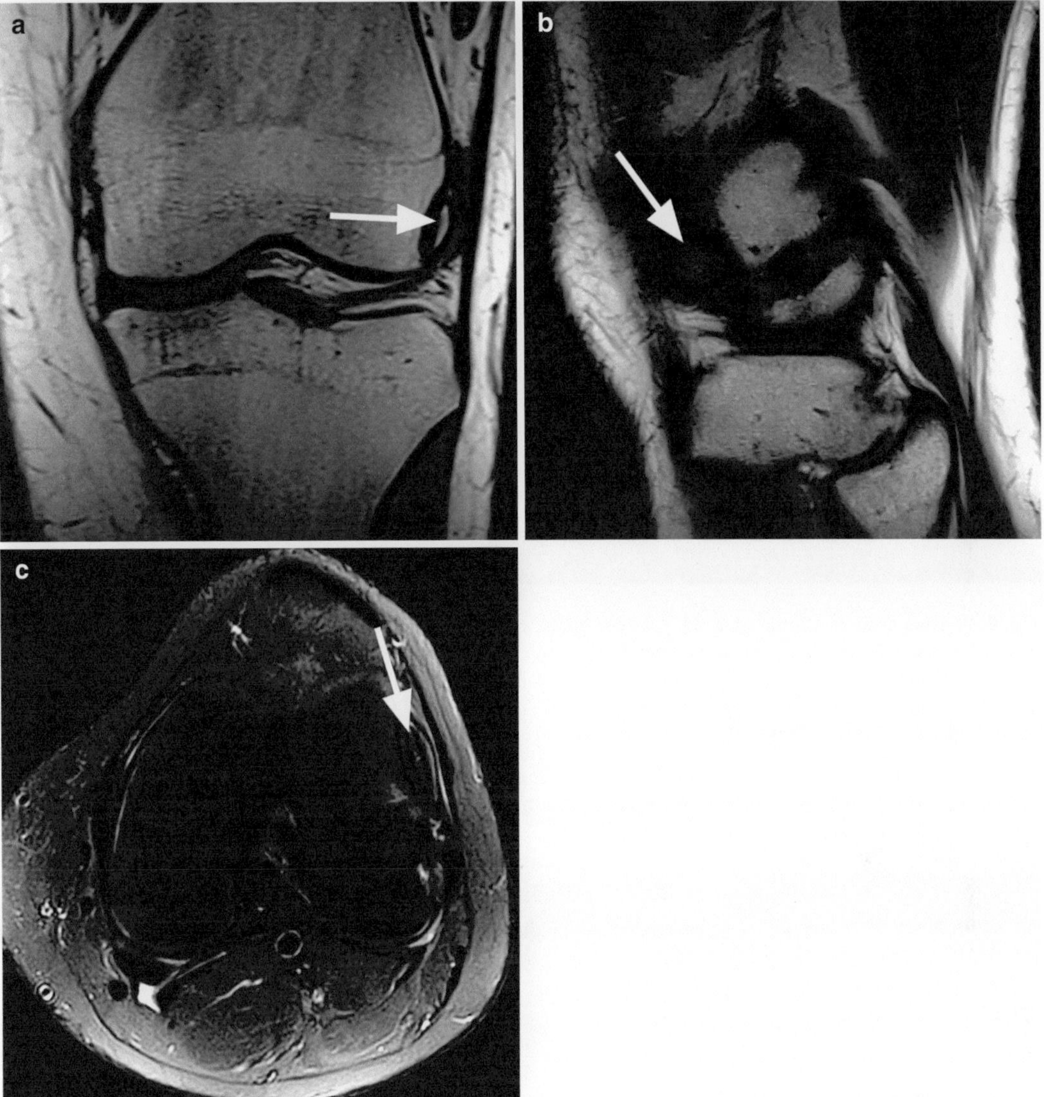

Fig. 8.19 Detached bone fragment in a 21 year old female 3 years after knee injury. Coronal T1-weighted image (**a**), sagittal proton-density (PD) image (**b**), and axial proton-density (PD) fat-suppressed image (**c**) show a bone fragment detached from the lateral femoral condyle (*arrows*). The chronicity of the condition is demonstrated by the synovial reaction around the lesion and the absence of bone marrow edema

MRI demonstrates periarticular inflammation and tendon and ligament inflammation as well as complications such as ruptures of the tendons, presence of "rice-bodies" bursitis, osteonecrosis, and stress fractures [25, 26].

Although rheumatoid arthritis and the seronegative spondyloarthropathies share similar pathological changes, several findings can narrow the differential diagnosis [12]. In rheumatoid arthritis, there are symmetrical abnormalities, and the extent of subchondral erosions and the degree of synovial inflammation are more prominent. However, intra-articular rheumatoid nodules are rarely seen [27]. The rheumatoid nodules are solitary or multiple nodules that appear as inhomogeneous isointense or hypointense lesions on T1-weighted images and inhomogeneous isointense or hyperintense on T2-weighted

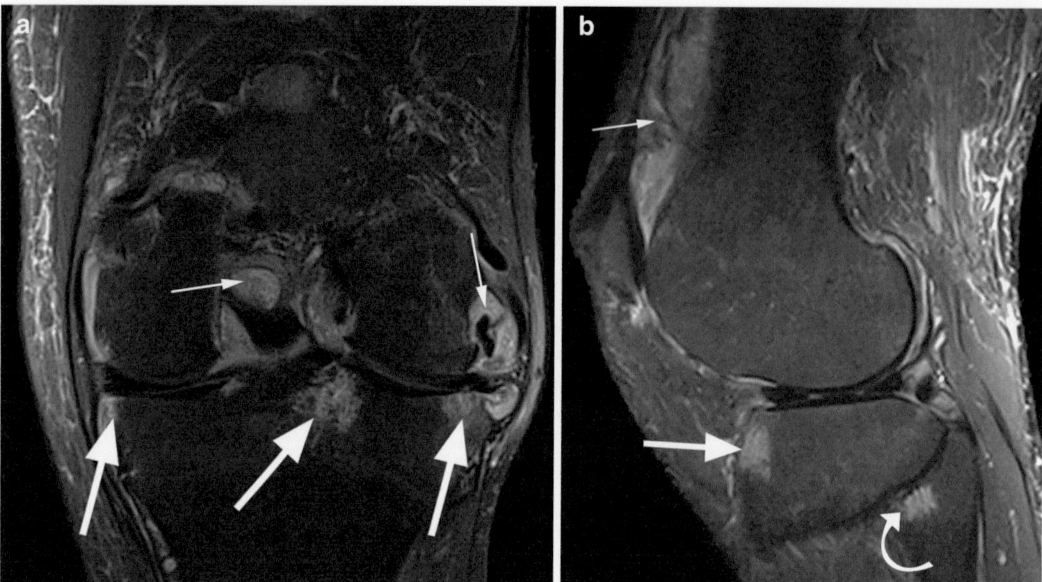

Fig. 8.20 Rheumatoid arthritis in a 45 year old male. Coronal proton-density (PD) fat-suppressed image (**a**) shows small innumerable nodules within the synovial membrane (*small arrows*). Subchondral erosions are seen in the tibial subchondral bone (*large arrows*). Sagittal T2-weighted fat-suppressed image (**b**) also shows subchondral bone marrow edema of the anterior tibial plateau (*large arrow*), synovitis (*small arrow*), and erosion of the fibular head (*curved arrow*)

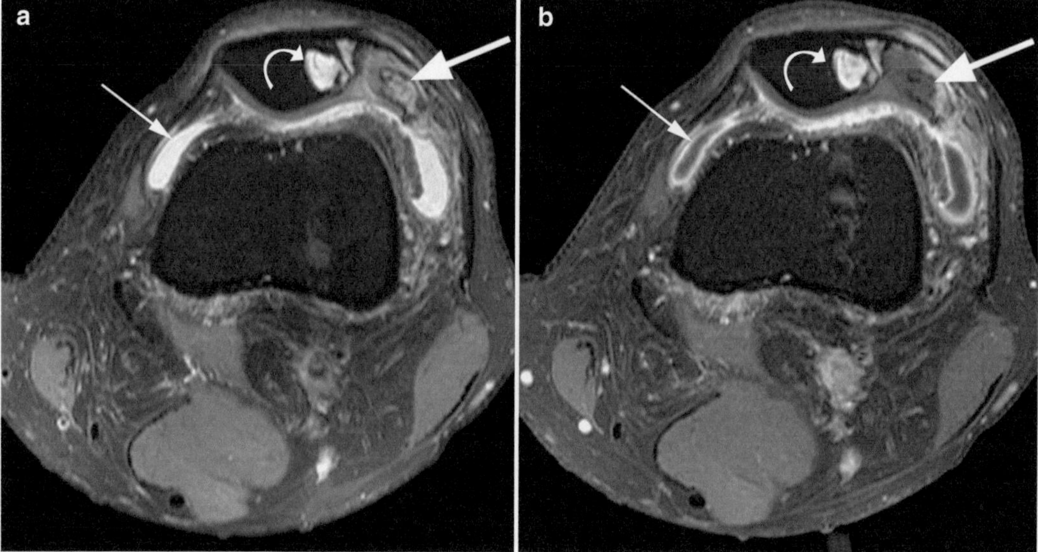

Fig. 8.21 Acute gout in a 55 year old male. Axial proton-density (PD) fat-suppressed image (**a**) and axial T1-weighted fat-suppressed postcontrast image (**b**) show the gout tophus of relatively high signal intensity on a fat-suppressed image (*large arrow* in **a**) but without enhancement after contrast administration (*large arrow* in **b**). Subchondral cysts are seen within the adjacent patella (*curved arrows* in **a**, **b**) resulting from repetitive gout attacks. The synovia is thickened and joint effusion is present (*small arrows* in **a**, **b**)

Table 8.3 Etiology and MRI appearance of intra-articular bodies [12]

Etiology/structure	MRI findings
Cartilage/meniscus (Fig. 8.18)	Similar signal intensity with joint cartilage/meniscus; MR images should be carefully scrutinized for donor site; the size of the body should match the size of the donor site
Bone (Fig. 8.19)	Signal intensity of bone marrow; MR images should be carefully scrutinized for donor site
Osteochondral fragment	Cortical bone of low signal intensity on all MR sequences with attached cartilage of intermediate signal intensity on T1- and T2-weighted; may mirror the defect at the donor site
Inflammatory synovitis (including tuberculosis) (Fig. 8.20)	Intermediate- to low-signal-intensity small innumerable nodules along the synovial membrane (rice bodies)
Gout (Fig. 8.21)	Soft tissue tophi of monosodium urate crystal deposits with inhomogeneous T2-weighted signal intensity; enhances after i.v. contrast administration
Primary synovial osteochondromatosis	Multiple circumscribed nodules of metaplastic hyaline cartilage (range from 2.0 mm to more than 1.0 cm); the signal intensity varies according to the maturity of the nodules and the presence of calcifications within the nodules; may present as conglomerate mass
Pigmented villonodular synovitis	Conglomerate or scattered nodules within the joint; low signal intensity on T1-weighted images and low to high signal intensity on T2-weighted images; "blooming" on gradient-echo images due to iron deposition
Hemophilic arthropathy	Similar appearance with pigmented villonodular synovitis
Metallic foreign bodies	Filling defects with susceptibility artifacts
Intra-articular gas	Low-signal-intensity globular filling defects with "blooming" on gradient-echo images

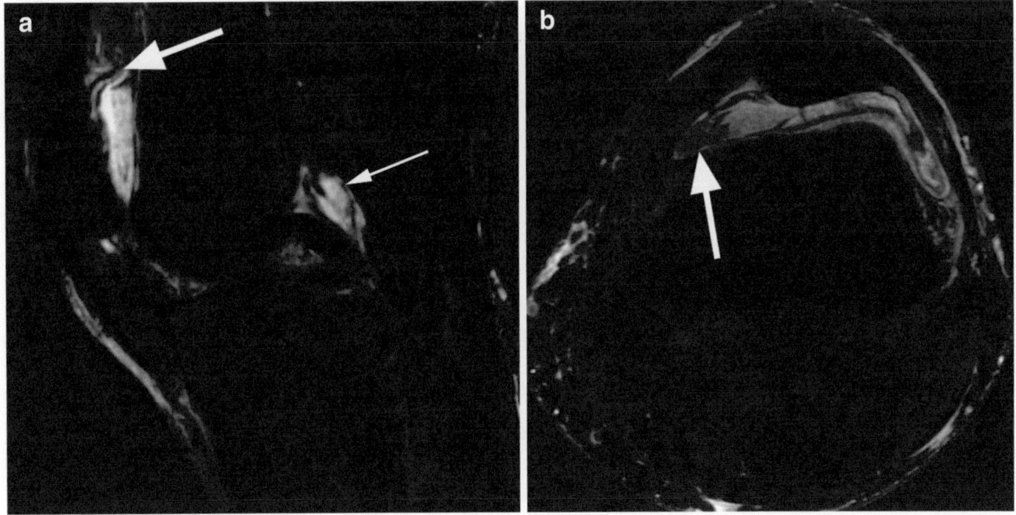

Fig. 8.22 Chronic synovitis in a 65 year old male. Sagittal T2-weighted fat-suppressed image (**a**) and axial proton-density (PD) fat-suppressed image (**b**) show a synovium with a thickness of more than 3 mm but without a clear delineation from the joint fluid (*large arrows* in **a**, **b**). Note the diffuse involvement of the entire synovium including the posterior recess (*small arrow* in **a**)

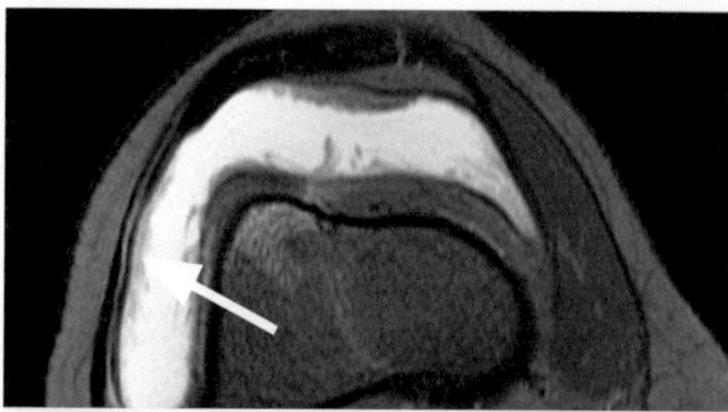

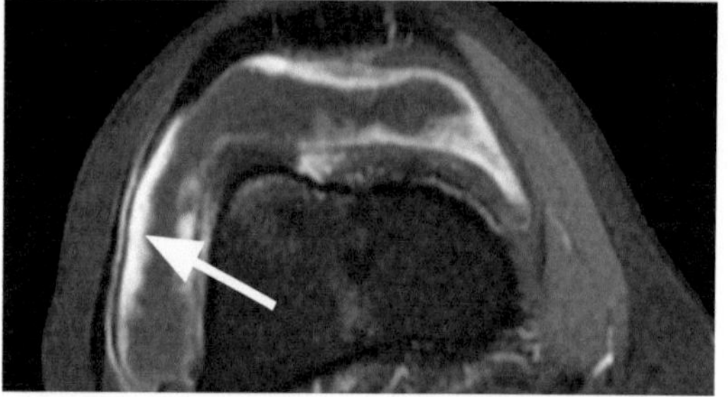

Fig. 8.23 Acute synovitis in a 25 year old female. Axial proton-density (PD) fat-suppressed image (**a**) shows synovial hypertrophy and irregularity (*arrow*). Axial T1-weighted fat-suppressed postcontrast image (**b**) shows an increased enhancement and enables a superior delineation of the hypertrophied synovial membrane (*arrow*) from the joint effusion

images compared with muscles (Fig. 8.24). They may enhance homogeneously or heterogeneous predominantly in the periphery. In ankylosing spondylitis and other seronegative spondyloarthropathies, the knee joint is involved in 30 % of the patients with long-standing disease, and the bone marrow edema has a perientheseal distribution that is not commonly seen in patients with rheumatoid arthritis [12, 28]. The osseous fusion is also more common in seronegative spondyloarthropathies. Overall, however, differential diagnosis remains difficult on MR images, and in the clinical routine, one might not be disappointed when a final diagnosis cannot be made with 100 % confidence.

Synovitis in Osteoarthritis

Synovial proliferation and joint effusion in osteoarthritis is the result of ligament injuries, loose bodies, cartilage deterioration, and meniscal damage (Fig. 8.25) [29, 30]. Synovitis is present even in the early phase of osteoarthritis, and there is evidence that synovial proliferation is not only

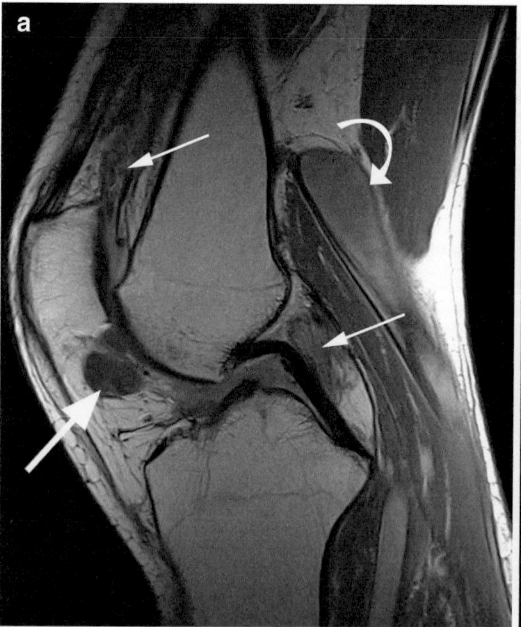
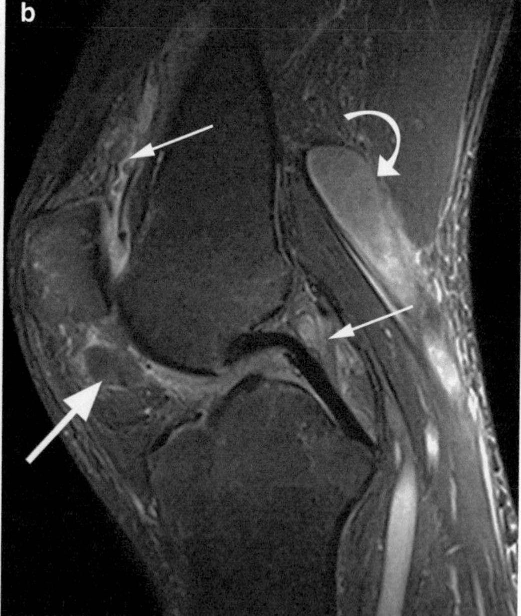

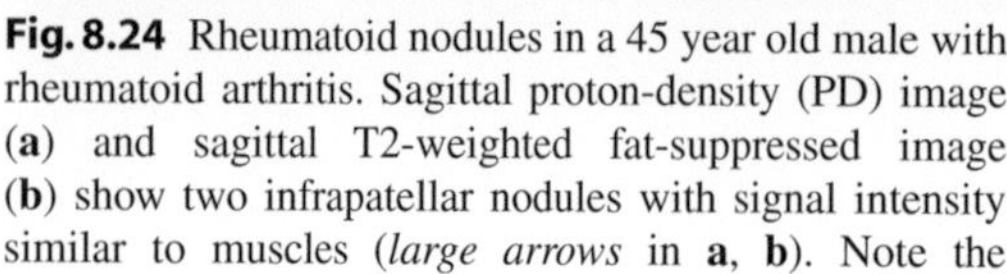

Fig. 8.24 Rheumatoid nodules in a 45 year old male with rheumatoid arthritis. Sagittal proton-density (PD) image (**a**) and sagittal T2-weighted fat-suppressed image (**b**) show two infrapatellar nodules with signal intensity similar to muscles (*large arrows* in **a**, **b**). Note the synovitis in the suprapatellar bursa and central recesses (*small arrows* in **a**, **b**) as well as the inflammation of the Baker's cyst (*curved arrow* in **a**, **b**) which appears with inhomogeneous signal intensity and diffuse pericystic changes

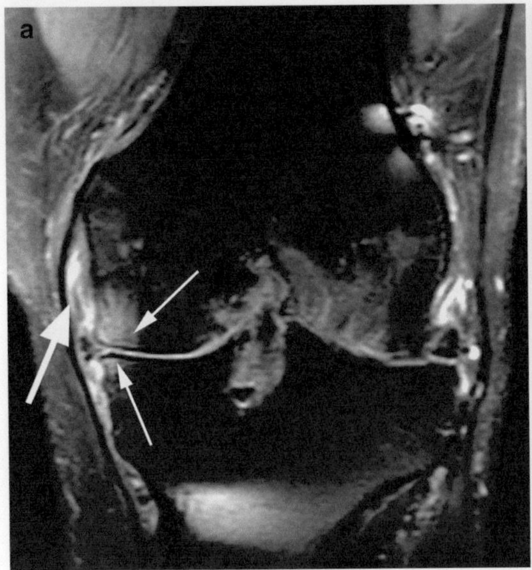
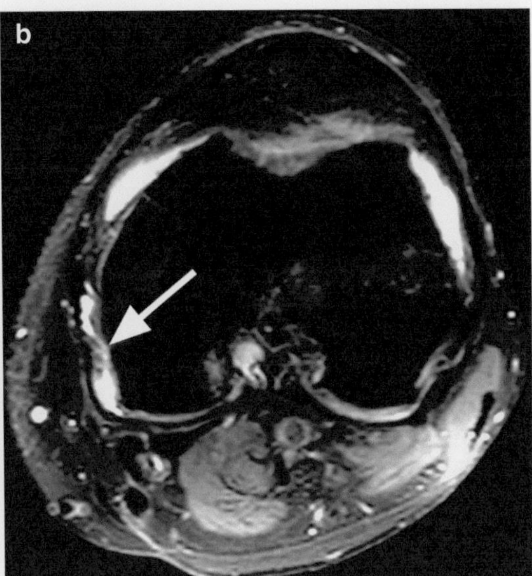

Fig. 8.25 Chronic medial collateral bursitis in a 45 year old male with advanced medial knee osteoarthritis. Coronal proton-density (PD) fat-suppressed image (**a**) and axial proton-density (PD) fat-suppressed image (**b**) show the presence of fluid between the superficial and the deep layers of the medial collateral ligament (MCL) (*large arrows* in **a**, **b**). Note the subchondral edema and the cartilage absence in the medial compartment (*small arrows* in **a**)

a secondary phenomenon but that it also plays a role in progression of cartilage loss [29]. Synovial inflammation is believed to contribute to pain in patients with knee osteoarthritis, and several studies have indeed shown that high-grade synovitis in patients with knee osteoarthritis is statistically associated with pain [29, 31].

Infectious Synovitis

The imaging findings in infectious synovitis are nonspecific, and MRI cannot differentiate septic from nonseptic arthritis. The clinical history is key for differential diagnosis. Early detection of infectious synovitis is crucial in the treatment management and in preventing bone deformities. Thus, if there is clinical suspicion for infection, MR should be performed immediately and any destructive monoarticular process should be regarded as infection until proven otherwise [12]. There are several MRI findings that suggest an infectious etiology. These include synovial thickening, soft tissue edema, and extensive bone marrow edema with enhancement involving both sides of articulation and bone erosions (Fig. 8.26) [32, 33]. Inhomogeneous joint effusion with septa and debris or the presence of synovial or

bone abscess is highly correlated with septic arthritis (Fig. 8.26). The evolution and the variation of the imaging findings can help narrowing down the differential diagnosis. In bacterial arthritis, there is a rapid evolution with extensive erosions, whereas in tuberculosis, the evolution is slow and the granulation inflammatory tissue extends in the subchondral bone (pannus) [12].

Hemosiderotic Synovitis

Hemosiderotic synovitis occurs in hemophiliac males because of chronic intra-articular hemorrhage. The knee joint is particularly often involved, and the patients develop osteoarthritis and complain of pain and stiffness of the joint [34, 35]. Due to repetitive hemorrhage, the synovium becomes thickened owing to intrasynovial fibrous scarring [34]. The absorption of hemosiderin by the synovial membrane leads to inflammation and hypertrophy with pannus formation extending throughout the cartilage into the subchondral bone. MR imaging identifies the thickened synovium and hemarthrosis as well as subchondral cysts and erosions (Fig. 8.27). The thickened synovium is best appreciated on post-contrast T1-weighted images. On gradient-echo

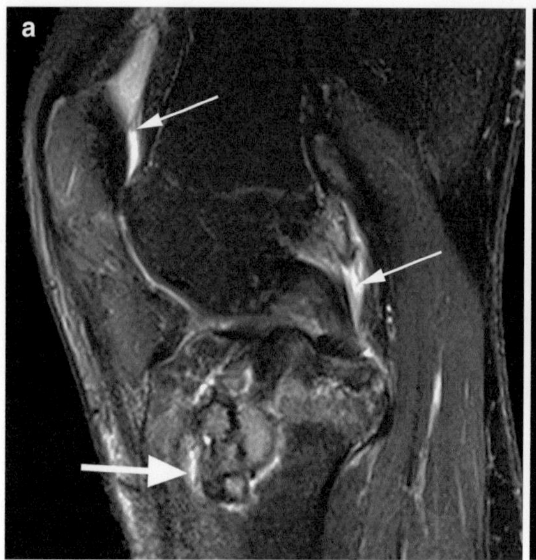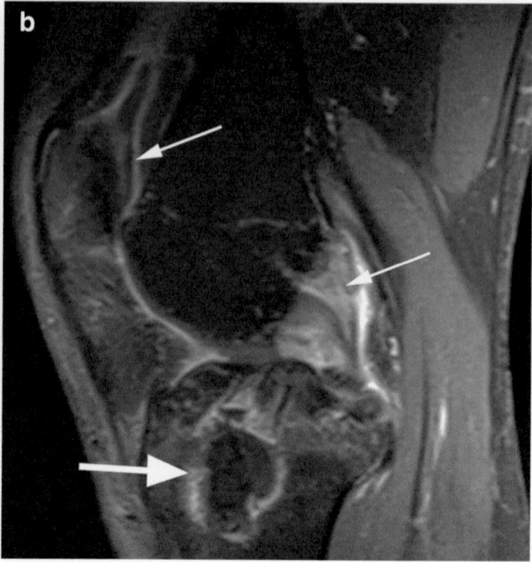

Fig. 8.26 Infectious arthritis in a 32 year old female after anterior cruciate (ACL) reconstruction. Sagittal T2-weighted fat-suppressed image (**a**) and sagittal T1-weighted fat-suppressed postcontrast image (**b**) show an abscess of the tibial plateau (*large arrows* in **a** and **b**). The synovia is thickened and shows increased enhancement of the synovial membrane in the suprapatellar bursa and the pericruciate area (*small arrows* in **a** and **b**)

sequences, blooming artifacts are characteristic for the hemosiderin-laden synovium and helpful for detection in early phases of the disease [36]. Hemosiderotic synovitis can be found also in patients with intrasynovial hemangiomas for which the knee joint is the most frequently involved site [37].

Arthridities and Metabolic Diseases
Gout

Gout is a rheumatological disorder characterized by urate crystal deposition within the joint. The tophi vary from a few millimeters to 5 cm and can be localized in the capsule, the synovium, the articular cartilage, the subchondral bone, and the periarticular soft tissue. In the acute phase, there is thickening of the synovia and effusion, and the tophi are isointense or hypointense to muscle on T1-weighted images and variable low to high signal intensity on T2-weighted images depending on the edema and granulation tissue (Fig. 8.21). After repetitive attacks, subchondral erosions and small subchondral cysts may be seen reflecting intraosseous deposits of tophi [38]. The most specific imaging modality for urate deposition is dual-energy CT which can confirm or rule out gout disease with near 100 % accuracy [39].

Calcium Pyrophosphate Dihydrate Crystal Deposition (CPPD) or Pseudogout

Calcium pyrophosphate dihydrate crystal deposition is the result of crystal deposition in the synovium, the cartilage, the menisci, the periarticular tissue, and the intervertebral disk. It can be idiopathic or may be associated with other metabolic disorders, including hyperparathyroidism, gout, hypomagnesemia, Wilson's disease, acromegaly, hemochromatosis, and hypophosphatasia [40]. The acute form commonly affects the knee, and MR imaging reveals thickening of the synovium with calcium deposits, joint effusion, and calcified low-signal-intensity loose bodies. In the chronic form, MR imaging shows an accelerated form of a destructive arthritis. Cartilage and meniscal calcifications are better seen on gradi-

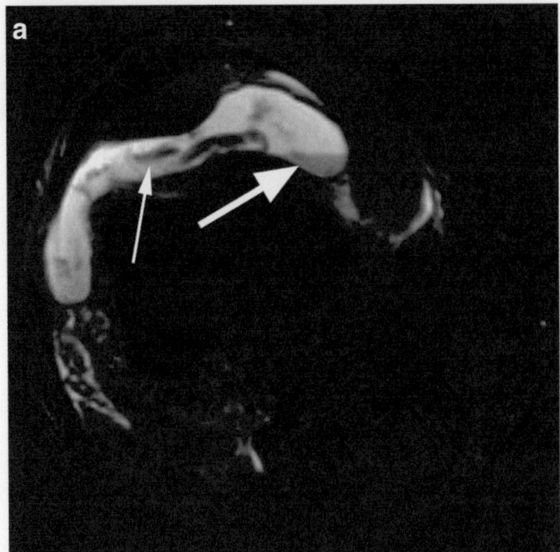

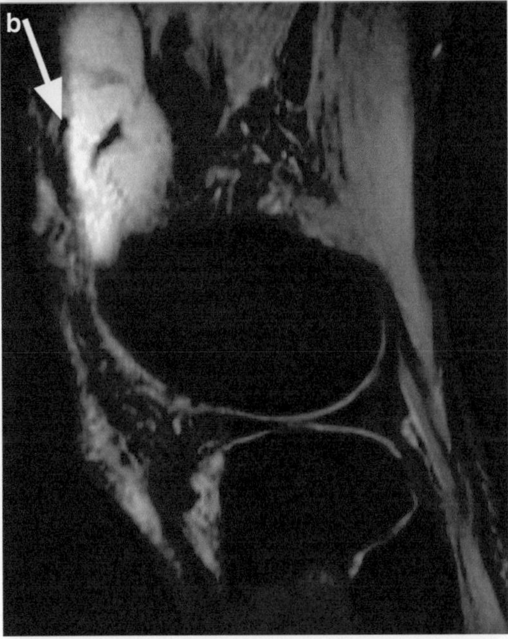

Fig. 8.27 Hemosiderotic synovitis in a 29 year old hemophiliac male. Axial proton-density (PD) fat-suppressed image (**a**) shows hemarthrosis with double-layer appearance. The inferior level is represented by cellular debris of intermediate signal intensity (*large arrow*). The synovium is thickened owing to intrasynovial fibrous scarring (*small arrow*). Sagittal T2-weighted fat-suppressed image (**b**) demonstrates a small area of hemosiderin-laden synovium (*arrow*)

ent-echo sequences because of the blooming arti-facts. Calcifications of low signal intensity on all

MR sequences are commonly encountered in the periarticular soft tissue.

Basic Calcium Phosphate Crystal Deposition (Hydroxyapatite)

Hydroxyapatite deposition is the most common deposition disease and most frequently affects the shoulder. Crystal deposition may be identified on MR imaging due to intra-articular foreign bodies, calcified tendons insertions, cartilage destruction, and subchondral cysts and erosions. In some cases, deposition near the origin or insertion of tendons may simulate a malignant bone neoplasm [41].

Amyloidosis

Amyloid deposition involves the synovial membrane, which shows focal nodules or bulky masses [2]. Amyloid arthropathy has been well documented as a complication in long-term dialysis patients and usually occurs at least 5 years after treatment [12]. MR imaging identifies the nodules which have a signal intensity that is in between that of cartilage and muscle. Subchondral cysts and small erosions are also often present.

8.2.4   Bursitis

Bursitis may be acute or chronic and may be caused by local or systemic processes such as trauma, overuse, infection, inflammatory arthropathy, and tumors. Thickening of the synovial membrane and effusion make the bursa visible on MR images as fluid collections with low signal on T1-weighted images and high signal on T2-weighted images in acute cases. In chronic cases, the inflamed bursa appears as an inhomogeneous mass mainly due to thickening, calcifications, and hemorrhage [3]. Diffuse inflammation of the soft tissue in the vicinity of bursitis may be present. Most of the bursae around the knee are only visible in pathological conditions, and the clinical symptoms and the etiology may differ between different bursae (Table 8.4). However, to establish a correct diagnosis is important for the differentiation from other intra- or extra-articular disorders and for avoiding unneces-

Table 8.4 Etiology and clinical manifestations of bursitis [3, 42–49]

	Etiology of bursitis	Clinical symptoms
Suprapatellar bursitis (Fig. 8.28)	Synovitis, infections, trauma, inflammatory and degenerative joint disorders, tumors; isolated bursitis is uncommon	Anterior knee pain; soft tissue mass may be palpated
Prepatellar bursitis (Fig. 8.29)	Overuse injury or trauma; occupational kneeling or crawling (housemaid's knee, carpet layer's knee)	Focal pain and swelling anterior to patella
Superficial infrapatellar or pretibial bursitis (Fig. 8.30)	Trauma or occupational overuse (clergyman's knee)	Pain anterior to tibial tubercle
Deep infrapatellar bursitis (Fig. 8.29)	Extensor mechanism overuse; runners and jumpers	Anterior knee pain; may mimic patellar tendinitis
Gastrocnemius-semimembranosus bursa	*See* Baker's cyst	*See* Baker's cyst
Iliotibial bursitis	Overuse injury in runners	Anterolateral knee pain; may mimic iliotibial tendinitis
Lateral collateral ligament-biceps femoris bursitis	Trauma	Pain and swelling along the lateral side
Medial collateral bursitis (Fig. 8.25)	Genu valgum, trauma, osteoarthritis, osteophytic spurs, rheumatoid disorders, flatfoot deformity; horseback riding, motorcycling	Pain along the medial side over the medial collateral ligament; palpable nodule at the medial side of the knee
Pes anserinus bursitis (Fig. 8.31)	Rheumatoid arthritis or osteoarthritis especially in overweight middle-aged to elderly women; runners	Vague medial knee pain; tenderness and swelling along the proximal medial tibia; may mimic meniscal or medial collateral ligament injury
Medial collateral ligament-semimembranosus bursitis	Repetitive or acute trauma; valgus stress	Focal pain along the posteromedial knee at the level of knee joint

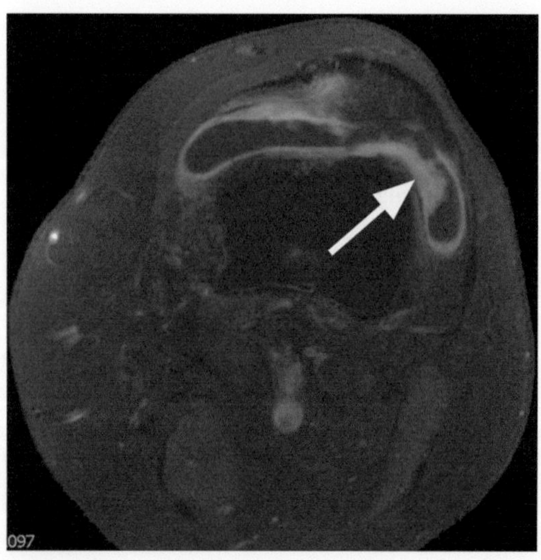

Fig. 8.28 Acute suprapatellar bursitis in a 46 year old patient with knee arthritis. Axial T1-weighted fat-suppressed postcontrast image shows irregular thickening and increased enhancement of the synovial membrane (*arrow*)

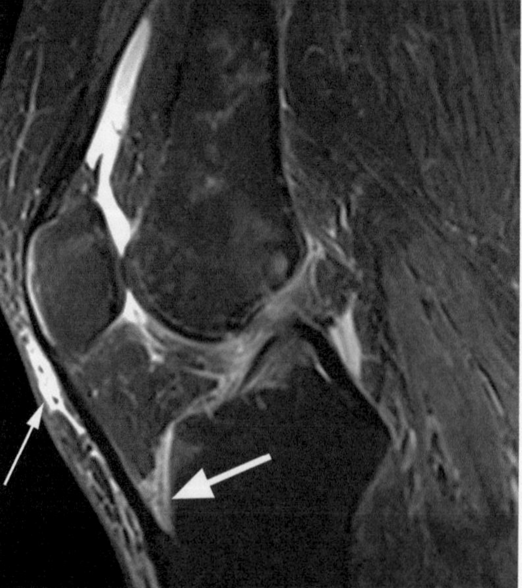

Fig. 8.29 Prepatellar bursitis and deep infrapatellar bursitis in a 56 year old male. Sagittal T2-weighted fat-suppressed image shows inflammation of the deep infrapatellar bursa (*large arrow*) and fluid collection in the prepatellar bursa (*small arrow*)

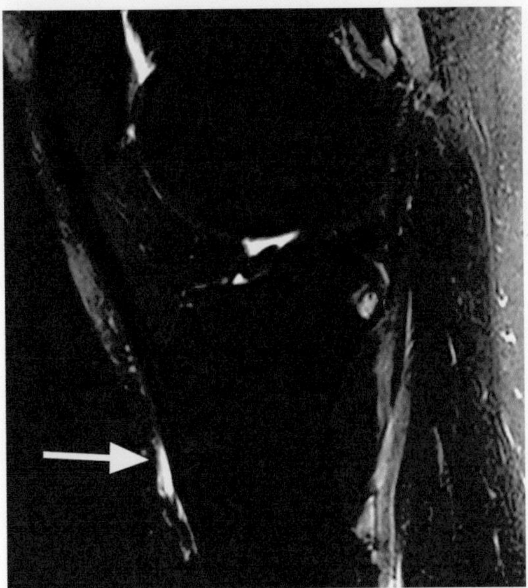

Fig. 8.30 Superficial pretibial bursitis in a 36 year old female. Sagittal T2-weighted fat-suppressed image shows fluid collection anterior to the tibial tubercle (*arrow*)

sary arthroscopy. Within the fluid accumulation of the bursae, loose bodies may be identified. Predominant locations are the suprapatellar bursa and the gastrocnemius-semimembranosus bursa.

Adventitial Bursitis

In contrast to the inherent anatomic bursae, there are also bursae which develop secondarily as a result of the increased friction between a normal tendon, muscle, or ligament and a pathologic point such as osteochondroma. Adventitial bursitis may appear also between orthopedic hardware and normal anatomical knee structures.

8.2.5   Synovial Cysts

Synovial cysts are juxta-articular fluid collections lined by synovial cells that may or may not communicate with the joint and may extend in any direction [44, 50]. The presence of the synovial lining allows the distinction from other cystic lesion, and its presence makes the disorders that affect the knee synovium affect the synovial cysts as well (inflammatory synovitis, metabolic synovitis, hemorrhage, synovial osteochondromatosis).

Synovial cysts are often discovered incidentally in routine MRI examinations. The most specific type of synovial cyst is the popliteal (Baker's) cyst.

Popliteal (Baker's) Cyst

The term popliteal cyst refers to the fluid collection in the gastrocnemius-semimembranosus bursa. The cyst communicates with the knee joint and with the medial gastrocnemius bursa. The incidence of popliteal cyst on MRI reported in the literature ranges from 5 to 38 % and is significantly higher in patients over 50 years [51–54]. There is a high association between joint effusion and osteoarthritis and the popliteal cyst. Several internal derangements of the knee coexist with popliteal cyst even in the absence of joint effusion [52]. Tears of the posterior horn of the medial meniscus, lateral meniscal tears, bilateral meniscal tears, and anterior cruciate ligament tears are associated with popliteal cyst [3]. Patients may be asymptomatic or may complain with palpable mass in the popliteal fossa, posterior knee pain, calf claudication due to compression of the popliteal artery, or symptoms of nerve compression [54, 55]. On MR imaging, uncomplicated simple popliteal cyst appears as lobulated multilocular hypointense on T1-weighted images and hyperintense on T2-weighted images fluid mass between semimembranosus and gastrocnemius tendons that may extend over a variable distance superiorly or inferiorly (Fig. 8.32). In the case of complicated popliteal cyst, the MR imaging appearance is inhomogeneous demonstrating foci of hemorrhage and calcifications. Rupture of the cyst is identified as diffuse fluid of high signal T2-weighted intensity in the surrounding muscles and in the subcutaneous tissue (Fig. 8.33).

8.2.6   Ganglion Cysts

Ganglion cysts are tumor-like lesions surrounded by a dense capsule of connective tissue and are found in locations that are under constant stress. They are filled with mucoid material because of mucoid cystic degeneration in collagenous structures [56]. The ganglia are classified into intra-

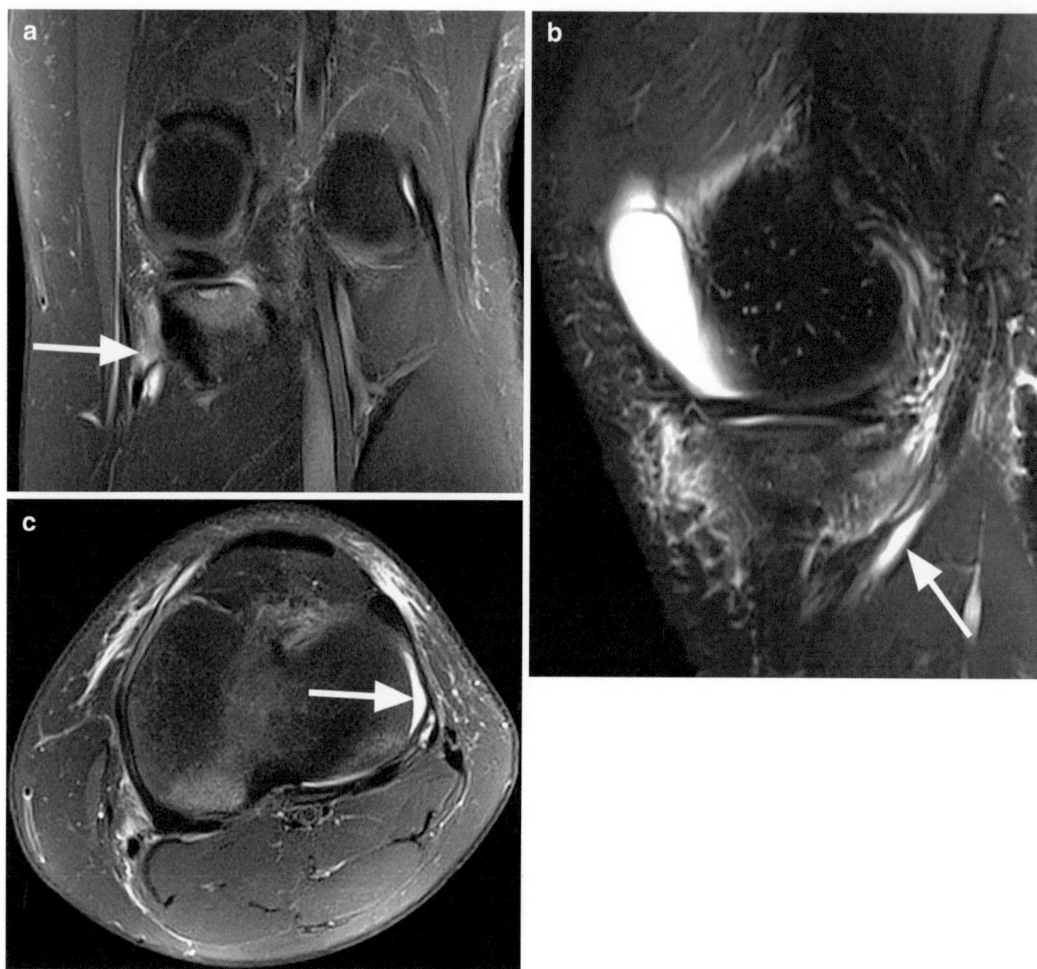

Fig. 8.31 Pes anserinus bursitis in a 47 year old female. Coronal proton-density (PD) fat-suppressed image (**a**), sagittal T2-weighted fat-suppressed image (**b**), and axial proton-density (PD) fat-suppressed image (**c**) show fluid collection in the pes anserinus bursa (*arrows*)

articular, extra-articular, and periosteal ganglia [3]. On MR imaging, they all appear as well-delineated rounded mass of hypointensity or intermediate signal intensity on T1-weighted images, of high signal intensity on T2-weighted images (compared to skeletal muscle), and with peripheral enhancement on postcontrast fat-suppressed T1-weighted images.

Intra-articular Ganglion Cysts

Intra-articular ganglion cysts are an uncommon finding (Fig. 8.34). A prevalence of 0.2–1.9 % on knee imaging or arthroscopy is reported [57–61]. They are extrasynovial and intracapsular and rarely communicate with the joint. Usually, they are associated with the cruciate ligaments, the infrapatellar fat pad, and the posterior capsule. No association was described with cruciate ligament tears. The clinical symptoms are pain, tenderness, limitation of motion, clicking, and palpable mass depending on the location [58–61]. Mucoid degeneration of the ligaments and ganglion cysts likely represents manifestations of the same pathology (Fig. 8.35) [62]. The ganglion cysts associated with the anterior cruciate ligament are fusiform and tend to extend along the ligament, whereas the cysts associated with posterior cruciate ligament or the infrapatellar fat

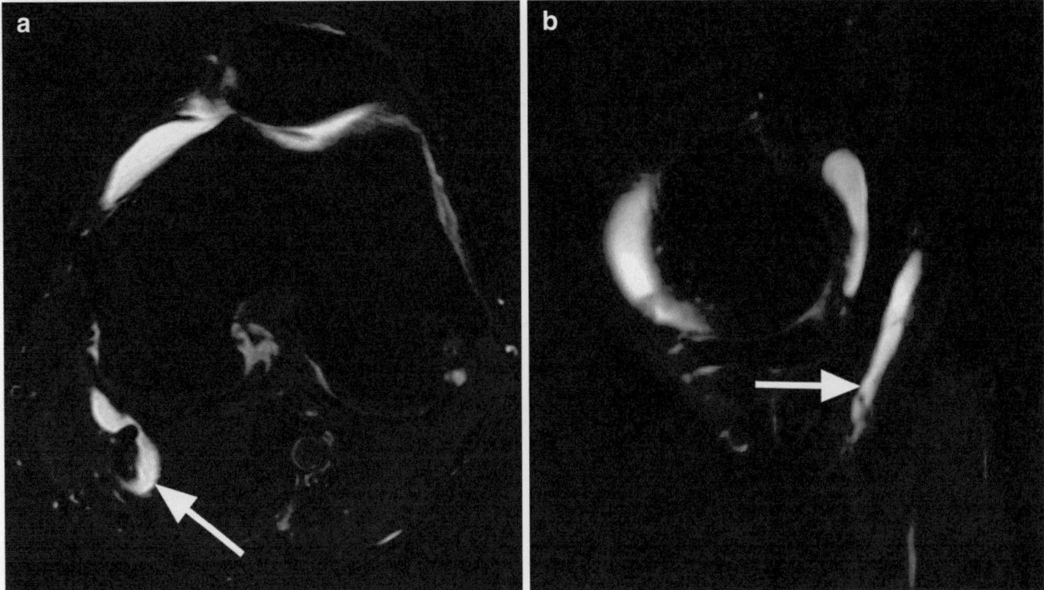

Fig. 8.32 Uncomplicated popliteal or Baker's cyst in a 49 year old male. Axial proton-density (PD) fat-suppressed image (**a**) and sagittal T2-weighted fat-suppressed image (**b**) show the fluid collection in the gastrocnemius-semimembranosus bursa (*arrows*). Baker's cyst may extend superior or inferior along the semimembranosus and gastrocnemius tendons

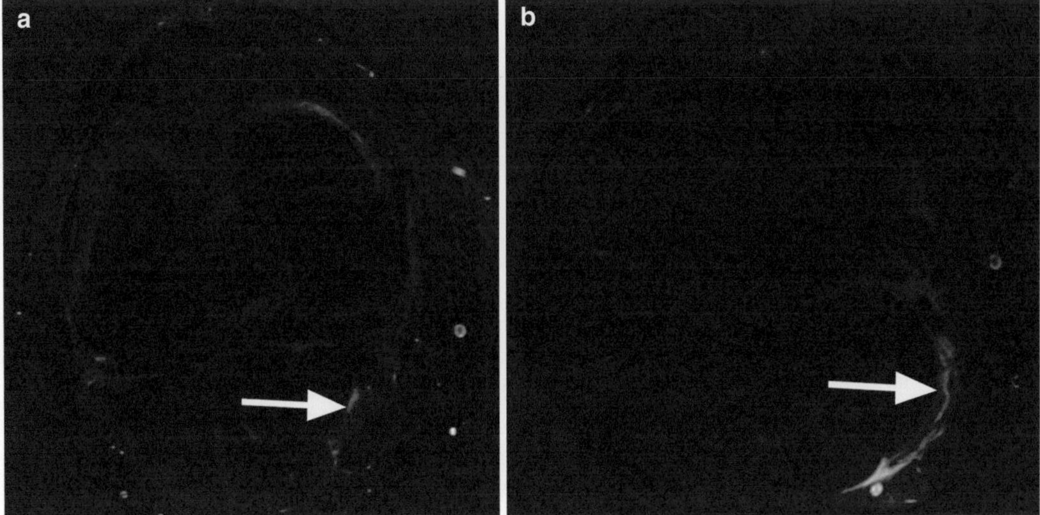

Fig. 8.33 Complicated popliteal or Baker's cyst in a 53 year old male. Two axial proton-density (PD) fat-suppressed images (**a**, **b**) show diffuse collection which extends distally along the medial gastrocnemius muscle (*arrows*) suggestive for rupture of the Baker's cyst

pad are more often multiloculated (Fig. 8.36) [63]. Ganglion cysts within the infrapatellar fat pad are most often located anterior to the anterior horn of the lateral meniscus.

Intraosseous ganglion cysts are located in the epiphyses of the bones and are associated with mucoid degeneration and ganglion cyst of cruciate ligaments [62]. They are

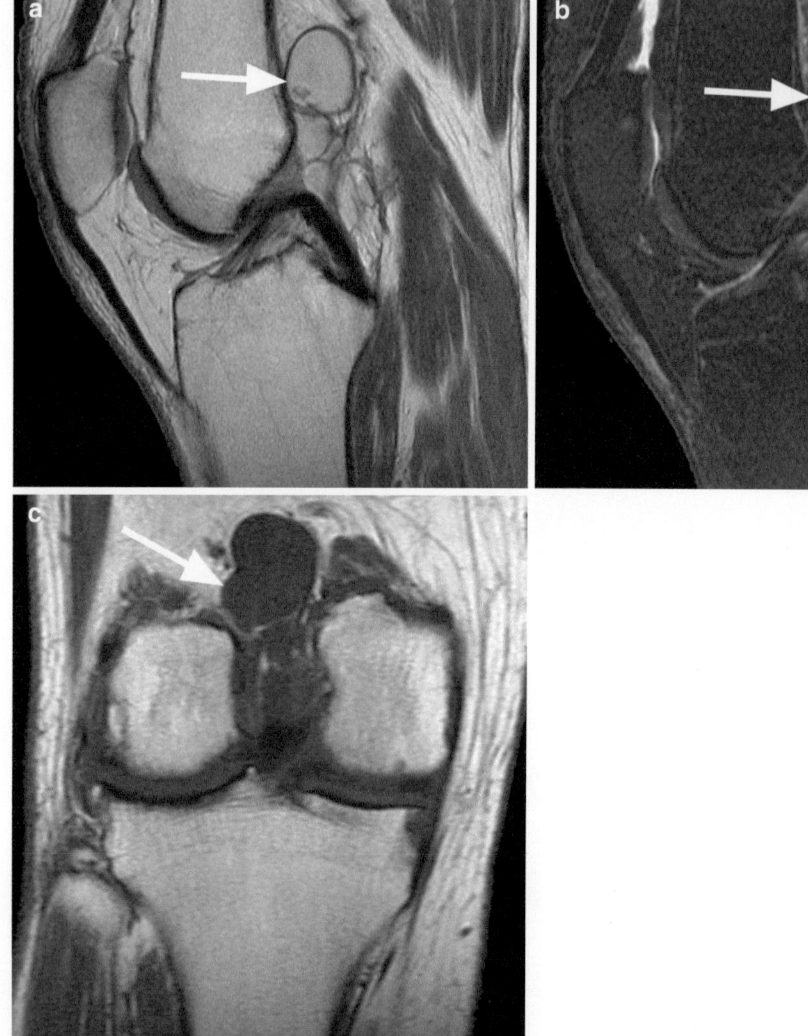

Fig. 8.34 Popliteal ganglion cyst in 71 year old female. Sagittal proton-density (PD)image (**a**), sagittal T2-weighted fat-suppressed image (**b**) and coronal T1-weighted image (**c**) show an intraarticular lobulated and septate cystic mass located in the popliteal fossa (*arrows*)

well-delineated unilocular or multilocular (Fig. 8.37).

Extra-articular Ganglion Cyst

Extra-articular ganglion cysts may arise from joint capsule, tendon sheath, ligaments, muscles, or bursae. Although they rarely communicate with the joint, the detection of a possible communication is important in planning the surgery

[44]. Bone erosions and dissection along the tissue planes may occur [44, 57].

Periosteal Ganglion Cyst

Periosteal ganglion cysts are very rare, occur more frequently in men, and are the result of mucoid degeneration of the periosteum [3]. They produce erosions and reactive periosteal reaction with symptoms such as pain and swelling

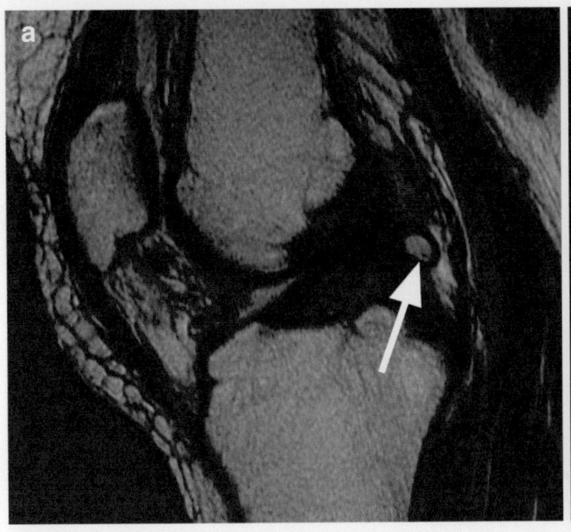

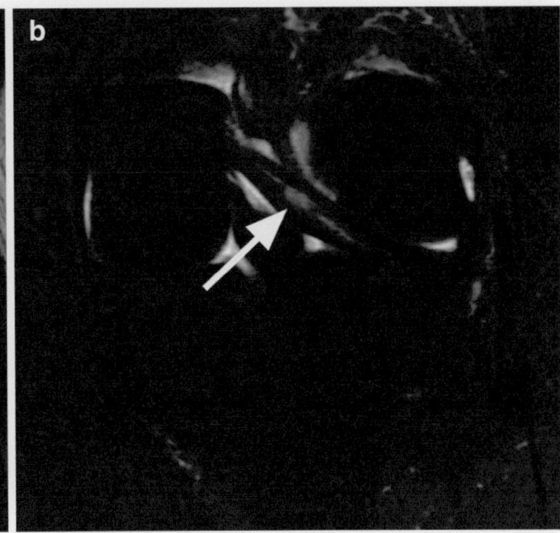

Fig. 8.35 Mucoid degeneration of the Wrisberg ligament in a 43 year old male. Sagittal proton-density (PD) image (**a**) and coronal proton-density (PD) fat-suppressed image (**b**) show a ganglion cyst of the Wrisberg ligament (*arrows*) resulting from mucoid degeneration of the ligament

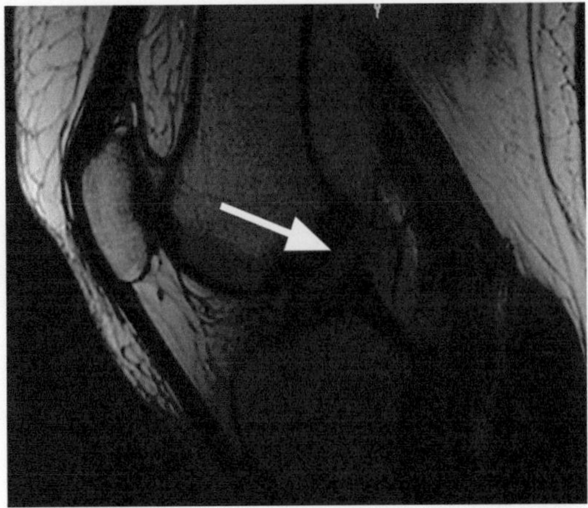

Fig. 8.36 Ganglion cyst of the anterior cruciate ligament (ACL) in a 53 year old female. Sagittal proton-density (PD) image shows a fusiform ganglion cyst of the anterior cruciate ligament (*arrow*)

[64, 65]. The most common location is in close proximity of the pes anserinus, in the proximal tibial shaft [64, 65].

8.2.7 Synovial Plica Syndrome

Plica syndrome is defined as a painful impairment of knee function in which the only finding is the presence of thickened plica [4]. The plica syndrome is a rather obscured and unappreciated pathological entity [66]. Trauma, a sudden increase in athletic activity, synovial foreign bodies, or any form of synovitis may lead to inflammation of synovial plica. The result is fibrosis and thickening of the synovial fold that may impinge against intra-articular structures, often creating localized cartilage pathology of the femoropatellar joint [66]. These result in pain, snapping, or pseudolocking during knee flexion. The infrapatellar and the mediopatellar plica syndromes are the most common. A symptomatic plica may be palpable especially when the hypertrophied plica resembles a soft tissue mass [67, 68]. Because of the anterior pain, especially in the mediopatellar plica syndrome, the symptoms may mimic the clinical findings of a medial

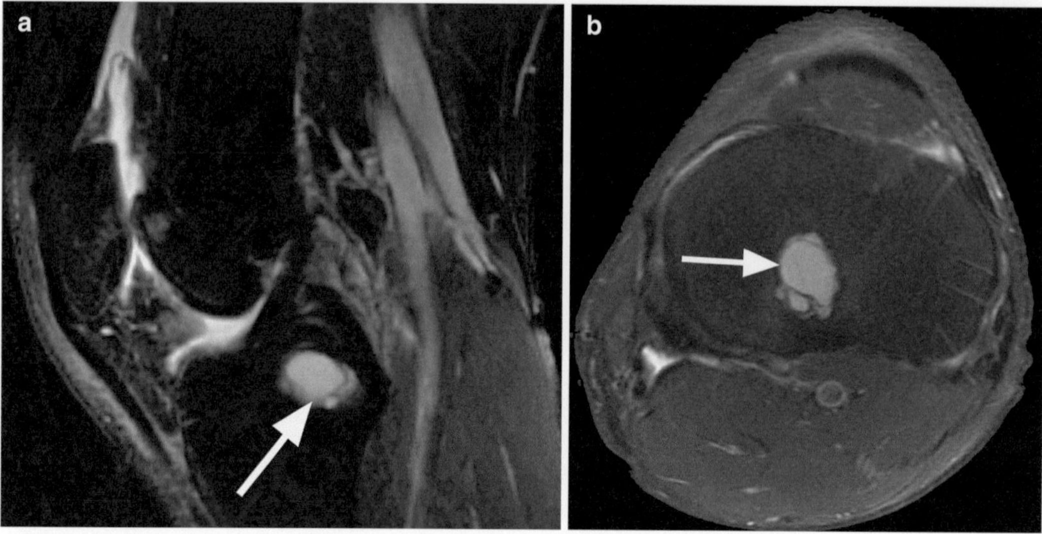

Fig. 8.37 Intraosseous ganglion cysts in a 49 year old male. Sagittal T2-weighted fat-suppressed image (**a**) and axial proton-density (PD) fat-suppressed image (**b**) show an intraosseous cystic lesion of the proximal tibial epiphysis (*arrows*)

meniscus tear [4]. Pathological plica appears on MR images as a thickened low-signal band or a small mass and is easily identified especially when joint fluid is present (Fig. 8.13). In chronic cases, cartilage damages or erosions may be seen in the femoropatellar joint. For any form of plica syndrome, a conservative treatment should be considered as the first choice especially in young patients.

Table 8.5 Classification of synovial tumor-like lesions and synovial tumors

Benign	Malignant
Synovial osteochondromatosis	Synovial sarcoma
Pigmented villonodular synovitis (PVNS)	Synovial chondrosarcoma
Localized nodular synovitis	Metastases
Lipoma arborescens	
Synovial hemangioma	

8.2.8 Synovial Tumor-Like Lesions and Synovial Tumors
(Table 8.5)

Synovial Osteochondromatosis

Primary synovial osteochondromatosis is an uncommon benign synovial disorder characterized by formation of round metaplastic cartilaginous subsynovial nodules or osseous loose bodies in joints, tendon sheaths, or bursae. The nodules may contain calcifications, cartilage and bone, or only cartilage (synovial chondromatosis) [69–71]. There is no association between synovial osteochondromatosis and previous trauma, and the knee is the most affected joint. Clinically it manifests with pain, swelling, and limitation of motion [72]. Osteochondromatosis appears on MR imaging as soft tissue mass with internal nodules variable in size (from 2.0 mm to 1.0 cm). The presence of joint effusion is a typical sign in all forms of osteochondromatosis. The nodular lesions that are exclusively cartilaginous are hypointense or isointense to the muscle on T1-weighted images and of high signal on T2-weighted images. Uncalcified lesions are sometimes difficult to distinguish from the joint effusion on unenhanced images, but on postcontrast fat-suppressed T1-weighted MR images, the nodules show enhancement and are easy to differentiate from the synovial fluid. The presence of calcifications or bone within the nodules leads to an inhomogeneous MRI appearance with low-signal-intensity foci (calcifications) or high-signal-intensity lesion on T1-weighted images showing signal suppression on fat-saturated images (fatty marrow in bony lesions) (Fig. 8.38) [73]. Subchondral erosions may also be seen but typically in more aggressive forms of the disease. Intra-articular cartilaginous or osse-ous loose bodies with joint effusion and hypertrophy of synovial membrane may be seen in idiopathic epiphyseal osteonecrosis, osteochondral fracture, and osteochondritis dissecans. This particular condition is referred by some authors as *secondary synovial osteochondromatosis with loose bodies* [74].

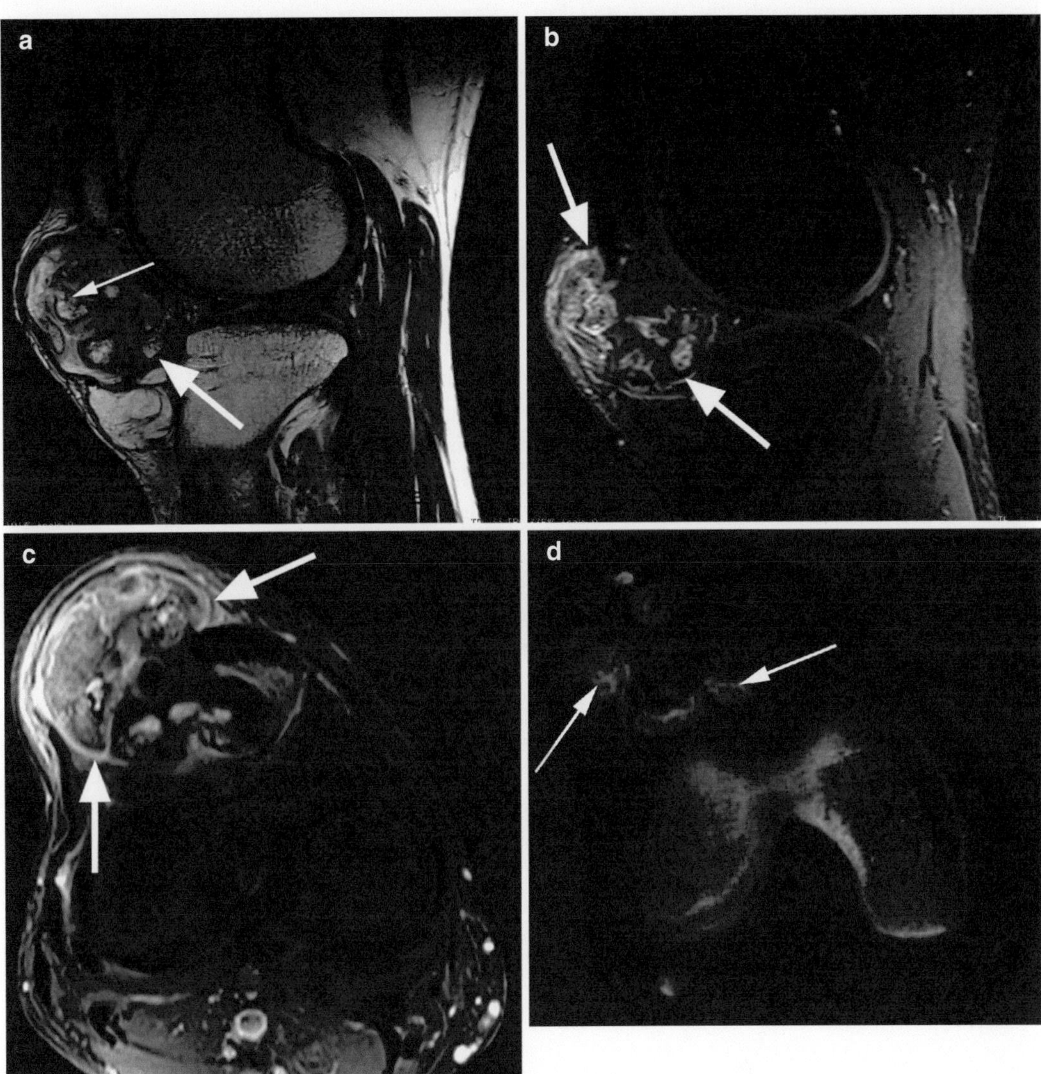

Fig. 8.38 Primary synovial osteochondrosarcoma in a 55 year old male. Sagittal proton-density (PD) image (**a**) shows an intraarticular well delineated mass (*large arrow*) in the infrapatellar fat pad. The lesion is highly inhomogeneous with a large amount of calcified cartilage (*small arrow*). After contrast administration, sagittal (**b**) and axial (**c**) T1-weighted fat-supressed images show inhomogeneous enhancement (*arrows* in **a** and **b**). CT image (**d**) demonstrates the calcified cartilage within the tumor (*arrows* in **g**). A definite differential diagnosis between osteochondrosarcoma and osteochondroma is practically imposible based only on the imaging findings

Pigmented Villonodular Synovitis (PVNS)

Pigmented villonodular synovitis is a benign slow-growing proliferative disorder that produces localized or diffuse nodular thickening of the synovial membrane. The disease is locally invasive, and the localized intra-articular form occurs almost exclusively in the knee [26]. The diffuse intra-articular form usually affects the large joint, most commonly the knee and hip [26]. Hemosiderin deposition is common in all forms of disease, but the extent of hemosiderin is much more prominent in diffuse intra-articular forms [75]. The disease may also occur extra-articularly in a bursa (pigmented villonodular bursitis) or tendon sheath (pigmented villonodular tenosynovitis) [75]. The disease affects males and females equally, and the age of presentation is between the second and fifth decade of life. The patients complain of acute episodes of pain and swelling and functional mechanical symptoms like locking and catching. In the focal or nodular form of PVNS, MR imaging may reveal low-signal-homogeneous-intensity solitary mass on T1-weighted images with moderate contrast enhancement. Small hyperintense T1-weighted of xanthomatous foci may be also present. On T2-weighted images, the nodules are inhomogeneous low signal intensity as a result of hemosiderin deposit (Fig. 8.39). In the diffuse form of the disease, MRI shows heterogeneous diffuse plaque-like thickening with villonodular appearance of intermediate to low signal intensity on T1-weighted images, low signal intensity on T2-weighted images, and hyperintense on T1-weighted postcontrast images. Associated large joint effusion is common, but the cartilage is preserved and subchondral erosions may be seen only in late phases. Although, the definitive diagnosis is made by biopsy, the MR imaging findings are virtually pathognomonic for pigmented villonodular synovitis [76].

Localized Nodular Synovitis (Synovial Giant Cell Tumor)

Localized nodular synovitis (synovial giant cell tumor) is a benign neoplasm characterized histologically by proliferating histiocytes bearing lipids and hemosiderin with a variable number of multinuclear giant cells [77]. The knee is the preferred synovial joint affected, and patients may complain with anterior knee pain, meniscal symptoms, and locking [77, 78]. MR imaging is the best diagnosis tool and shows a mass lesion of low or intermediate high signal intensity on T1-weighted images, intermediate or moderate high signal intensity on T2-weighted images, and moderate enhancement on postcontrast T1-weighted images (Fig. 8.40). On gradient-echo MR images, blooming artifacts may appear

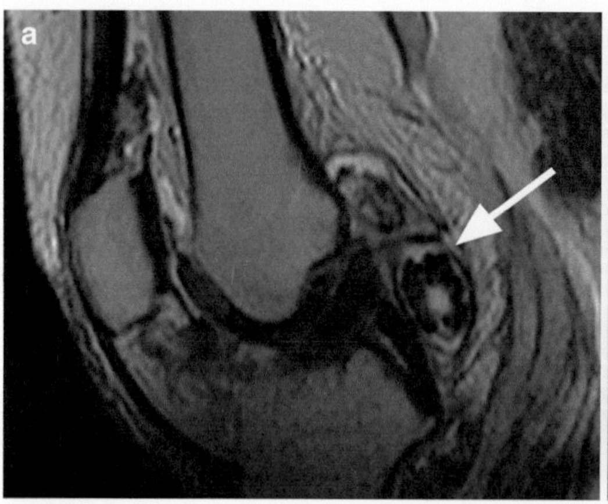

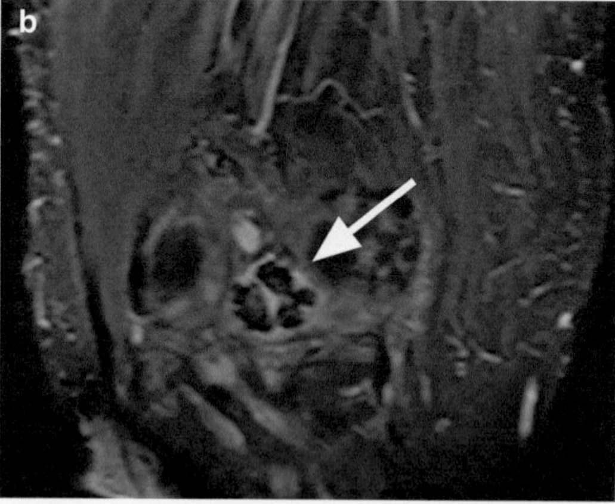

Fig. 8.39 Intra-articular pigmented villonodular synovitis in a 50 year old female. Sagittal proton-density (PD) image (**a**) and coronal proton-density (PD) fat-suppressed image (**b**) show a low-signal inhomogeneous solitary mass in the posterior synovial recess (*arrows*). Note the low signal intensity of hemosiderin deposition which is prominent in the intra-articular forms compared with the extra-articular forms

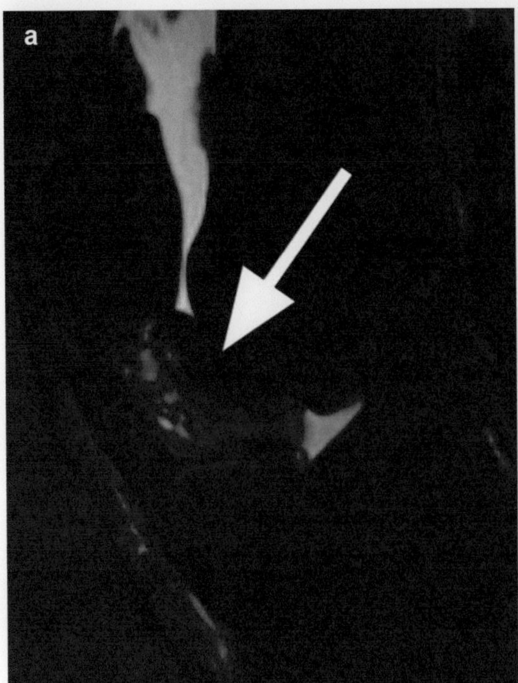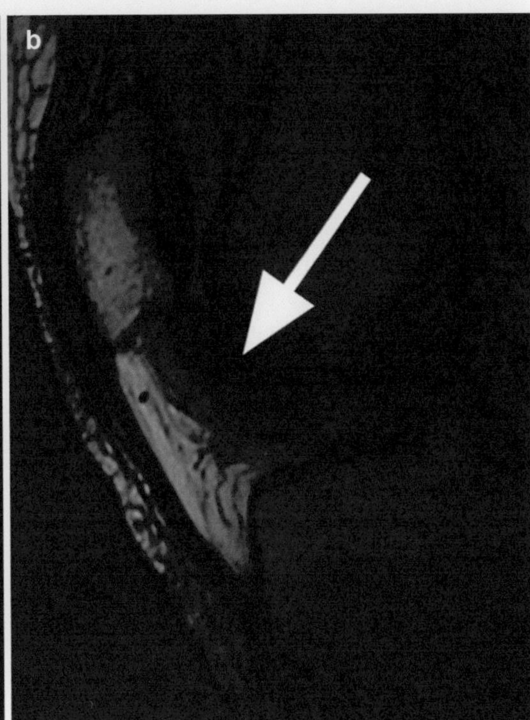

Fig. 8.40 Localized nodular synovitis (synovial giant cell tumor) in a 21 year old female. Sagittal T2-weighted fat-suppressed image (**a**) and sagittal proton-density (PD) image (**b**) show a mass lesion of low signal intensity located into the infrapatellar fat pad (*arrows*)

because of the presence of hemosiderin. The lesion is most commonly located within the infrapatellar fat pad and suprapatellar bursa.

Lipoma Arborescens (Villous Lipomatous Proliferation of the Synovial Membrane or Diffuse Synovial Lipoma)

Lipoma arborescens is one of the rarest benign synovial disorders and is characterized by fatty infiltration of the synovial membrane. It affects preferentially adult men [74]. The lesions can be multifocal and bilateral and can appear as high-signal-intensity fatty intra-articular mass on T1- and T2-weighted images (see Fig. 7.34). The synovial membrane is usually inflamed and enhances after contrast administration.

Synovial Hemangioma

Synovial hemangioma is vascular malformation that affects mainly children and young adults [79]. The lesion may be localized or diffuse and it manifests with pain and swelling. MR imaging may show an isointense T1-weighted to muscles lesion with dilated, tortuous vessels with signal flow void. The lesion enhances variably after contrast administration. Synovial hemangiomas may bleed and the MR imaging findings in these cases mimic hemosiderotic synovitis.

Synovial Sarcoma

Synovial sarcoma accounts for approximately 5 % of all soft tissue sarcomas with the vast majority representing secondary involvement by the tumor from immediate structures of the joint [80, 81]. One third of the cases occur in the lower extremity and are the most common soft tissue malignancy of the lower extremity in the 6- to 25-year age range [81]. The knee joint is the most common involved joint (88 %) [82]. There is a lack of specific findings on MR imaging that makes this entity to be considered in the differential diagnosis if imaging findings are not specific for another entity [82]. Usually, the tumor appears as a cystic inhomogeneous well-delineated lobulated and septated mass with peripheral and septal enhancement [83, 84]. The tumor is in the proximity of the joint or within the joint and may be in contiguity with the bone or invading the bone [85]. Other MR imaging findings include calcifications, foci of hemorrhage, fluid-fluid levels, and the triple signal intensity appearance [85]. Calcifications are usually seen on radiographs and are present in up to 32 % of the cases [86]. The triple signal intensity appearance is seen on T2-weighted images and is defined by the presence of hyperintense, isointense, and hypointense lesions relative to the fat signal intensity translating the mixture of solid, cystic, fibrous, and hemorrhagic content [85].

Synovial Chondrosarcoma

Synovial chondrosarcoma is extremely rare and is not clear whether arises de novo or from malignant degeneration of synovial osteochondromatosis [79]. The MRI appearance is similar to synovial osteochondromatosis, and, therefore, there are no reliable distinguishing MRI findings between the two entities (Fig. 8.38). Distant metastases usually appear in the lung [87].

Synovial Metastases

Lung cancer is the most common cancer that metastasizes in the joints, and the knee joint is most frequently affected [88]. The result is a metastatic arthritis that can involve all structures of the knee joint: the synovium, cartilage, and bone. The diagnosis is made with biopsy or cytology of the joint effusion [79, 88].

8.3 MRI Impression

1. Joint effusion (within suprapatellar bursa, within recesses, within popliteal tendon sheath)
2. Hemarthrosis
3. Lipohemarthrosis (usually indicator of bone fracture)
4. Intra-articular bodies (specify the origin of the bodies):
   - Cartilage
   - Bone
   - Osteochondral fragment
   - Small nodules (in inflammatory synovitis)
   - Tophi in gout
   - Small hyaline cartilage (primary synovial osteochondromatosis)
   - Scattered nodules with "blooming" artifacts (pigmented villonodular synovitis or hemophilic arthropathy)
   - Metallic foreign bodies (correlation with clinical history)
   - Intra-articular gas
5. Synovitis (thickness >2–3 mm)
   - Inflammatory (associated bone marrow edema, erosions)
   - Osteoarthritis (associated cartilage loss, subchondral cysts)
   - Synovial thickening, bone marrow edema, erosions suggesting infectious synovitis
   - Hemosiderotic synovitis
   - Synovitis with crystal deposition (gout, calcium pyrophosphate dehydrate crystal deposition, hydroxyapatite)
   - Amyloid deposition
6. Bursitis (location of the involved bursa)
   - Complicated bursitis (loose bodies, calcifications, hemorrhage, soft tissue inflammation)
7. Adventitial bursitis – specify the cause of bursitis (osteochondroma, orthopedic hardware)
8. Synovial cyst (location)
   - Uncomplicated
   - Complicated (loose bodies, calcifications, hemorrhage, rupture, nerve or artery compression)
9. Ganglion cyst (intra-articular/extra-articular/periosteal)
10. Synovial plica thickening (suprapatellar, infrapatellar, mediopatellar, lateral patellar)
11. Synovial mass (correlated with clinical history)
    - Osteochondromatosis
    - Pigmented villonodular synovitis
    - Localized synovitis
    - Lipoma
    - Hemangioma
    - Sarcoma
    - Chondrosarcoma
    - Metastases

References

1. Steinberg PJ, Hodde KC. The morphology of synovial lining of various structures in several species as observed with scanning electron microscopy. Scanning Microsc. 1990;4(4):987–1019; discussion 1019–20.
2. Fenn S, Datir A, Saifuddin A. Synovial recesses of the knee: MR imaging review of anatomical and pathological features. Skeletal Radiol. 2009;38(4):317–28.
3. Beaman FD, Peterson JJ. MR imaging of cysts, ganglia, and bursae about the knee. Radiol Clin North Am. 2007;45(6):969–82, vi.
4. Garcia-Valtuille R, et al. Anatomy and MR imaging appearances of synovial plicae of the knee. Radiographics. 2002;22(4):775–84.
5. Doppman JL. Baker's cyst and the normal gastrocnemio-semimembranosus bursa. Am J Roentgenol Radium Ther Nucl Med. 1965;94:646–52.
6. Resnick D, et al. Proximal tibiofibular joint: anatomic-pathologic-radiographic correlation. AJR Am J Roentgenol. 1978;131(1):133–8.
7. Guerra Jr J, et al. Pictorial essay: gastrocnemio-semimembranosus bursal region of the knee. AJR Am J Roentgenol. 1981;136(3):593–6.
8. Johnson RL, De Smet AA. MR visualization of the popliteomeniscal fascicles. Skeletal Radiol. 1999;28(10):561–6.
9. Munshi M, et al. MR imaging, MR arthrography, and specimen correlation of the posterolateral corner of the knee: an anatomic study. AJR Am J Roentgenol. 2003;180(4):1095–101.
10. Perdikakis E, Skiadas V. MRI characteristics of cysts and "cyst-like" lesions in and around the knee: what the radiologist needs to know. Insights Imaging. 2013;4(3):257–72.
11. Boles CA, Martin DF. Synovial plicae in the knee. AJR Am J Roentgenol. 2001;177(1):221–7.
12. Chung CB, Boucher R, Resnick D. MR imaging of synovial disorders of the knee. Semin Musculoskelet Radiol. 2009;13(4):303–25.
13. Schweitzer ME, et al. Knee effusion: normal distribution of fluid. AJR Am J Roentgenol. 1992;159(2):361–3.
14. Hall FM. Radiographic diagnosis and accuracy in knee joint effusions. Radiology. 1975;115(1):49–54.
15. McCarthy D. Synovial fluid. In: McCarthy O, editor. Arthritis and allied conditions. 11th ed. Philadelphia: Lea & Febiger; 1989. p. 70–1.
16. Martin DJ, et al. Recurrent hemarthrosis associated with gout. Clin Orthop Relat Res. 1992;277:262–5.
17. Blyth T, et al. Subsynovial vascular abnormality causing recurrent hemarthrosis in an 84-year-old man. J Rheumatol. 1995;22(3):552–3.
18. Ryu KN, et al. Evolving stages of lipohemarthrosis of the knee. Sequential magnetic resonance imaging findings in cadavers with clinical correlation. Invest Radiol. 1997;32(1):7–11.
19. Gylys-Morin VM, et al. Knee in early juvenile rheumatoid arthritis: MR imaging findings. Radiology. 2001;220(3):696–706.
20. Hill CL, et al. Knee effusions, popliteal cysts, and synovial thickening: association with knee pain in osteoarthritis. J Rheumatol. 2001;28(6):1330–7.
21. Saddik D, McNally EG, Richardson M. MRI of Hoffa's fat pad. Skeletal Radiol. 2004;33(8):433–44.
22. Crema MD, et al. Peripatellar synovitis: comparison between non-contrast-enhanced and contrast-enhanced MRI and association with pain. The MOST study. Osteoarthritis Cartilage. 2013;21(3):413–8.
23. Sugimoto H, et al. Early-stage rheumatoid arthritis: diagnostic accuracy of MR imaging. Radiology. 1996;198(1):185–92.
24. Frick MA, Wenger DE, Adkins M. MR imaging of synovial disorders of the knee: an update. Radiol Clin North Am. 2007;45(6):1017–31, vii.
25. Narvaez JA, et al. MR imaging assessment of clinical problems in rheumatoid arthritis. Eur Radiol. 2002;12(7):1819–28.
26. Jaganathan S, et al. Spectrum of synovial pathologies: a pictorial assay. Curr Probl Diagn Radiol. 2012;41(1):30–42.
27. Huang TL, et al. Intra-articular rheumatoid nodule of the knee joint associated with recurrent subluxation of the patella. A case report. J Bone Joint Surg Am. 1979;61(3):438–40.
28. McGonagle D, Gibbon W, Emery P. Classification of inflammatory arthritis by enthesitis. Lancet. 1998;352(9134):1137–40.
29. Crema MD, et al. Magnetic resonance imaging assessment of subchondral bone and soft tissues in knee osteoarthritis. Rheum Dis Clin North Am. 2009;35(3):557–77.
30. Roemer FW, et al. The association of meniscal damage with joint effusion in persons without radiographic osteoarthritis: the Framingham and MOST osteoarthritis studies. Osteoarthritis Cartilage. 2009;17(6):748–53.
31. Hill CL, et al. Synovitis detected on magnetic resonance imaging and its relation to pain and cartilage loss in knee osteoarthritis. Ann Rheum Dis. 2007;66(12):1599–603.
32. Erdman WA, et al. Osteomyelitis: characteristics and pitfalls of diagnosis with MR imaging. Radiology. 1991;180(2):533–9.
33. Graif M, et al. The septic versus nonseptic inflamed joint: MRI characteristics. Skeletal Radiol. 1999;28(11):616–20.
34. Stein H, Duthie RB. The pathogenesis of chronic haemophilic arthropathy. J Bone Joint Surg Br. 1981;63B(4):601–9.
35. Luck JV Jr, Kasper CK. Surgical management of advanced hemophilic arthropathy. An overview of 20 years' experience. Clin Orthop Relat Res. 1989;(242):60–82. http://www.ncbi.nlm.nih.gov/pubmed/2650951.
36. Rand T, et al. Magnetic resonance imaging in hemophilic children: value of gradient echo and contrast-enhanced imaging. Magn Reson Imaging. 1999;17(2):199–205.
37. Devaney K, Vinh TN, Sweet DE. Synovial hemangioma: a report of 20 cases with differential diagnostic considerations. Hum Pathol. 1993;24(7):737–45.

38. Monu JU, Pope Jr TL. Gout: a clinical and radiologic review. Radiol Clin North Am. 2004;42(1):169–84.
39. Bongartz T, et al. Dual-energy CT for the diagnosis of gout: an accuracy and diagnosis yield study. Ann Rheum Dis doi:10.1136/annrheumdis-2013-205095
40. Ahn JK, et al. Idiopathic calcium pyrophosphate dihydrate (CPPD) crystal deposition disease in a young male patient: a case report. J Korean Med Sci. 2003;18(6):917–20.
41. Hayes CW, et al. Calcific tendinitis in unusual sites associated with cortical bone erosion. AJR Am J Roentgenol. 1987;149(5):967–70.
42. Stuttle FL. The no-name and no-fame bursa. Clin Orthop. 1959;15:197–9.
43. Kerlan RK, Glousman RE. Tibial collateral ligament bursitis. Am J Sports Med. 1988;16(4):344–6.
44. Janzen DL, et al. Cystic lesions around the knee joint: MR imaging findings. AJR Am J Roentgenol. 1994;163(1):155–61.
45. Forbes JR, Helms CA, Janzen DL. Acute pes anserine bursitis: MR imaging. Radiology. 1995;194(2):525–7.
46. Rothstein CP, et al. Semimembranosus-tibial collateral ligament bursitis: MR imaging findings. AJR Am J Roentgenol. 1996;166(4):875–7.
47. LaPrade RF, Hamilton CD. The fibular collateral ligament-biceps femoris bursa. An anatomic study. Am J Sports Med. 1997;25(4):439–43.
48. LaPrade RF. The anatomy of the deep infrapatellar bursa of the knee. Am J Sports Med. 1998;26(1):129–32.
49. De Maeseneer M, et al. MR imaging of the medial collateral ligament bursa: findings in patients and anatomic data derived from cadavers. AJR Am J Roentgenol. 2001;177(4):911–7.
50. Steiner E, et al. Ganglia and cysts around joints. Radiol Clin North Am. 1996;34(2):395–425, xi–xii.
51. Fielding JR, Franklin PD, Kustan J. Popliteal cysts: a reassessment using magnetic resonance imaging. Skeletal Radiol. 1991;20(6):433–5.
52. Miller TT, et al. MR imaging of Baker cysts: association with internal derangement, effusion, and degenerative arthropathy. Radiology. 1996;201(1):247–50.
53. Marti-Bonmati L, et al. MR imaging of Baker cysts – prevalence and relation to internal derangements of the knee. MAGMA. 2000;10(3):205–10.
54. Labropoulos N, Shifrin DA, Paxinos O. New insights into the development of popliteal cysts. Br J Surg. 2004;91(10):1313–8.
55. Robertson CM, Robertson RF, Strazerri JC. Proximal dissection of a popliteal cyst with sciatic nerve compression. Orthopedics. 2003;26(12):1231–2.
56. McCarthy CL, McNally EG. The MRI appearance of cystic lesions around the knee. Skeletal Radiol. 2004;33(4):187–209.
57. Burk Jr DL, et al. Meniscal and ganglion cysts of the knee: MR evaluation. AJR Am J Roentgenol. 1988; 150(2):331–6.
58. McLaren DB, Buckwalter KA, Vahey TN. The prevalence and significance of cyst-like changes at the cruciate ligament attachments in the knee. Skeletal Radiol. 1992;21(6):365–9.
59. Nokes SR, Koonce TW, Montanez J. Ganglion cysts of the cruciate ligaments of the knee: recognition on MR images and CT-guided aspiration. AJR Am J Roentgenol. 1994;162(6):1503.
60. Kang CN, et al. Intra-articular ganglion cysts of the knee. Arthroscopy. 1999;15(4):373–8.
61. Sumen Y, et al. Ganglion cysts of the cruciate ligaments detected by MRI. Int Orthop. 1999;23(1):58–60.
62. Bergin D, et al. Anterior cruciate ligament ganglia and mucoid degeneration: coexistence and clinical correlation. AJR Am J Roentgenol. 2004;182(5): 1283–7.
63. Kim MG, et al. Intra-articular ganglion cysts of the knee: clinical and MR imaging features. Eur Radiol. 2001;11(5):834–40.
64. McCarthy EF, et al. Periosteal ganglion: a cause of cortical bone erosion. Skeletal Radiol. 1983;10(4):243–6.
65. Abdelwahab IF, et al. Periosteal ganglia: CT and MR imaging features. Radiology. 1993;188(1):245–8.
66. Schindler OS. 'The Sneaky Plica' revisited: morphology, pathophysiology and treatment of synovial plicae of the knee. Knee Surg Sports Traumatol Arthrosc. 2014;22(2):247–62.
67. Apple JS, et al. Synovial plicae of the knee. Skeletal Radiol. 1982;7(4):251–4.
68. Trout TE, Bock H, Resnick D. Suprapatellar plicae of the knee presenting as a soft-tissue mass. Report of five patients. Clin Imaging. 1996;20(1):55–9.
69. Villacin AB, Brigham LN, Bullough PG. Primary and secondary synovial chondrometaplasia: histopathologic and clinicoradiologic differences. Hum Pathol. 1979;10(4):439–51.
70. Apte SS, Athanasou NA. An immunohistological study of cartilage and synovium in primary synovial chondromatosis. J Pathol. 1992;166(3):277–81.
71. Sviland L, Malcolm AJ. Synovial chondromatosis presenting as painless soft tissue mass–a report of 19 cases. Histopathology. 1995;27(3):275–9.
72. Milgram JW. Synovial osteochondromatosis: a histopathological study of thirty cases. J Bone Joint Surg Am. 1977;59(6):792–801.
73. McKenzie G, Raby N, Ritchie D. A pictorial review of primary synovial osteochondromatosis. Eur Radiol. 2008;18(11):2662–9.
74. O'Connell JX. Pathology of the synovium. Am J Clin Pathol. 2000;114(5):773–84.
75. Murphey MD, et al. Pigmented villonodular synovitis: radiologic-pathologic correlation. Radiographics. 2008;28(5):1493–518.
76. Hughes TH, et al. Pigmented villonodular synovitis: MRI characteristics. Skeletal Radiol. 1995;24(1): 7–12.
77. Nau T, et al. Giant-cell tumor of the synovial membrane: localized nodular synovitis in the knee joint. Arthroscopy. 2000;16(8):E22.
78. Yoo JH, Yang BK, Park JM. Localized nodular synovitis of the knee presenting as anterior knee pain: a case report. Knee. 2007;14(5):398–401.
79. Sheldon PJ, Forrester DM, Learch TJ. Imaging of intraarticular masses. Radiographics. 2005;25(1):105–19.

80. McKinney CD, Mills SE, Fechner RE. Intraarticular synovial sarcoma. Am J Surg Pathol. 1992;16(10): 1017–20.
81. Kransdorf MJ. Malignant soft-tissue tumors in a large referral population: distribution of diagnoses by age, sex, and location. AJR Am J Roentgenol. 1995;164(1): 129–34.
82. Bui-Mansfield LT, O'Brien SD. Magnetic resonance appearance of intra-articular synovial sarcoma: case reports and review of the literature. J Comput Assist Tomogr. 2008;32(4):640–4.
83. Ayoub KS, et al. Synovial sarcoma arising in association with a popliteal cyst. Skeletal Radiol. 2000;29(12): 713–6.
84. Namba Y, et al. Intraarticular synovial sarcoma confirmed by SYT-SSX fusion transcript. Clin Orthop Relat Res. 2002;395:221–6.
85. Jones BC, Sundaram M, Kransdorf MJ. Synovial sarcoma: MR imaging findings in 34 patients. AJR Am J Roentgenol. 1993;161(4):827–30.
86. Cadman NL, Soule EH, Kelly PJ. Synovial sarcoma; an analysis of 34 tumors. Cancer. 1965;18:613–27.
87. Taconis WK, van der Heul RO, Taminiau AM. Synovial chondrosarcoma: report of a case and review of the literature. Skeletal Radiol. 1997;26(11):682–5.
88. Thompson KS, et al. Synovial metastasis: diagnosis by fine-needle aspiration cytologic investigation. Diagn Cytopathol. 1996;15(4):334–7.

Nicolae Bolog, Gustav Andreisek, and Erika Ulbrich

9.1 Anatomy and Normal MRI Appearance

The muscle groups around the knee have an anti-gravity role and offer knee stabilization during standing position and stability in a variety of different positions. They can be classified based on their anatomic location as well as on their function. The muscles of the thigh and lower leg are comprised of compartments defined as distinct anatomical spaces bordered by fascia or bone. The knowledge of the anatomical boundaries of the compartments is important especially when describing the extension of the soft tissue tumors (e.g., extra- or intracompartmental). The anterior compartment of the thigh is represented by the quadriceps muscle, the sartorius, and the tensor fascia latae. The posterior compartment includes the hamstring muscles (the semitendinosus, the semimembranosus, and the biceps femoris). The medial compartment contains the gracilis and the adductor muscles. The gastrocnemius muscles are included together with the soleus muscle in the superficial posterior compartment of the lower leg.

Functionally, the muscles can be divided into four groups, which produce knee flexion (biceps femoris, semitendinosus, semimembranosus, gracilis, sartorius, and popliteus muscle), knee extension (quadriceps femoris and tensor fasciae latae), internal rotation (popliteus, semitendinosus, semimembranosus, sartorius, gracilis, and medial head of gastrocnemius muscle), or lateral rotation (biceps femoris and the lateral head of the gastrocnemius muscle). Another possibility is to distinguish the muscles around the knee based on their topography. This approach enables an easier interpretation of the MR examination with the muscles classified into three groups: the anterior, the posteromedial, and the posterolateral group.

The normal MR signal intensity of the muscles around the knee is, as with all muscles, intermediate between the signal intensity of fat and cortical bone (Fig. 9.1). The MRI signal intensity differences between the hyperintense thin intermuscular fat planes and the muscle tissue enable the separation between individual muscles or groups of muscles. The tendons appear mainly as hypointense structures in most MR sequences (Fig. 9.1).

9.1.1 The Anterior Muscle Group

The anterior muscle group of the knee or the quadriceps group includes *the vastus lateralis, the vastus medialis, the vastus intermedius,* and *the rectus femoris* (Fig. 9.2). The quadriceps muscle and tendon extend the lower leg and play an important role in patellar stability. The muscle is also an important part of the extensor mechanism of the knee, which also includes the medial and lateral patellar retinaculum, patellofemoral and patellotibial ligaments, the patellar tendon, the prepatellar structures, the Hoffa's fat pad, and the tibial tubercle.

N.V. Bolog et al., *MRI of the Knee: A Guide to Evaluation and Reporting*,
DOI 10.1007/978-3-319-08165-6_9, © Springer International Publishing Switzerland 2015

The proximal insertion of the rectus femoris is the anterior inferior iliac spine. The vastus lateralis inserts proximally to the greater

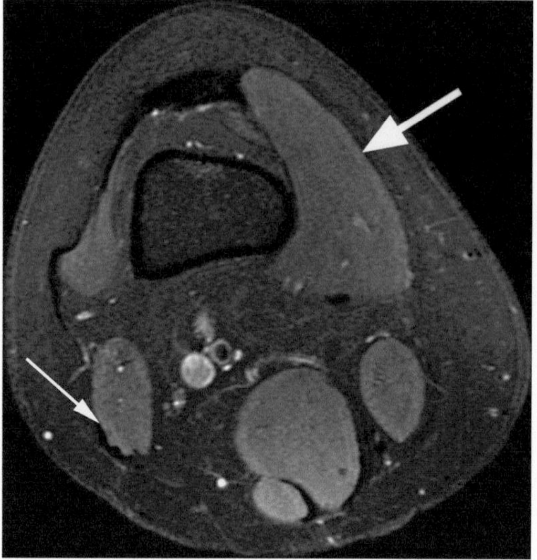

Fig. 9.1 Normal MRI appearance of muscles and tendons in a 33 year old female. Axial proton-density (PD) fat-suppressed image shows the intermediate signal intensity of the muscle (between the signal intensity of fat and cortical bone) (*large arrow* indicating the vastus medialis muscle). The tendons appear as hypointense structures (*small arrow* indicating the tendon of the biceps femoris)

femoral trochanter and the vastus medialis inserts to the femoral intertrochanteric line. The vastus intermedius has its proximal insertion along the proximal anterolateral two thirds of the femoral diaphysis. Distally, the four muscular elements of the quadriceps converge and fuse 2 cm above the patella to form the quadriceps tendon and inserts on the superior pole of the patella [1]. On MR imaging, the normal quadriceps tendon has a striated appearance with two or three layers in most of the cases (Fig. 9.3) [2]. The superficial layer is formed by the rectus femoris, the intermediate layer is represented by the vastus medialis and vastus lateralis, and the deep layer is formed by the vastus intermedius. The tendon can very rarely be identified on MR images as a homogeneously hypointense structure [1, 2].

9.1.2 The Posteromedial Muscle Group

The posteromedial group of muscles consists of the *sartorius*, *gracilis*, *semitendinosus*, *semimembranosus*, and *medial gastrocnemius*.

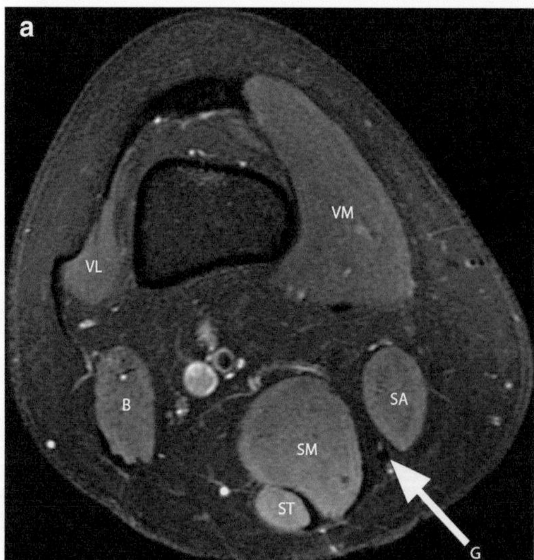

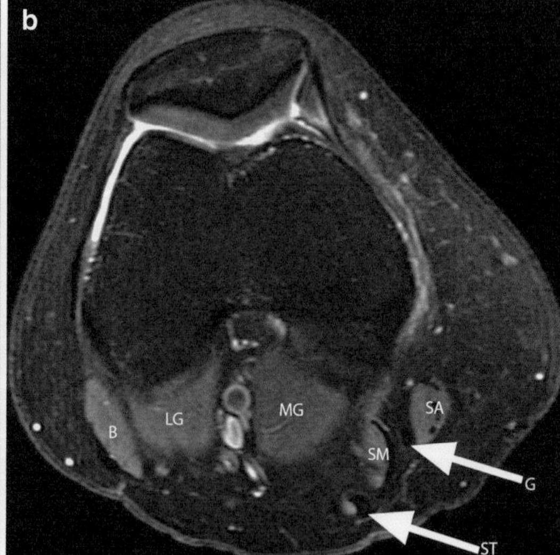

Fig. 9.2 Axial proton-density (PD) fat-suppressed image 8 cm above the joint line (**a**) and 3 cm above the joint line (**b**) shows the vastus medialis (*VM*) and vastus lateralis (*VL*). The posteromedial group of muscles consists of the sartorius (*SA*), gracilis (*G*), semitendinosus (*ST*), semimembranosus (*SM*), and medial gastrocnemius (*MG*). The biceps femoris muscle and tendon (*B*) and the lateral head of the gastrocnemius muscle (*LG*) are part of the posterolateral muscle group

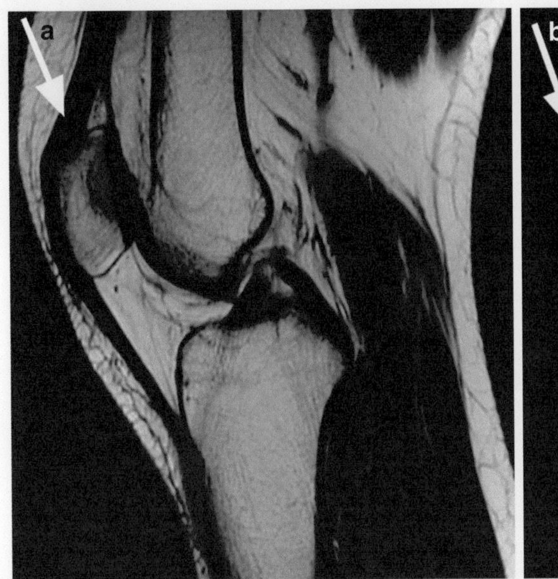
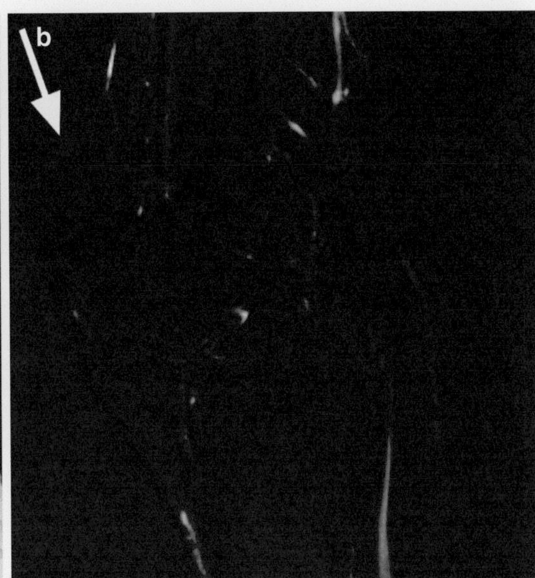

Fig. 9.3 Normal appearance of the quadriceps tendon in a 33 year old female. Sagittal proton-density (PD) image (**a**) and sagittal T2-weighted fat-suppressed image (**b**) show the three-layer appearance of the tendon (*arrows*). The superficial layer is formed by the rectus femoris, the intermediate layer is represented by the vastus medialis and vastus lateralis, and the deep layer is formed by the vastus intermedius

The proximal insertions of the *sartorius*, *gracilis*, and *semitendinosus* are the anterior superior iliac spine (sartorius), inferior pubic ramus (gracilis), and ischial tuberosity (semitendinosus). The semitendinosus tendon has a common ischial insertion with the biceps femoris muscle. The distal parts of the sartorius, gracilis, and semitendinosus tendons converge into the *pes anserinus* and insert to the proximal anteromedial tibia. The sartorius muscle is the most medially located muscle (Fig. 9.2). Lateral to the former is the gracilis muscle and its tendon (Fig. 9.2). The semitendinosus muscle is located posterolateral to the gracilis muscle and posterior to the semi-membranosus muscle (Fig. 9.2). Between the pes anserinus and the medial collateral ligament, there is the pes anserinus bursa, which typically does not communicate with the knee joint. The three muscles and the pes anserinus contribute to knee flexion and internal rotation.

The semimembranosus muscle is the largest of the posteromedial group and originates from the ischial tuberosity and extends to the posterome-dial tibial condyle below the articular surface. The proximal, ischial insertion of the semimembranosus is located just lateral to the common insertion of the semitendinosus and biceps femoris. The three muscles are known as the hamstring complex or the hamstring muscles. They extend the thigh and flex and rotate the lower leg. At the level of the knee joint, the semi-membranosus tendon reinforces the posterome-dial corner of the knee. On axial MR images, the semimembranosus muscle is located between the medial head of the gastrocnemius muscle and the gracilis muscle (Fig. 9.2). Between the semi-membranosus tendon and the medial collateral ligament of the knee, there is the medial collateral-semimembranosus bursa. Between the semimembranosus muscle and tendon and the medial head of the gastrocnemius muscle, there is the gastrocnemius-semimembranosus bursa. The semimembranosus muscle flexes the knee and contributes to internal rotation.

The medial head of the gastrocnemius muscle plays also an important role in reinforcing the posteromedial corner of the knee. It inserts to the medial condyle and posterior surface of the femur and extends to the Achilles tendon (Fig. 9.4). The medial posterior femoral recess (the medial

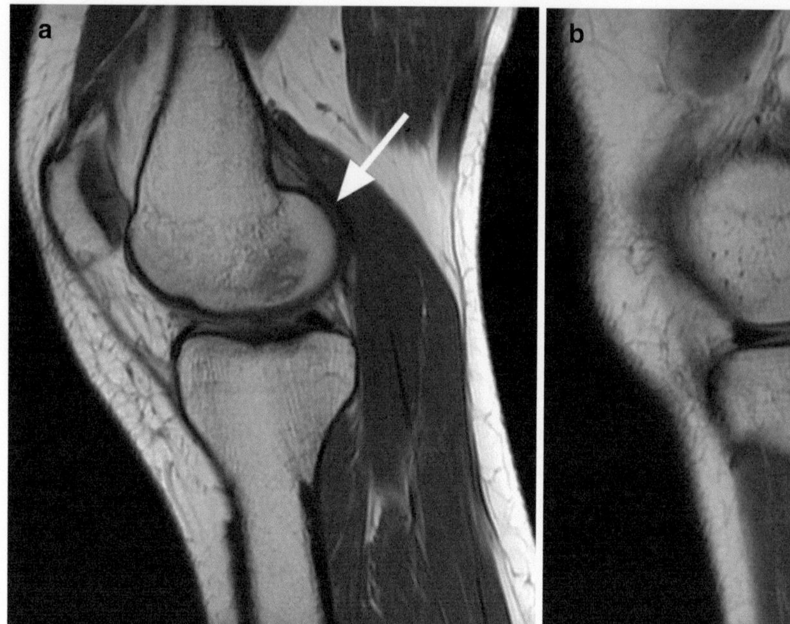

Fig. 9.4 Proximal insertions of medial and lateral gastrocnemius muscles. Sagittal proton-density (PD) image through the medial compartment (**a**) shows the medial tendon and musculotendinous junction of the medial gastrocnemius muscles (*arrow*). Sagittal proton-density (PD) image through the lateral compartment (**b**) shows the tendon of the lateral gastrocnemius muscles (*arrow*)

gastrocnemius bursa) is located between the posterior horn of the medial meniscus and the knee capsule and the medial head of the gastrocnemius muscle, respectively. This bursa may or may not communicate with the knee joint. The gastrocnemius muscle flexes the lower leg and contributes to internal rotation.

9.1.3 The Posterolateral Muscle Group

The posterolateral group is formed by the *iliotibial band, biceps femoris, popliteus, plantaris, and the lateral head of the gastrocnemius muscle* (Fig. 9.2).

The iliotibial band or the iliotibial tract represents a thickening of the fascia lata, which extends from the outer margin of the anterior iliac crest down to the Gerdy's tubercle and to the head of the fibula (Fig. 9.5). A portion of fascia lata known as the anterior longitudinal expansion merges with the anterior quadriceps aponeurosis, forms the intermediate layer of the lateral

retinaculum, and attaches to the patella [3]. The fascia lata is considered an anterolateral knee stabilizer and is tense in both flexion and extension of the knee [4].

The biceps muscle is one of the three muscles that form the hamstring complex. The long head of the biceps femoris inserts proximally together with the semitendinosus muscle on the ischial tuberosity. The short head of the biceps has its proximal insertion on the linea aspera and the lateral supracondylar line. Distally, the biceps muscle joins the lateral collateral ligament and forms a conjoined tendon that inserts on the fibular head (Fig. 9.6). The biceps tendon is seen on axial MR images posterior to the iliotibial band and the lateral collateral ligament (Fig. 9.6). Between the biceps tendon and the lateral collateral ligament, the lateral collateral ligament-biceps femoris bursa is constantly described [5]. The biceps femoris contributes to the lateral stabilization of the knee and to the external rotation of the tibia.

The popliteus muscle inserts on the lateral femoral condyle above the superior margin of the lateral meniscus, distal and anterior to the lateral

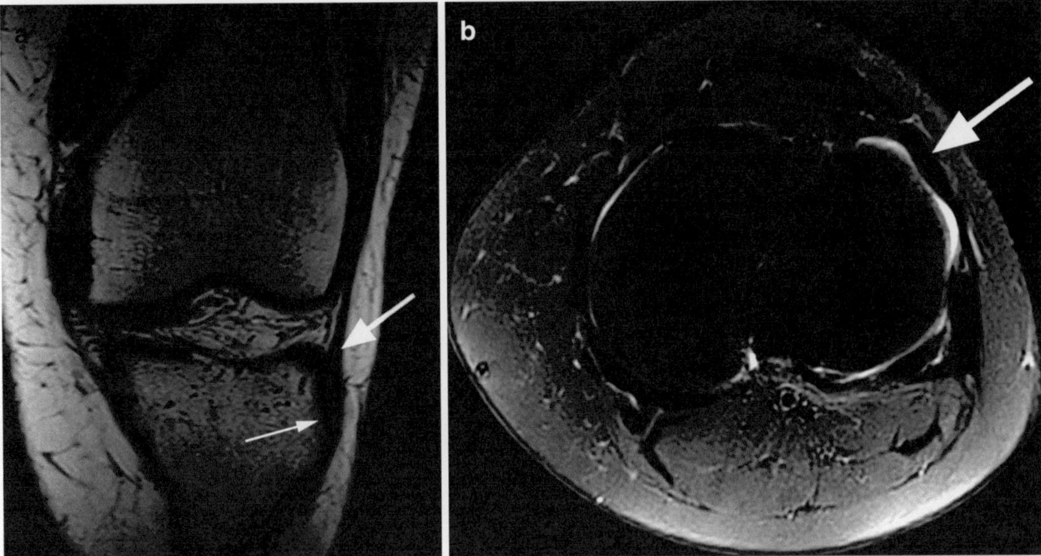

Fig. 9.5 Iliotibial band in a 27 year old female. Coronal T1-weighted image (**a**) and axial proton-density (PD) fat-suppressed image (**b**) show the distal iliotibial band (*large arrow* in **a**, **b**) and the insertion on the Gerdy's tubercle (*small arrow* in **a**)

collateral ligament (Fig. 9.7) [6, 7]. Two separate bundles are described at the proximal attachment: the posterior superficial bundle and the anterior deep bundle. Laterally, the muscle joins the arcuate ligament of the knee capsule (Fig. 9.8). The tendon passes through a hiatus in the coronary ligament, crosses obliquely deep to the lateral collateral ligament, and becomes extra-articular. It inserts to the posteromedial surface of the tibial metaphysis (Fig. 9.7). The tendon is surrounded by the popliteal bursa [8]. At the proximal insertion, the tendon creates a sinusoidal indentation of the cartilage at the border of the lateral femoral condyle called sulcus statarius of Furst, and the tendon slides into this sulcus during flexion [6].

The popliteus muscle alone is responsible for knee flexion and tibial internal rotation of the tibia at the beginning of flexion. Also the popliteal tendon is an important structure of the posterolateral corner of the knee that limits posterior translation, varus angulation, and external rotation [9]. The muscle is connected to the lateral meniscus and the proximal aspect of the fibula. The connection between the medial part of the muscle and the lateral meniscus is ensured by the

posterosuperior and anteroinferior popliteo-meniscal fascicles (Fig. 9.9). The popliteofibular ligament attaches the popliteus tendon to the fibular head and has a thickness similar to the lateral collateral ligament (Fig. 9.10).

The plantaris muscle has the origin on the lateral supracondylar line of the femur (Fig. 9.11), and its long distal tendon inserts on the posteromedial part of the calcaneus. The muscle has a role in flexion of the lower leg at the knee joint.

The lateral head of the gastrocnemius inserts on the lateral femoral condyle and posterior surface of the femur (Fig. 9.4) and extends to the Achilles tendon. Between the lateral head of the gastrocnemius muscle and the posterior horn of the lateral meniscus and the knee capsule, the lateral posterior femoral recess or bursa is present. Besides the role of flexion of the lower leg at the knee joint, it also contributes to lateral rotation.

9.1.4 Anomalous Knee Muscles

Anomalous Gastrocnemius Muscles

Anomalous gastrocnemius variations are very rare and may involve the medial or the lateral

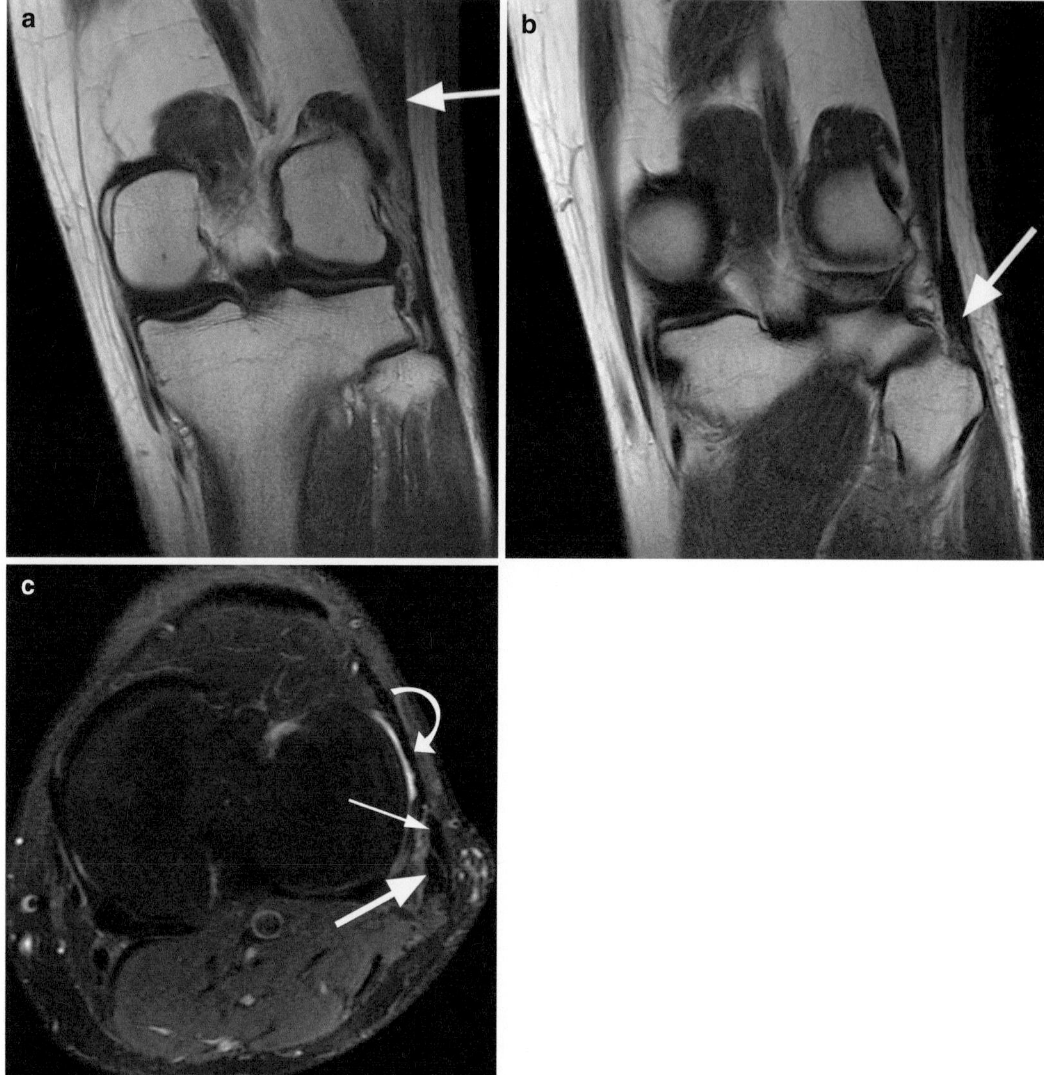

Fig. 9.6 Distal biceps tendon in a 40 year old male. Two coronal proton-density (PD) images through the posterior joint (**a**, **b**) show the distal tendon (*arrow* in **a**) and the insertion on the fibular head (*arrow* in **b**). At the insertion the tendon forms a conjoined tendon with the lateral collateral ligament (LCL). Axial proton-density (PD) fat-suppressed image (**c**) shows that the biceps tendon (*large arrow*) is seen posterior to the lateral collateral ligament (LCL) (*small arrow*) and to the iliotibial band (*curved arrow*)

head of the gastrocnemius. On the medial side, a known variation is a third gastrocnemius head. On the lateral side, possible variations include the origin and the number of muscle bundles.

The medial variation is commonly known as *the third head of the gastrocnemius muscle*. It has been described in adults in the setting of popliteal artery entrapment syndrome [10, 11]. If present, the anomaly refers to an accessory third gastrocnemius head which is more medial than the normal medial head.

A medial accessory origin of a segmental bundle of the lateral gastrocnemius head has also been described [12]. In this case, the accessory gastrocnemius bundle originates from the iliotibial tract [12]. *In medial accessory anomalous origin of the lateral gastrocnemius head*, an accessory bundle

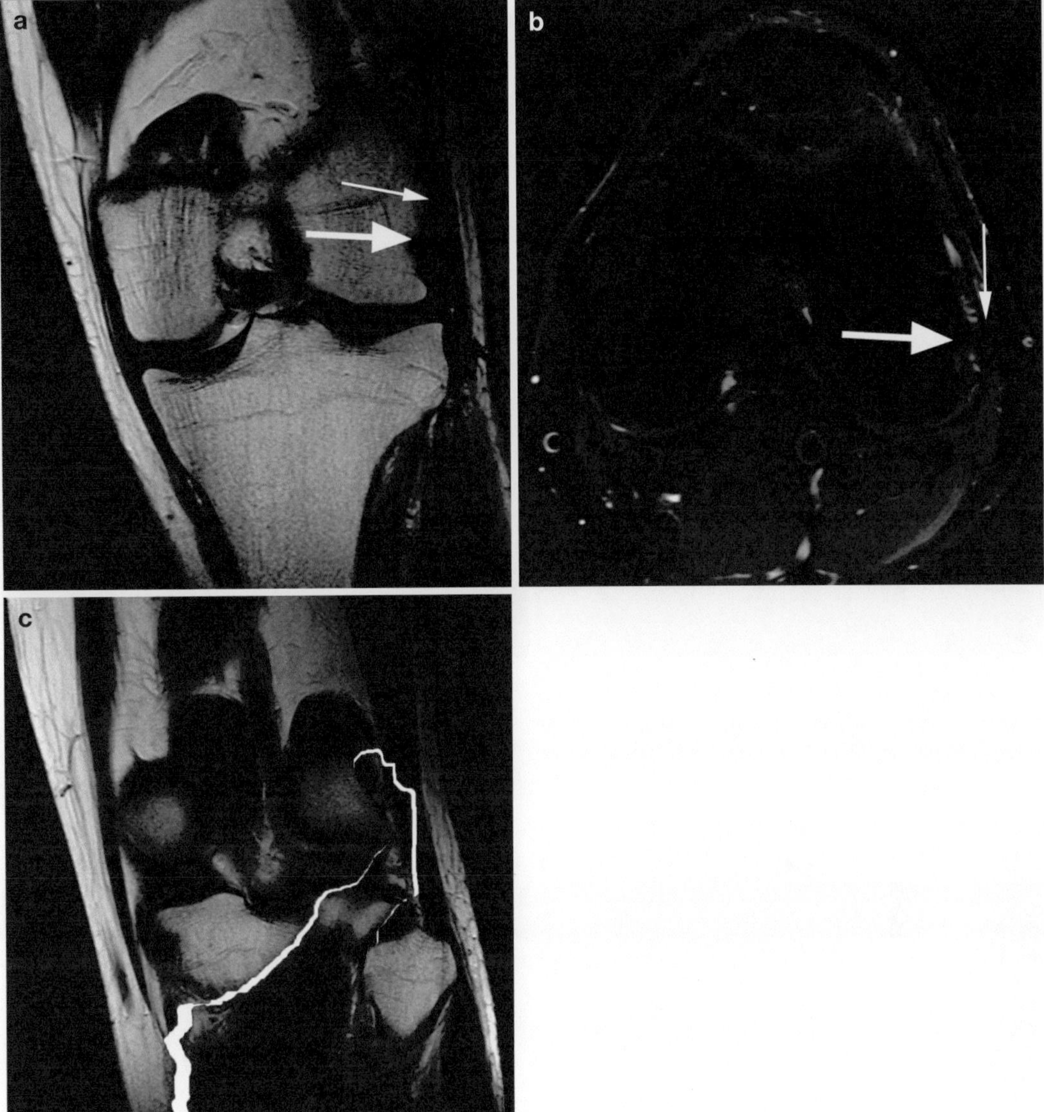

Fig. 9.7 Popliteus muscle in a 40 year old male. Coronal proton-density (PD) image (**a**) and axial proton-density (PD) fat-suppressed image (**b**) show the proximal insertion to the lateral femoral condyle (*large arrows* in **a**, **b**). The insertion is distal and anterior to the lateral collateral ligament (*small arrows* in **a**. **b**). Coronal proton-density (PD) image (**c**) shows the normal area of the popliteus muscle including its distal part adjacent to the posteromedial surface of the tibial metaphysis

originates from the posterior and medial aspect of the lateral femoral condyle, lateral to popliteal vessels, which then merges with the medial aspect of the lateral head of the gastrocnemius.

On MR imaging, the variations of the gastrocnemius are best identified on axial images. It remains particularly difficult to assess the anomalies on coronal or sagittal planes. Almost half of the patients may present chronic nontraumatic pain with no additional MR imaging findings [12]. Thus, in cases where no other findings are present, one might always think about normal anatomical variants. The etiology of the pain may be ischemic due to popliteal artery entrapment or due to compression and/or impaired nerve function. For the latter, evaluation of the tibial and peroneal nerve is mandatory.

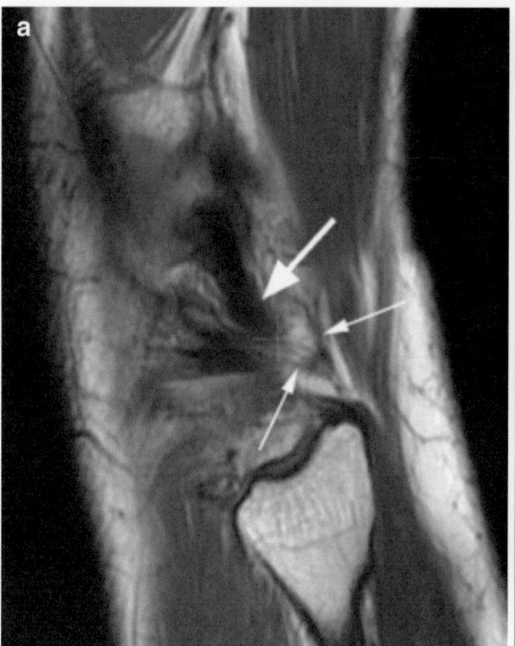

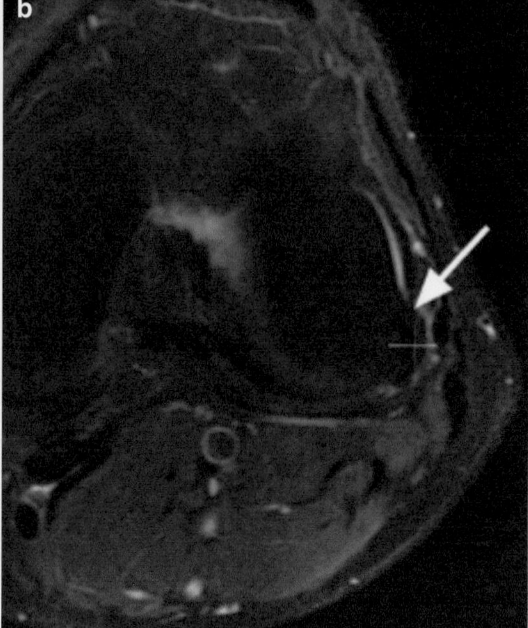

Fig. 9.8 Popliteus muscle and arcuate ligament in a 40 year old male. Sagittal proton-density (PD) image (**a**) and axial proton-density (PD) fat-suppressed image (**b**) show the popliteal tendon (*large arrows* in **a, b**) joining and the arcuate ligament (*small arrow* in **a**) at the level of posterolateral capsule (cross in **a, b**)

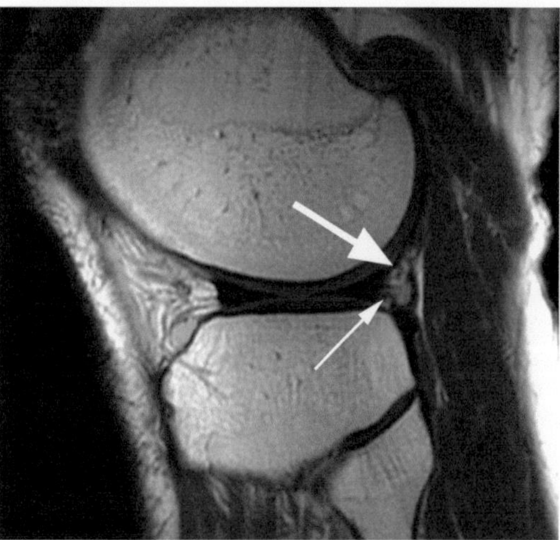

Fig. 9.9 Popliteomeniscal fascicles in a 56 year old male. Sagittal proton-density (PD) image shows the connection between the popliteus muscle and the lateral meniscus ensured by the posterosuperior (*large arrow*) and anteroinferior popliteomeniscal fascicles (*small arrow*)

Tensor Fascia Suralis Muscle

The tensor fascia suralis muscle originates in the majority of cases from the distal semitendinosus muscle and inserts into the posterior fascia of the lower leg, into the medial head of the gastrocnemius, or via a long and thin tendon onto the Achilles tendon [13, 14]. The muscle is situated superficially between the semimembranosus and semitendinosus.

Accessory Popliteus Muscle

This accessory muscle has a common origin with the lateral head of the gastrocnemius and inserts distally to the posteromedial capsule [14]. The muscle is seen on axial MR images within the popliteal fossa anterior to the popliteal vessels and nerves and may be of clinical significance in the cases of vascular compression.

9.2 MRI Pathological Findings

9.2.1 Traumatic Injuries: General Findings

MR imaging is the best imaging choice for the assessment of the muscles and tendons around

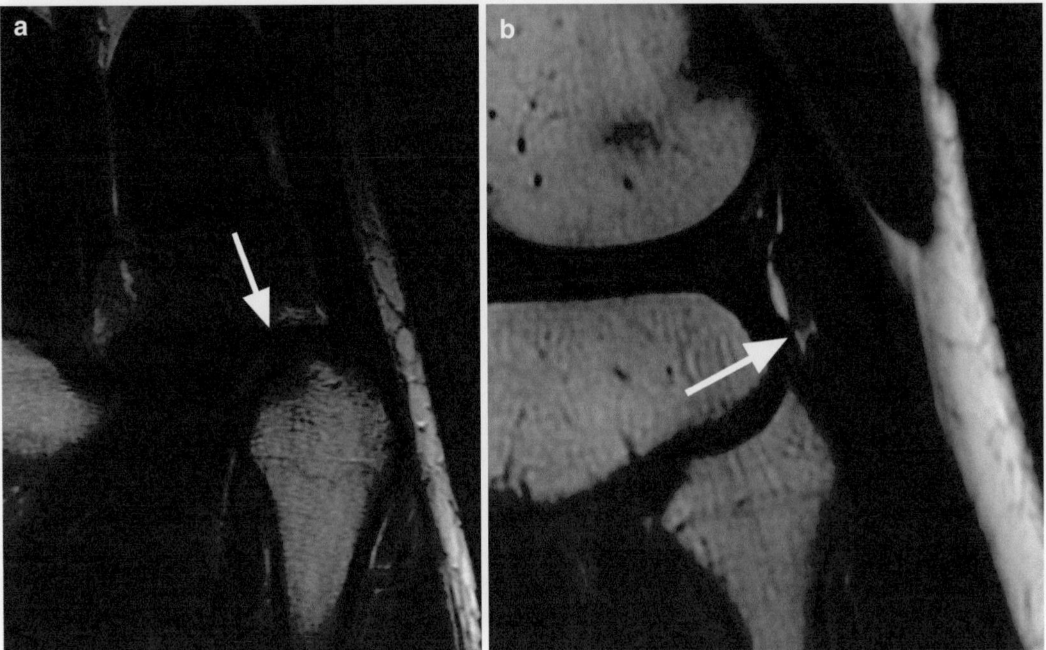

Fig. 9.10 Popliteofibular ligament in a 40 year old male. Coronal proton-density (PD) image (**a**) and sagittal proton-density (PD) image (**b**) show the popliteofibular ligament (*arrows*) connecting the popliteus tendon to the fibular head

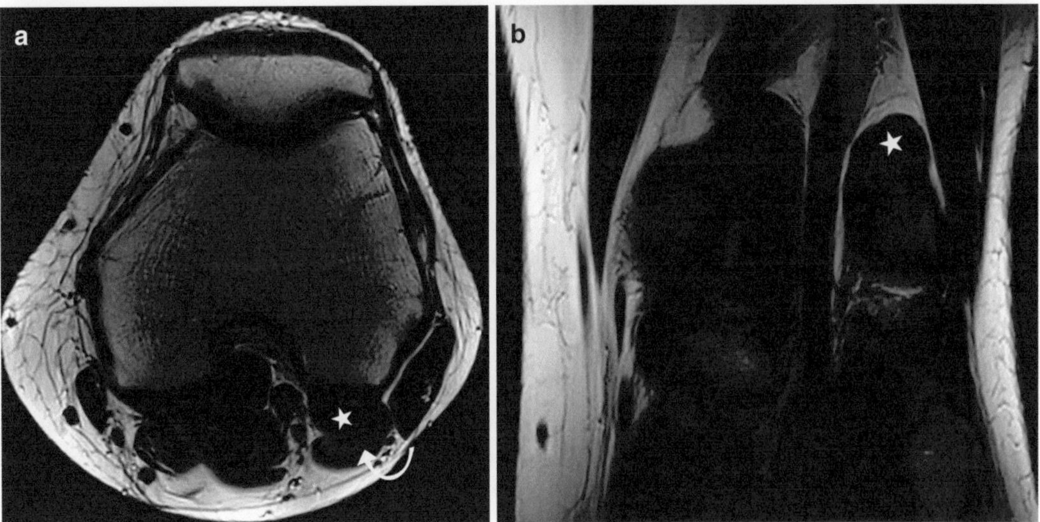

Fig. 9.11 Plantaris muscle in a 25 year old female. Axial proton-density (PD) image (**a**) and coronal proton-density (PD) image (**b**) show the plantaris muscle (*star* in **a**, **b**) originating from the posterior lateral femoral condyle. The muscle is situated at its origin anterior to the lateral gastrocnemius muscle (*curved arrow* in **a**)

the knee. In acute trauma cases, it is used to target the location, the extension, and the severity of muscle lesions. Placing a skin marker before examination (e.g., a vitamin E capsule) enables the radiologist to correlate the imaging findings with the clinical pain. A correct diagnosis is crucial for a reliable prognosis. The most common muscle injuries are contusions (direct injuries),

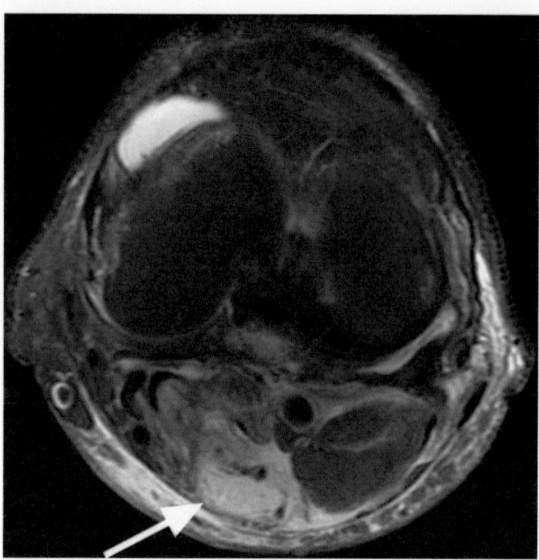

Fig. 9.12 Hematoma of the medial gastrocnemius muscle in a 51 year old male after direct muscle injury. Axial proton-density (PD) fat-suppressed image shows an ill-defined hyperintense area with fiber discontinuity indicating the intramuscular hematoma (*arrow*)

strains or tears (indirect injuries), and tendinous avulsions.

Muscular Contusions (Direct Lesions)

Muscular contusions are direct acute muscle injuries characterized by lacerations or contusions due to external forces [15, 16]. The most frequently injured muscles are the exposed rectus femoris and the vastus intermedius. Lesions can be clinically graded into mild, moderate, and severe [17]. The patient presents with pain and swelling and, occasionally, with a palpable mass. Contusions may lead to diffuse predominantly intramuscular hemorrhage with the muscle fibers displaced and compressed with or without longitudinal discontinuity. Contusions can lead to severe complications such as acute compartment syndrome, active bleeding, or large hematoma [18]. On MR imaging, the lesions appear as an ill-defined hyperintense area on T2-weighted images with or without fiber discontinuity (Fig. 9.12) or as a well-circumscribed intramuscular hematoma (Fig. 9.12). Intramuscular hematoma displays a homogeneous intermediate-signal-intensity pattern on T1-weighted images

slightly higher than that of the normal muscle. Rarely, T1-weighted hyperintense foci of hemorrhage may be seen. On T2-weighted images, acute or subacute hematoma appears as a high-signal-intensity mass (Fig. 9.12). In chronic phases, hematoma appears as an inhomogeneous well-circumscribed lesion on T1-weighted images with hyperintense foci and peripheral hypointense hemosiderin. After contrast administration, chronic hematomas may enhance at the periphery. On T2-weighted images and T2*-weighted images, hematomas are inhomogeneous and hyperintense with areas of low signal intensity and susceptibility artifacts due to blood degradation and heterotopic calcifications. Chronic intramuscular hematomas may mimic the appearance of soft tissue tumors (e.g., sarcomas). Intramuscular hematomas often resorb over a period of 6–8 weeks [19].

A complication associated with severe contusions is *myositis ossificans*, a benign proliferation of bone and cartilage in the area of contusion [16]. The reported incidence of myositis ossificans is between 9 and 17 % and should be suspected in any patient in which the symptoms worsen after 2–3 weeks accompanied by loss of functionality and persistent swelling [16, 17, 20]. Early-on myositis ossificans lesions consist of a non-ossified core of benign fibroblasts and myofibroblasts, with a minor component of osteoid and mature lamellar bone at the periphery [21]. In intermediate phases, myositis ossificans lesions are found to be surrounded by mature lamellar bone with no fibroblasts in the central portion [21]. Late-phase myositis ossificans lesion consists exclusively of mature lamellar bone. Intralesional hemorrhage, inflammation, and fibrosis or inflammation of the surrounding tissue may be present (Fig. 9.13) [21].

The bone component of myositis ossificans is identified on radiographs as early as 3 weeks after the injury [20]. On MR imaging, myositis ossificans appears in early and intermediate phases as an inhomogeneous high-signal-intensity mass on T2-weighted images with surrounding edema that can be present within 8 weeks of the onset of symptoms [21]. During

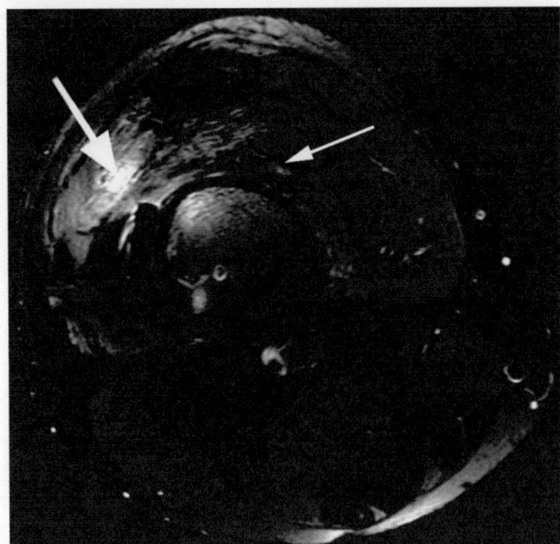

Fig. 9.13 Late-phase myositis ossificans of the quadriceps muscle in a 38 year old male. Axial proton-density (PD) fat-suppressed image shows a fibrotic indeterminate mass with hemorrhage (*large arrow*) and mature lamellar bone (*small arrow*)

these phases, it mimics a tumor. Curvilinear low-signal-intensity lesion corresponding to bone tissue may be seen within the mass. In late-phase myositis ossificans, the lesion is intermediate signal intensity on T2-weighted and T1-weighted images with peripheral low signal intensity due to calcification. Areas of fatty signal intensity and areas of decreased signal intensity due to bone formation may be seen within the lesion [21].

Strains/Tears (Indirect Lesions)

Strain is a biomechanical term, which can be used indiscriminately for anatomically and functionally different muscles and tendons [18]. However, there is no general agreement between radiologists and practitioners regarding the terminology and the definition of muscle strains and tears, and this aspect may lead to a high rate of inaccurate diagnosis or misunderstanding [18]. Use of the same classification and terminology between radiologists and clinicians is crucial to avoid premature return to full activity and the risk of reinjury [22]. We suggest the following classification system, which is based on the distinction between functional and structural muscle

disorders, but encourage all radiologists to discuss its use with the referring clinicians (Table 9.1).

The functional muscle injuries are distinct clinical entities, which lead to painful limitation for the patients or athletes. The functional injuries include *fatigue-induced muscle disorder* and *delayed onset of muscle soreness.* Although the disorders are below the sensibility of standard MR imaging techniques, they are a risk factor for structural lesions [18]. It should be noted however that in some of these disorders, dedicated MR techniques, such as muscle spectroscopy, muscle diffusion (tensor) imaging, arterial spin labeling (ASL), or intravoxel incoherent motion (IVIM) imaging, might be able to show abnormalities in the future. For now, however, these techniques are only used for research and not applicable in the clinical routine.

The term *tear* is used for *structural muscle injuries* and macroscopically damages to the muscle structure. They are easily demonstrated on MR imaging, and they can be classified based on the affected diameter of the muscle (Table 9.1). The lesions lead to loss of continuity of muscle fibers and bundles. As a result, there is a loss of contractile properties of the muscle [18].

MR imaging can aid in the investigation of acute muscle injuries in predicting recovery time based on the size, the location, and the grade of the acute traumatic muscle lesion, and all these MRI findings should be described in the MRI report in detail. Since there are no consensus guidelines or agreed-upon MRI and clinical criteria for safe return to sport following muscle injuries, the detailed MR imaging findings are generally used to assist in determining prognosis for initial injury rather than a screening for return to activity [23].

Tendinous Avulsions (Indirect Lesions)

Tendinous avulsions are indirect injuries that implies the detachment of a bone fragment from pulling away the tendon from its insertion (Fig. 9.20). Avulsions fractures around the knee are discussed in Chap. 11.

Table 9.1 Classification and MR imaging of acute muscle injuries

Classification		Definition	Clinical manifestations	MR imaging
Functional disorders	Fatigue-induced muscle disorder	Increase of muscle tone due to overexertion	Aching muscle; can provoke pain at rest	Negative
	Delayed-onset muscle soreness	More generalized pain following unaccustomed movements	Acute pain; pain at rest after activity	Negative or diffuse high-signal-intensity edema[a]
Structural lesions or tears	Minor partial tear (Figs. 9.14 and 9.15)	Injury involving a maximum diameter of less than a muscle fascicle/bundle	Sharp pain at time of injury	Fiber disruption; diffuse edema[b] and possible small intramuscular hematoma[c]
	Moderate partial tear (Fig. 9.16)	Injury involving more than a muscle fascicle/bundle	Sharp pain at time of injury; possible defect at palpation	Significant fiber disruption; may include fiber retraction; diffuse edema[b] and intramuscular hematoma[c]
	Subtotal muscle/tendon tear (Fig. 9.17)	Tear involving more than 50 % of the muscle or tendon diameter	Dull pain at time of injury; large defect at palpation	Discontinuity involving more than 50 % of the muscle or tendon diameter; possible wavy tendon and retraction; intramuscular hematoma[c]
	Complete muscle/tendon tear (Figs. 9.18 and 9.19)	Complete disruption of the muscle or tendon	Dull pain at time of injury; possible fall at time of accident; palpable defect	Complete discontinuity of the muscle or tendon; wavy tendon and muscle retraction; intramuscular hematoma[c]

Modified after Mueller-Wohlfahrt et al. [18]

[a]Diffuse hyperintense muscle on T2-weighted images

[b]Ill-defined, feathery hyperintensity on T2-weighted images intermuscular and between the muscle fibers/bundles

[c]Intramuscular diffuse or well-delineated intermediate-signal-intensity lesion on T1-weighted images and high signal intensity on T2-weighted images

9.2.2 Traumatic Injuries: Clinical and Imaging Findings of Specific Muscles Around the Knee

Anterior Muscle Group Injuries (Quadriceps Muscle and Tendon)

Partial or complete tear of the quadriceps occurs frequently in sports activities and may appear anywhere in the distal part of the muscle. Most commonly, it involves the tendon of the vastus intermedius and the myotendinous junction of the rectus femoris muscle. Repetitive trauma or strong deceleration may result in tears of the quadriceps tendon above the patellar insertion or acute avulsion at the patellar insertion [24]. Spontaneous tears occur in degenerated or weakened quadriceps muscle tendons (Fig. 9.21). Underlying causes include gout, diabetes, hyperparathyroidism, and collagen vascular diseases [25].

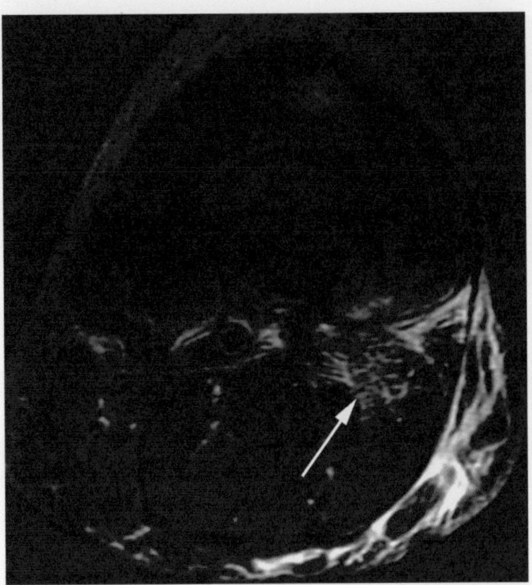

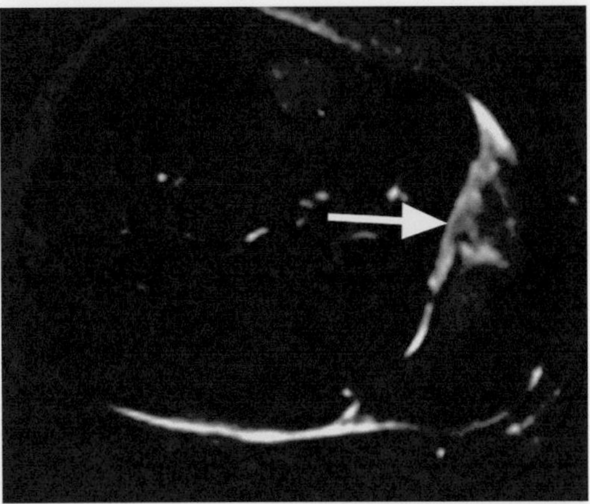

Fig. 9.16 Moderate partial tear of the medial gastrocnemius muscle. Axial T2-weighted fat-suppressed image shows diffuse high-signal-intensity changes which involve more than a muscle fascicle/bundle (*arrow*)

Fig. 9.14 Minor partial tear of the biceps muscle in a 48 year old female. Axial proton-density (PD) fat-suppressed image shows diffuse edema in the muscle (*arrow*) without fiber discontinuity and without hematoma

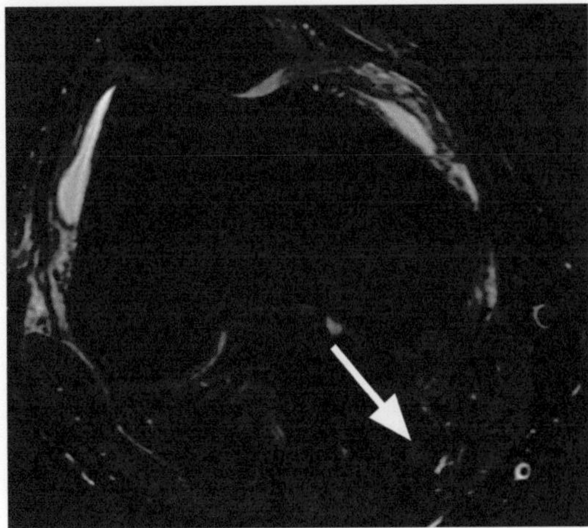

Fig. 9.15 Minor partial tear of the semimembranosus muscle in a 45 year old female. Axial proton-density (PD) fat-suppressed image shows a small hematoma in the semimembranosus muscle (*arrow*) involving less than a muscle fascicle

Posteromedial Muscle Group Injuries

The distal tendons of the *sartorius, gracilis, and semitendinosus* muscles converge into a common insertion constituting the so-called pes anserinus. The sartorius muscle is commonly susceptible to injuries due to its superficial location [25]. *Pes anserinus tendino-bursitis* is a syndrome characterized by spontaneous medial knee pain with tenderness in the inferomedial aspect of the joint [26]. The syndrome may appear in runners as well as in patients with rheumatoid arthritis or osteoarthritis. Diabetes mellitus is also a known predisposing factor for this syndrome [26].

Injuries to the *semimembranosus tendon* (Fig. 9.15) can lead to muscle or tendon tears or to avulsion fractures at the insertion. Semimembranosus tendon tears are commonly associated with tears of the origin of the medial head of the gastrocnemius tendon especially in patients with posteromedial instability [25]. Avulsion injury of the insertion of the semimembranosus tendon results from a valgus stress to the knee and is usually associated with anterior cruciate ligament tears and tears of the posterior horn of the medial meniscus [27].

Traumatic injuries to *the medial head of the gastrocnemius muscle* may appear in combination with a rupture of the soleus and/or plantaris muscle or can be isolated and are then referred to as "tennis leg" [25, 28, 29]. The injuries are usually located at the proximal or midportion of the lower leg.

Posterolateral Muscle Group Injuries

Iliotibial band syndrome (iliotibial friction syndrome) is the most common cause of lateral knee symptoms in runners, with an incidence from 1.6

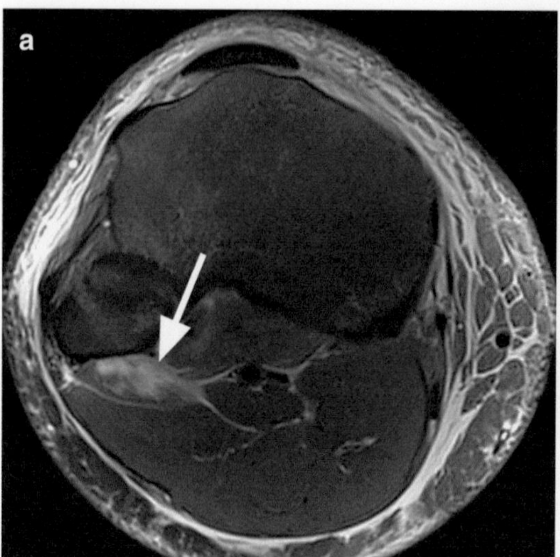

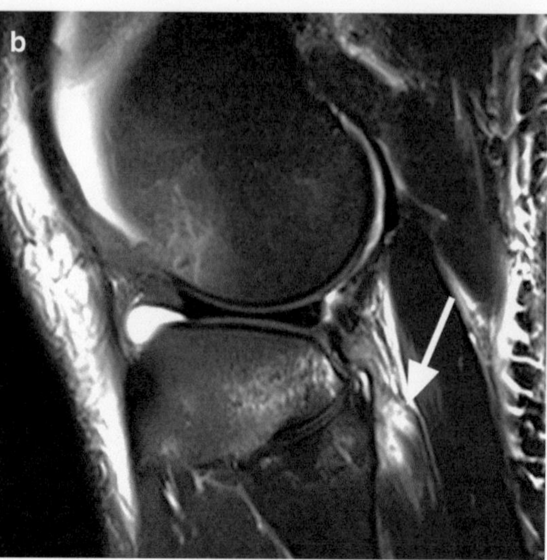

Fig. 9.17 Subtotal soleus muscle in a 21 year old male. Axial proton-density (PD) fat-suppressed image (**a**) and sagittal T2-weighted fat-suppressed image (**b**) show dif- fuse edema and hematoma (*arrow*) involving more than 50 % of the soleus muscle

to 12 % [30–34]. The syndrome was also reported in rowers, skiers, and soccer and hockey players [33, 35, 36]. The patient present initially with pain to the region of the distal iliotibial band and, as the condition worsens, with pain at rest [37]. The etiology is debatable. The most common theories include the friction of the iliotibial band against the lateral femoral condyle and chronic inflammation of the iliotibial bursa [37]. However, studies using histological examinations of cadaver knees and patients concluded that ilio- tibial band syndrome is a "fascia lata compres- sion syndrome" of the highly vascularized and innervated adipose tissue beneath the iliotibial band [38]. The MR imaging findings include poorly defined soft tissue edema of low signal intensity on T1-weighted images and high signal intensity on T2-weighted images in the fatty tis- sue deep to the iliotibial band (Fig. 9.22) [39]. The signal alteration may extend into the fatty tissue distal to the vastus lateralis and into the area between the iliotibial band and the biceps femoris muscle [39]. Thickening of the iliotibial band is seen especially in subacute and chronic stages. Circumscribed fluid collections are pres- ent in a minority of patients, but the differentiation

between this bursa-like reactive appearance and a true bursa is difficult [39, 40]. In some cases, dis- crete bone marrow edema involving the lateral femoral condyle adjacent to the iliotibial band can be identified on coronal MR images.

Being a lateral stabilizer of the knee, partial or complete tear of the iliotibial band may be seen on MR images in patients with acute posterolat- eral instability [25].

The mechanism of injury of the posterolateral corner of the knee is involved in *the biceps ten- don and popliteus tendon and muscle* injuries (e.g., direct varus force to the anteromedial aspect of the hyperextended knee). Isolated biceps ten- don (Fig. 9.23) and popliteal muscle injuries are very rare since almost 90 % of the patients with posterolateral injuries have multiligamentous injuries [41]. The popliteus tendon is involved in more than two thirds of the patients, and the biceps tendon is involved in more than one third of the patients with posterolateral corner injuries [41]. It is critical, however, to recognize all lesions of the structures that are involved in patients with posterolateral stability.

Injuries of the muscle and myotendinous junc- tion are the most common injuries of the popliteus

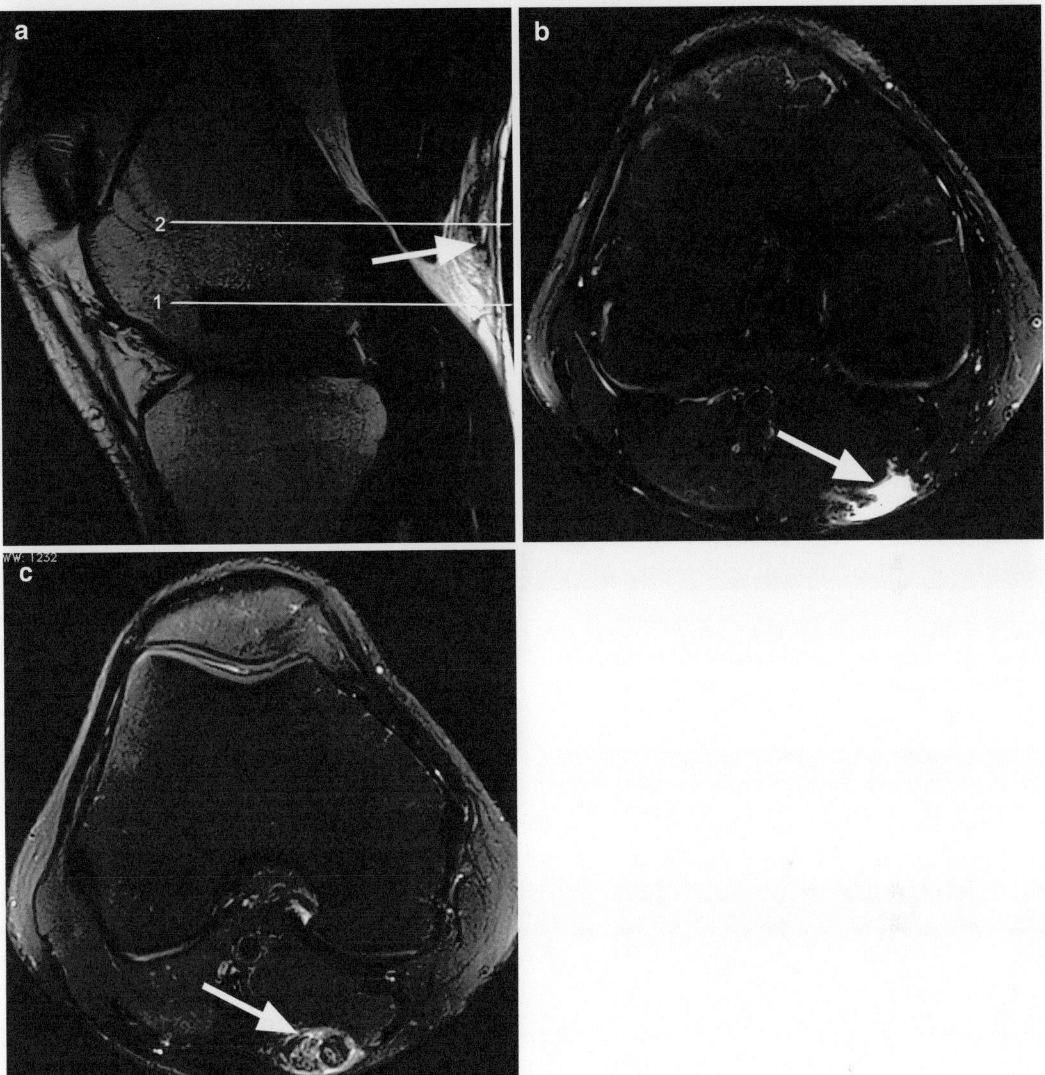

Fig. 9.18 Complete tear of the biceps tendon in a 25 year old male. Sagittal proton-density (PD) image (**a**) shows complete disruption of the biceps tendon with tendon retraction (*arrow*). Axial proton-density (PD) fat-suppressed image (**b**) through a plane caudally to the retracted tendon (*line* 1 in **a**) shows the presence of hematoma and the absence of the tendon at this level (*arrow*). Axial proton-density (PD) fat-suppressed image (**b**) obtained more cranially (*line* 2 in **a**) shows the retracted tendon with surrounding edema (*arrow*)

(Fig. 9.24) [42]. Avulsion fractures of the popliteus or the biceps tendon may be present, and the diagnosis is based on the identification of the donor site and the avulsed bone fragment. MR imaging is superior to radiographs and clearly demonstrates both the donor site and the bone fragment. This is especially useful in the cases in which the differential diagnosis between avulsion of the biceps tendon or the arcuate sign is equivocal on radiography (Fig. 9.20) [43].

Rupture of *the plantaris muscle* usually occurs at the myotendinous junction with or without an associated hematoma. A proximal injury of the plantaris muscle may occur as an isolated injury

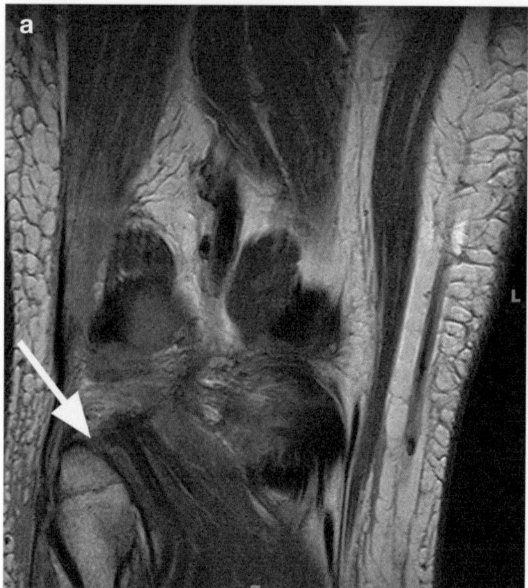
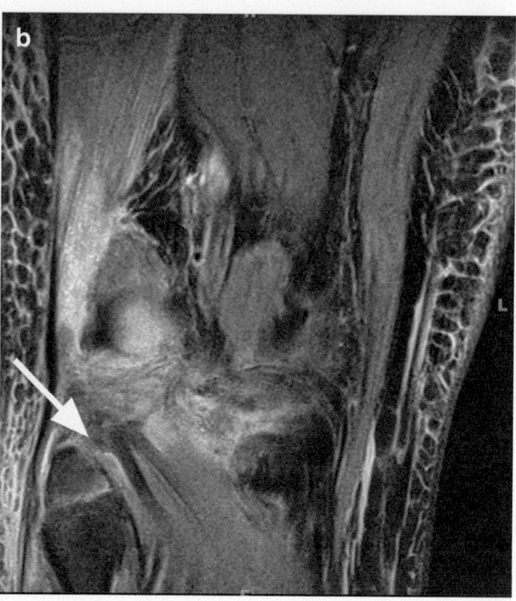

Fig. 9.19 Tear of popliteofibular ligament. Coronal proton-density (PD) image (**a**) and coronal T2-weighted fat-suppressed image (**b**) show a complete tear of the popliteofibular ligament with small hematoma at the fibular insertion (*arrow*)

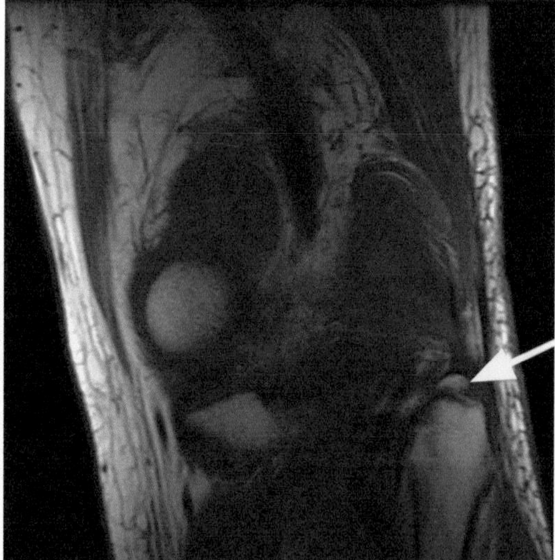

Fig. 9.20 The arcuate sign in a 51 year old male. Coronal proton-density (PD) image shows a detached bone fragment from the fibular head (*arrow*) resulting from biceps tendon avulsion

after a forceful contraction of the muscle, but in most of the cases, it is accompanied by partial tear of the medial head of the gastrocnemius muscle, tear of the anterior cruciate ligament, or posterolateral corner injuries [29].

Tears of *the lateral head of the gastrocnemius* muscle occur in patients with injuries that lead to posterolateral corner instability and are usually involved together with the popliteus tendon, biceps tendon, and plantaris muscle [25].

9.2.3 Intratendinous and Peritendinous Ganglion Cyst

Intratendinous ganglion cysts are uncommon lesions, but a correct diagnosis is necessary for differentiation from other pathologies and for a proper treatment modality [44]. Although ganglion cyst are usually painless, when symptomatic, they cause pain, local edema, and inflammation. Intratendinous ganglion cysts around the knee were reported in the tendon of the quadriceps muscle, semimembranosus muscle, and patellar tendon [44–46]. Repetitive trauma to the tendon with subsequent cystic degeneration or a congenital anomaly of the tendon in patients without trauma may be responsible for the intratendinous and peritendinous cyst

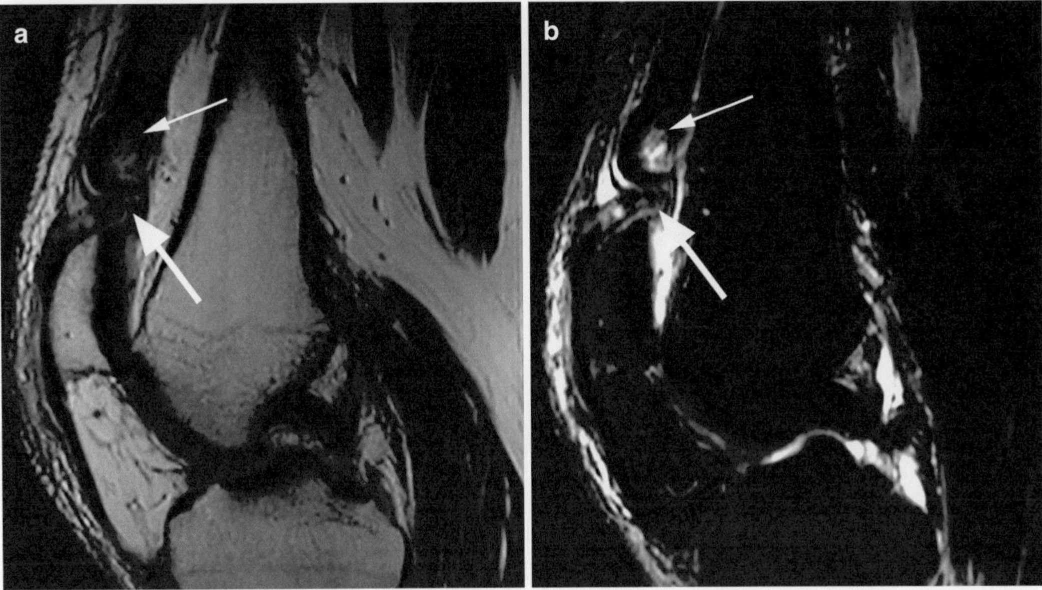

Fig. 9.21 Complete quadriceps tendon tear in a 63 year old male. Sagittal proton-density (PD) image (**a**) and sagittal T2-weighted fat-suppressed image (**b**) show a complete tear of the quadriceps tendon (*large arrow*). Note the degenerative changes of the tendon (*small arrow*) which indicates a weakened tendon

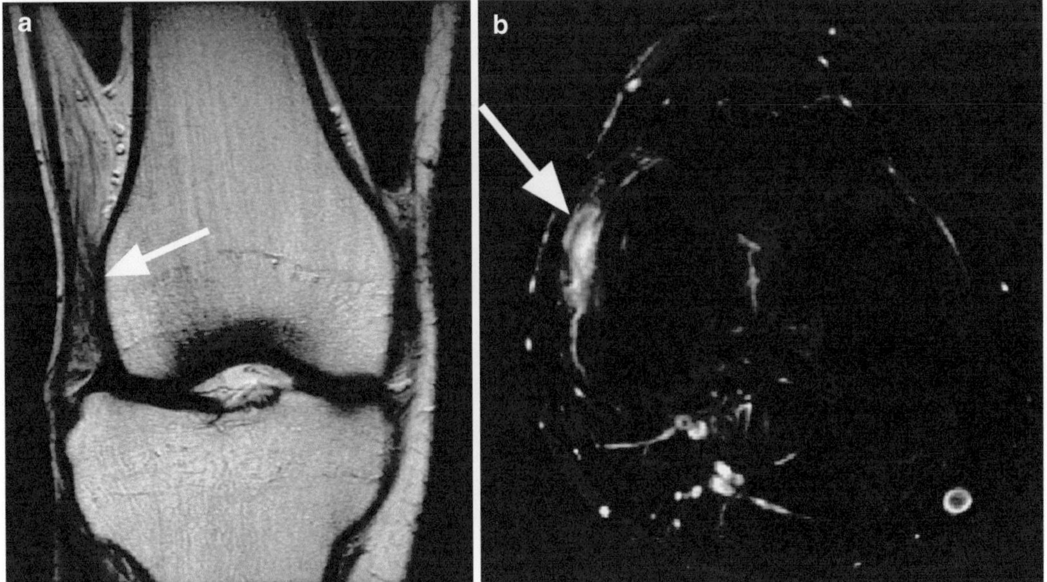

Fig. 9.22 Iliotibial band syndrome (iliotibial friction syndrome) in a 22 year old male. Coronal proton-density (PD) image (**a**) and axial proton-density (PD) fat-suppressed image (**b**) show a poorly defined soft tissue edema (*arrow*) in the fatty tissue between the iliotibial band and the femoral condyle

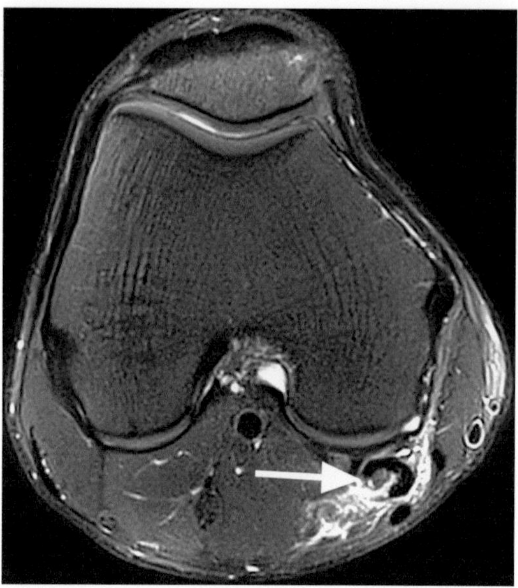

Fig. 9.23 Subtotal biceps tendon tear in a 31 year old male. Axial proton-density (PD) fat-suppressed image shows focal high-signal-intensity lesion which involves more than 50 % of the tendon diameter (*arrow*)

formation [47, 48]. On MR imaging, the cysts are well-delineated uni- or multilobulated lesions homogeneous hypointense on T1-weighted images and hyperintense on T2-weighted images. They may present internal septation and are located adjacent to the tendon.

9.3 MRI Impression

1. Anomalous muscle – description of insertion and position relative to neurovascular bundle
2. Muscle contusion or muscle tear – including the specific muscle or muscles, the extension of the lesion, and the grade (minor, moderate, or subtotal/complete tear)
3. Myositis ossificans – location and dimension
4. Intra- or peritendinous ganglion cyst – location and dimension

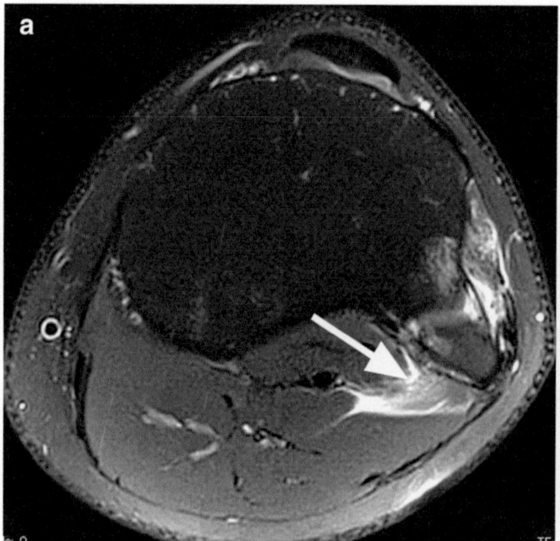
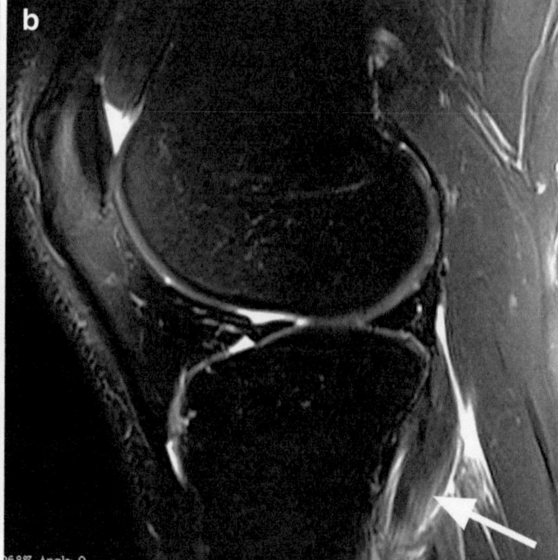

Fig. 9.24 Moderate partial tear of the musculotendinous junction of popliteus muscle in a 26 year old male. Axial proton-density (PD) fat-suppressed image (**a**), sagittal T2-weighted fat-suppressed image (**b**), and coronal proton-density (PD) fat-suppressed image (**c**) show diffuse edema involving more than a muscle fascicle but less than 50 % of the muscle thickness (*arrow*)

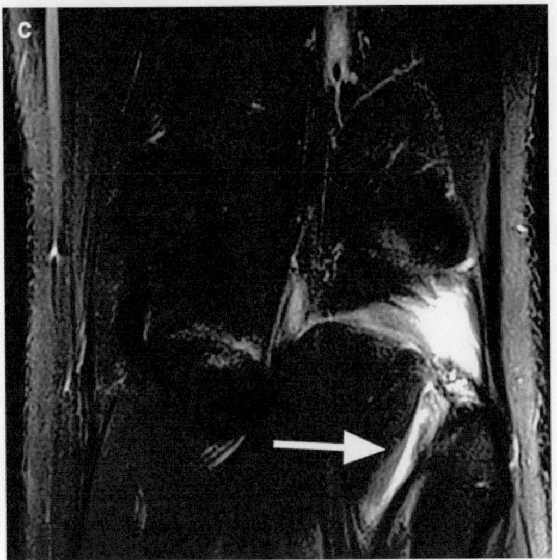

Fig. 9.24 (continued)

References

1. Waligora AC, Johanson NA, Hirsch BE. Clinical anatomy of the quadriceps femoris and extensor apparatus of the knee. Clin Orthop Relat Res. 2009;467(12): 3297–306.
2. Zeiss J, Saddemi SR, Ebraheim NA. MR imaging of the quadriceps tendon: normal layered configuration and its importance in cases of tendon rupture. AJR Am J Roentgenol. 1992;159(5):1031–4.
3. Fulkerson JP, Gossling HR. Anatomy of the knee joint lateral retinaculum. Clin Orthop Relat Res. 1980;153: 183–8.
4. Vieira EL, et al. An anatomic study of the iliotibial tract. Arthroscopy. 2007;23(3):269–74.
5. Munshi M, et al. MR imaging, MR arthrography, and specimen correlation of the posterolateral corner of the knee: an anatomic study. AJR Am J Roentgenol. 2003;180(4):1095–101.
6. Staubli HU, Birrer S. The popliteus tendon and its fascicles at the popliteal hiatus: gross anatomy and functional arthroscopic evaluation with and without anterior cruciate ligament deficiency. Arthroscopy. 1990;6(3):209–20.
7. Watanabe Y, et al. Functional anatomy of the posterolateral structures of the knee. Arthroscopy. 1993;9(1): 57–62.
8. Recondo JA, et al. Lateral stabilizing structures of the knee: functional anatomy and injuries assessed with MR imaging. Radiographics. 2000;20 Spec No:S91–102.
9. Bolog N, Hodler J. MR imaging of the posterolateral corner of the knee. Skeletal Radiol. 2007;36(8): 715–28.
10. Levien LJ. Popliteal artery entrapment syndrome. Semin Vasc Surg. 2003;16(3):223–31.
11. Macedo TA, et al. Popliteal artery entrapment syndrome: role of imaging in the diagnosis. AJR Am J Roentgenol. 2003;181(5):1259–65.
12. Kim HK, Laor T, Racadio JM. MR imaging assessment of the lateral head of the gastrocnemius muscle: prevalence of segmental anomalous origins in children and young adults. Pediatr Radiol. 2008;38(12):1300–5.
13. Tubbs RS, Salter EG, Oakes WJ. Dissection of a rare accessory muscle of the leg: the tensor fasciae suralis muscle. Clin Anat. 2006;19(6):571–2.
14. Sookur PA, et al. Accessory muscles: anatomy, symptoms, and radiologic evaluation. Radiographics. 2008; 28(2):481–99.
15. Beiner JM, Jokl P. Muscle contusion injuries: current treatment options. J Am Acad Orthop Surg. 2001;9(4): 227–37.
16. Kary JM. Diagnosis and management of quadriceps strains and contusions. Curr Rev Musculoskelet Med. 2010;3(1–4):26–31.
17. Ryan JB, et al. Quadriceps contusions. West Point update. Am J Sports Med. 1991;19(3):299–304.
18. Mueller-Wohlfahrt HW, et al. Terminology and classification of muscle injuries in sport: the Munich consensus statement. Br J Sports Med. 2013;47(6):342–50.
19. El-Khoury GY, et al. Imaging of muscle injuries. Skeletal Radiol. 1996;25(1):3–11.
20. Beiner JM, Jokl P. Muscle contusion injury and myositis ossificans traumatica. Clin Orthop Relat Res. 2002;403S:S110–S119.doi:10.1097/00003086-200210001-00013
21. Kransdorf MJ, Meis JM, Jelinek JS. Myositis ossificans: MR appearance with radiologic-pathologic correlation. AJR Am J Roentgenol. 1991;157(6):1243–8.
22. Malliaropoulos N, et al. Posterior thigh muscle injuries in elite track and field athletes. Am J Sports Med. 2010;38(9):1813–9.
23. Orchard J, Best TM, Verrall GM. Return to play following muscle strains. Clin J Sport Med. 2005;15(6): 436–41.
24. Sonin AH, et al. MR imaging appearance of the extensor mechanism of the knee: functional anatomy and injury patterns. Radiographics. 1995;15(2):367–82.
25. Bencardino JT, et al. Traumatic musculotendinous injuries of the knee: diagnosis with MR imaging. Radiographics. 2000;20 Spec No:S103–20.
26. Helfenstein Jr M, Kuromoto J. Anserine syndrome. Rev Bras Reumatol. 2010;50(3):313–27.
27. Chan KK, et al. Posteromedial tibial plateau injury including avulsion fracture of the semimembranous tendon insertion site: ancillary sign of anterior cruciate ligament tear at MR imaging. Radiology. 1999;211(3):754–8.
28. Menz MJ, Lucas GL. Magnetic resonance imaging of a rupture of the medial head of the gastrocnemius muscle. A case report. J Bone Joint Surg Am. 1991; 73(8):1260–2.
29. Helms CA, Fritz RC, Garvin GJ. Plantaris muscle injury: evaluation with MR imaging. Radiology. 1995;195(1):201–3.
30. Messier SP, et al. Etiology of iliotibial band friction syndrome in distance runners. Med Sci Sports Exerc. 1995;27(7):951–60.

31. Fredericson M, et al. Hip abductor weakness in distance runners with iliotibial band syndrome. Clin J Sport Med. 2000;10(3):169–75.
32. Ellis R, Hing W, Reid D. Iliotibial band friction syndrome–a systematic review. Man Ther. 2007;12(3): 200–8.
33. Lavine R. Iliotibial band friction syndrome. Curr Rev Musculoskelet Med. 2010;3(1–4):18–22.
34. Tenforde AS, et al. Overuse injuries in high school runners: lifetime prevalence and prevention strategies. PM R. 2011;3(2):125–31; quiz 131.
35. Devan MR, et al. A prospective study of overuse knee injuries among female athletes with muscle imbalances and structural abnormalities. J Athl Train. 2004;39(3):263–7.
36. Rumball JS, et al. Rowing injuries. Sports Med. 2005;35(6):537–55.
37. Strauss EJ, et al. Iliotibial band syndrome: evaluation and management. J Am Acad Orthop Surg. 2011; 19(12):728–36.
38. Fairclough J, et al. The functional anatomy of the iliotibial band during flexion and extension of the knee: implications for understanding iliotibial band syndrome. J Anat. 2006;208(3):309–16.
39. Muhle C, et al. Iliotibial band friction syndrome: MR imaging findings in 16 patients and MR arthrographic study of six cadaveric knees. Radiology. 1999;212(1): 103–10.
40. Martens M, Libbrecht P, Burssens A. Surgical treatment of the iliotibial band friction syndrome. Am J Sports Med. 1989;17(5):651–4.
41. Becker EH, Watson JD, Dreese JC. Investigation of multiligamentous knee injury patterns with associated injuries presenting at a level I trauma center. J Orthop Trauma. 2013;27(4):226–31.
42. Brown TR, et al. Diagnosis of popliteus injuries with MR imaging. Skeletal Radiol. 1995;24(7):511–4.
43. Gottsegen CJ, et al. Avulsion fractures of the knee: imaging findings and clinical significance. Radiographics. 2008;28(6):1755–70.
44. Vayvada H, et al. Giant ganglion cyst of the quadriceps femoris tendon. Knee Surg Sports Traumatol Arthrosc. 2003;11(4):260–2.
45. Kim SK, et al. Intratendinous ganglion cyst of the semimembranosus tendon. Br J Radiol. 2010;83(988): e79–82.
46. Jose J, O'Donnell K, Lesniak B. Symptomatic intratendinous ganglion cyst of the patellar tendon. Orthopedics. 2011;34(2):135.
47. Robertson DE. Cystic degeneration of the peroneus brevis tendon. J Bone Joint Surg Br. 1959;41-B(2): 362–4.
48. Pedrinelli A, et al. Anterior cruciate ligament ganglion: case report. Sao Paulo Med J. 2002;120(6): 195–7.

Nicolae Bolog, Gustav Andreisek, and Erika Ulbrich

10.1 Anatomy and Normal MRI Appearance

On MR imaging of the knee, the most important vascular and nervous structures that are identified are the popliteal neurovascular bundle and the common peroneal nerve. However, several structures around the knee are vascularized or innervated by arteries or nerves that are not within the field of view of a normal knee MRI examination. The vascularization and innervation of the knee structures are detailed in Table 10.1.

The popliteal neurovascular bundle consists of the popliteal artery, the popliteal vein, sural veins, and the tibial nerve. On "conventional" axial MR images, the neurovascular bundle is identified posterior to the intercondylar femoral fossa, between the lateral and the medial heads of the gastrocnemius (Fig. 10.1). The common peroneal nerve is located superficial and posterior to the lateral head of the gastrocnemius and adjacent to the medial margin of the biceps femoris (Fig. 10.1).

10.1.1 Arteries

The popliteal artery is the continuation of the femoral artery. It descends slightly lateral to the intercondylar fossa, anterior to the popliteal vein and the tibial nerve, and it ends at the inferior margin of the popliteus muscle where it divides into the anterior and posterior tibial arteries

(Fig. 10.2). Some authors use the term *tibial-peroneal trunk* for the arterial segment located between the origin of the anterior tibial artery which arises first and the origin of the posterior tibial artery and peroneal arteries [4, 5]. The length of the tibial-peroneal trunk is approximately 30 mm but can vary significantly [5]. Awareness of the anatomy of the popliteal artery, its variations, and its branches is important for radiologists and surgeons especially in complex traumatic injuries of the knee, such as dislocations, with a high likelihood for vascular involvement. The popliteal artery diameter is 7–8 mm and the length is approximately 190 mm [5]. Variants of branching pattern are rare. An important variant is *the aberrant anterior tibial artery* when the origin of the artery is high (proximal) and the tibial anterior artery courses inferiorly along the anterior surface of the popliteus muscle [6, 7]. The aberrant artery is at high risk of injury during surgery [6]. Another variant is the so-called trifurcation pattern. In this variant, the anterior tibial artery, the posterior tibial artery, and the peroneal arteries originate together from the popliteal artery [5].

The middle genicular artery originates from the anterolateral surface of the popliteal artery in the popliteal fossa, 3–5 cm proximal to the joint line either alone or having a common origin with the lateral genicular artery [8]. It is 3–5 cm long and is situated between the popliteal artery anteriorly and the knee capsule posteriorly [8]. The artery is accompanied by two venae comitantes.

N.V. Bolog et al., *MRI of the Knee: A Guide to Evaluation and Reporting*,
DOI 10.1007/978-3-319-08165-6_10, © Springer International Publishing Switzerland 2015

Table 10.1 The vascularization and innervation of the main knee structures [1–3]

Anatomical structure	Vascularization	Innervation
Anterior cruciate ligament	Vascular synovial envelope from the middle genicular artery	Tibial nerve; nociceptive and proprioceptive receptors
Posterior cruciate ligament	Mainly from the middle genicular artery; inferior medial and lateral genicular arteries also vascularize the ligament via the fat pad	Tibial nerve; nociceptive and proprioceptive receptors
Menisci	Perimeniscal plexus from branches of lateral and medial genicular arteries; blood reaches the outer 10–33 % of the body of menisci	Tibial nerve; nociceptors and mechanoreceptors reaching the outer 66 % of the meniscus
Cartilage	Devoid of vascularity	Devoid of innervation
Capsule	Poorly vascularized	Highly innervated: nociceptors and mechanoreceptors
Synovia	Highly vascularized from periarticular anastomotic plexus	Poorly innervated (insensitive to pain)
Muscles around the knee		
Quadriceps muscle and tendon	Descending genicular artery and both superior genicular arteries	Femoral nerve
Sartorius and semimembranosus	Descending genicular artery, branches of popliteal artery, and superior and inferior genicular arteries	Femoral nerve
Gracilis	Branches of popliteal artery and inferior genicular artery distally	Obturator nerve
Semitendinosus	Branches of popliteal artery and inferior genicular artery distally	Tibial nerve
Medial and lateral head of the gastrocnemius, popliteus	Popliteal artery (sural branches), medial and lateral inferior genicular arteries, posterior tibial artery, and peroneal artery	Tibial nerve
Biceps femoris	Popliteal artery (muscular branches)	Tibial nerve
Plantaris	Popliteal artery (sural branches), posterior tibial artery, and peroneal artery	Tibial nerve
Bones		
Patella	Five to six arteries forming an anastomotic network called Rete patellae; the descending genicular artery, superior and inferior genicular arteries, and anterior tibial recurrent artery contribute to this network	Femoral nerve through its vastus medialis and lateralis branches
Distal femur	Superior and inferior genicular arteries (lateral condyle) and medial genicular artery and popliteal artery (medial condyle)	Tibial nerve
Proximal tibia	Anterior and posterior tibial arteries	Tibial nerve
Tibiofibular joint	Anterior tibial artery	Common peroneal nerve

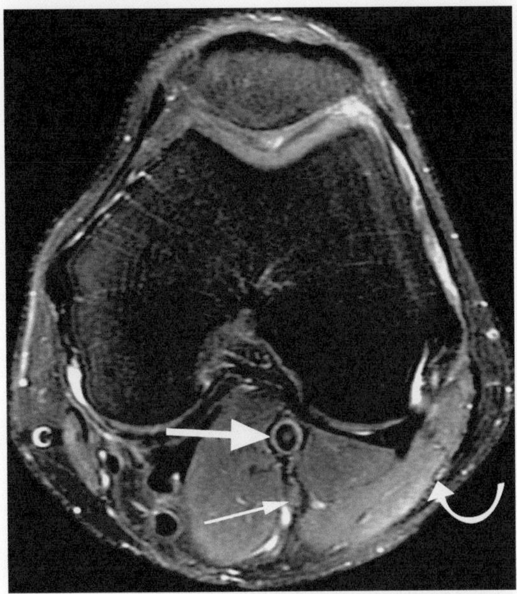

Fig. 10.1 The popliteal neurovascular bundle in a 40 year old male. Axial proton-density (PD) image shows the popliteal artery (*large arrow*), the tibial nerve (*small arrow*), and the common peroneal nerve (*curved arrow*)

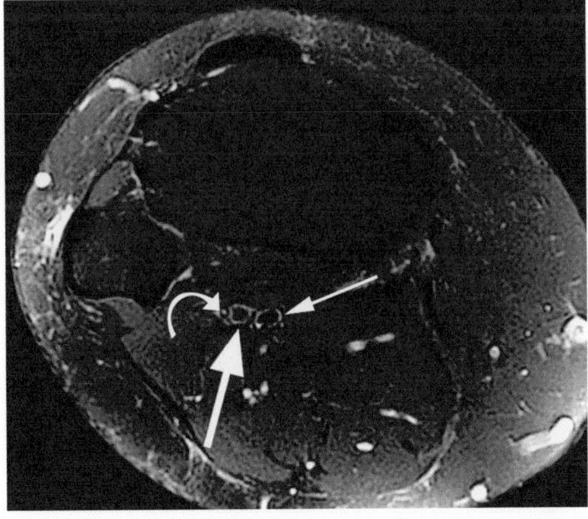

Fig. 10.2 The anterior and posterior tibial arteries in a 44 year old female. Axial proton-density (PD) image shows the anterior tibial artery (*large arrow*) and posterior tibial artery (*small arrow*). Note the popliteal vein adjacent to the anterior tibial artery (*curved arrow*)

The superior medial genicular artery originates primarily from the femoral artery. It descends under the semimembranosus and semitendinosus muscle above the medial head of the

gastrocnemius muscle and bifurcates into a superficial and a deep branch [9]. The deep branch joins the anterior tibial recurrent artery on the level of medial tibial plateau. It ends into and supplies the perimeniscal capillary plexus.

The superior lateral genicular artery arises from the popliteal artery beneath the lateral gastrocnemius muscle and passes under the biceps femoris tendon. It divides into a superficial and a deep branch and forms an anastomotic arch with the medial inferior genicular artery [9].

The inferior medial genicular artery originates from the popliteal artery closed to the origin of the anterior tibial artery [5]. It descends along the upper margin of the popliteus muscle, below the medial tibial plateau, and passes deep to the lateral collateral ligament.

The inferior lateral genicular artery originates from the anterior tibial artery deep to the lateral gastrocnemius muscle and runs laterally adjacent to the anterior aspect of the lateral tibial plateau and above the tibiofibular joint [5, 9]. The artery is situated deep to the lateral collateral ligament and biceps tendon.

The (medial and lateral) sural arteries originate just above the knee joint from the popliteal artery and distribute to the gastrocnemius, soleus, and plantaris muscles [9]. The sural artery is intimately connected to the sural nerve and supplies the skin of the lower and middle leg.

10.1.2 Veins

The popliteal vein is part of the deep vein system of the knee and collects the blood from the four anterior and posterior tibial veins. The popliteal vein is part of the popliteal neurovascular bundle and passes anteromedially in the distal thigh joining the deep femoral vein (Figs. 10.2 and 10.3).

The great saphenous vein is part of the superficial venous system of the leg and is situated within the subcutaneous tissue on the anteromedial aspect of the knee region (Fig. 10.4).

The sural veins and the genicular veins accompany the sural and genicular arteries.

Usually, there are five genicular veins which provide drainage to the knee.

10.1.3 Nerves

The tibial nerve is one of the two major branches of the sciatic nerve together with the common peroneal nerve. It branches off the sciatic nerve above the popliteal fossa where it is located lateral to the semimembranosus muscle. The tibial nerve descends between the medial and lateral heads of the gastrocnemius muscle and joins the neurovascular popliteal bundle. Within the neurovascular bundle, the tibial nerve is situated posterior to the popliteal artery and vein (Fig. 10.1). In the popliteal fossa, it divides into an articular branch to the knee, a cutaneous branch, and several branches to the calf muscles.

The common peroneal nerve descends from its origin, the sciatic nerve, posterior to the biceps femoris muscle and anterior to the tibial nerve and becomes more superficial at the knee line joint. At this level, the common peroneal nerve is located posterior to the biceps tendon and lateral to the lateral head of gastrocnemius muscle (Fig. 10.5). At the level of the proximal popliteal fossa, it divides into *the superficial perineal nerve and the deep peroneal nerve* which are both located posterior to the common peroneal nerve.

The nerves around the knee supply different groups of muscles of the leg. Knowing this distribution is important for the diagnosis of neuropathies based on indirect signs of muscles denervation (e.g., muscle atrophy) (Table 10.2).

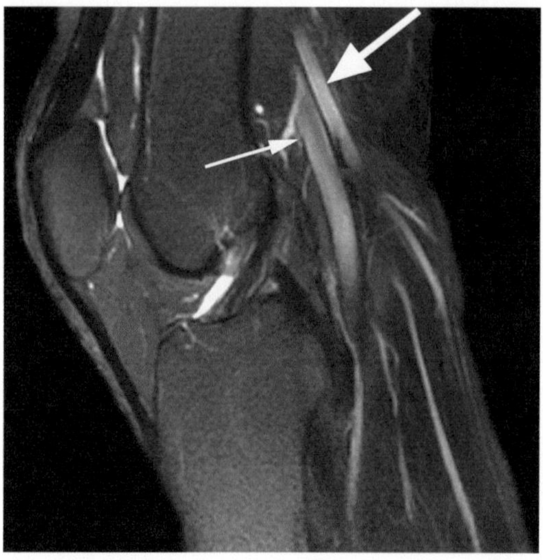

Fig. 10.3 The popliteal vein in a 40 year old male. Sagittal T2-weighted fat-suppressed image shows the popliteal vein (*large arrow*) posterior to the popliteal artery (*small arrow*)

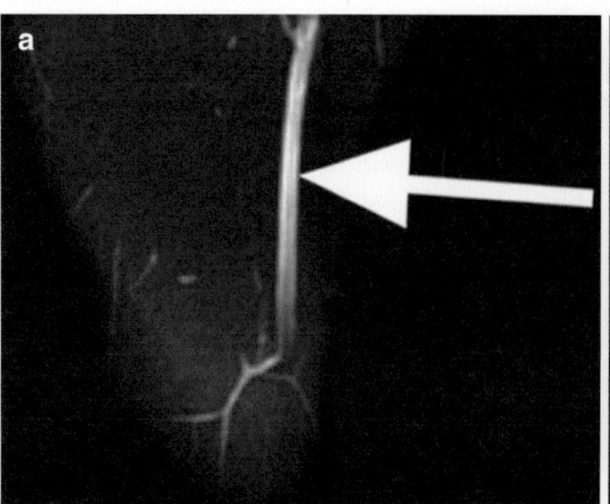

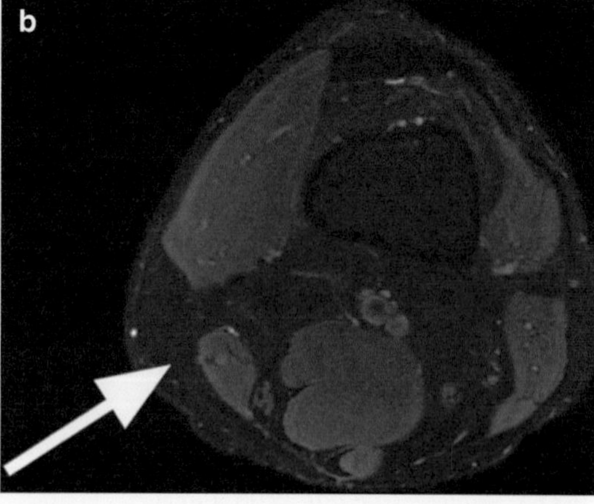

Fig. 10.4 The great saphenous vein in a 40 year old male. Sagittal T2-weighted fat-suppressed image (**a**) and axial proton-density (PD) image (**b**) show the great saphenous vein (*large arrows* in **a**, **b**) situated within the subcutaneous tissue on the medial aspect of the knee

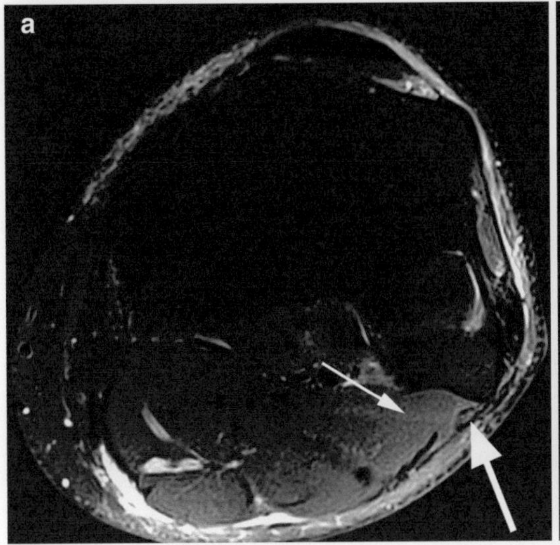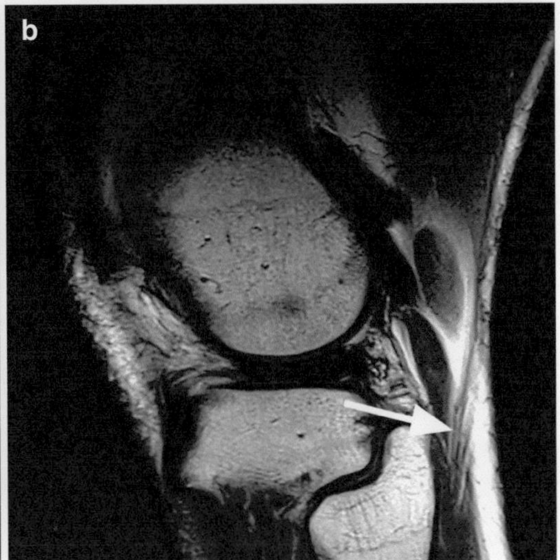

Fig. 10.5 The common peroneal nerve in 55 year old male. Axial proton-density (PD) fat-suppressed image (**a**) and sagittal proton-density (PD) image (**b**) show the common peroneal nerve (*large arrow* in **a**, **b**) posterior to the biceps tendon and lateral to the lateral head of gastrocnemius muscle (*small arrow* in **a**)

Table 10.2 Innervation of the muscles around the knee

Nerve	Muscles supplied
Tibial nerve	Posteromedial and posterolateral muscles of the knee:
	Long tendon of biceps muscle
	Popliteus muscle
	Gastrocnemius muscle (medial and lateral head)
	Plantaris muscle
	Soleus muscle
Superficial peroneal nerve	Lateral compartment of the leg:
	Peroneus brevis muscle
	Peroneus longus muscle
Deep peroneal nerve	Anterior compartment of the leg:
	Tibialis anterior muscle
	Extensor hallucis longus
	Extensor hallucis brevis

10.2 MRI Pathological Findings: Arteries

The main knee arteries can be affected by a variety of pathological conditions (Table 10.3). The affected patient population and the etiology of the pathological changes are often distinct, but the clinical signs and symptoms may frequently overlap [10]. MR imaging, including MR angiography, can be a "one-stop-shopping" examination due to the possibility of evaluating the muscle, ligamentous, and bone injuries as well as the vascular pathology in the same time. MR angiography has been shown to be equally effective as angiography in evaluating vascular injury of the knee with fewer complications than angiography [11]. A relatively new MR technique is time-resolved angiography, which provides dynamic imaging of the arterial and venous blood flow within one examination. The technique is based on rapid contrast-enhanced imaging and is based on an undersampling of the k-space with subsequent sharing of k-space information (view-sharing) to reconstruct a full volume data set. After image reconstruction, readers get realistic three-dimensional (3D) angiographic images, which show the arterial inflow, distribution, and venous drainage of the contrast agent. The image update rate defines the temporal resolution of the time-resolved MR angiography. While it is a compromise between image quality and speed, the temporal resolution can be as low as one 3D volume every second (1/s). Typical vendor acronyms for sequences are TREAT (Siemens), TRICKS (GE), and CENTRA (Philips).

Table 10.3 Knee arterial diseases [10, 12–17]

Pathological condition	Etiology	Clinical findings
Atherosclerosis and thrombosis	Endothelial injuries followed by atherosclerotic plaque formation	Intermittent claudication, rest pain, muscle atrophy
Embolism	Most often cardiac source Proximal arterial plaque	Clinical findings of acute ischemia including pain, pulselessness, paresthesia, and pallor
Aneurysm	Nonspecific Connective tissue diseases (e.g., Marfan's syndrome) Trauma Iatrogenic injury due to surgery (false aneurysm)	Asymptomatic in most of the cases; rarely, pain in the popliteal fossa
Artery entrapment syndrome	Abnormal relation to the normal or hypertrophic muscles or to fibrous structures	Arterial pulse that disappears in a particular knee or ankle position; claudication
Traumatic injuries (occlusion, dissection, arteriovenous fistula)	Trauma Iatrogenic injury due to surgery	The clinical findings may be confusing; angiography is mandatory in patients with suspected injuries
Hemangiomas	Benign proliferative tumors of the endothelial cells	Possible palpable and visible soft tissue mass if superficial
Vascular malformations	Errors of vascular morphogenesis	Possible palpable soft tissue mass if superficial; may grow in time

10.2.1 Atherosclerosis, Thrombosis, and Embolism

MR angiography (MRA) is a feasible diagnostic imaging option that provides all necessary information for choosing the therapeutic option in patients with peripheral atherosclerotic arterial disease. The popliteal artery is a very important artery for the evaluation of patients with peripheral ischemia because it is targeted for insertion of surgical bypass graft [18]. On MR angiography, popliteal arterial atherosclerosis appears as an irregular stenosis with or without collateral circulation. Post-stenotic dilation may be also present. The most important imaging findings in the diagnosis are the grade of the stenosis and the length of the involved segment. An imaging report should differentiate between a low-grade stenosis (<50 % narrowing) and a high-grade stenosis (>50 % narrowing). The latter is considered a hemodynamically significant lesion [18]. The length of the stenosis is also a significant criterion that influences the choice of treatment. Patients with more than 10 cm stenosis are less likely to benefit from angioplasty procedure [18].

In acute and severe arterial occlusion (embolism or thrombosis), MR angiography is usually not indicated since the patients need a rapid intervention. When is performed, MR imaging may show the enlargement of the vessel and diffuse perivascular edema (Fig. 10.6).

10.2.2 Aneurysms

Popliteal aneurysm is the most common peripheral aneurysm. It is often associated with aortic aneurysm and bilateral in 50–70 % of all cases [10, 19–21]. Popliteal aneurysms may be classified into true aneurysms and pseudoaneurysms false aneurysms. A true aneurysm is defined as a focal dilation of the artery greater than 2 cm in diameter or greater than 150 % of the normal arterial caliber (Fig. 10.7) [22, 23]. Atherosclerosis is the main etiology of true popliteal aneurysm. Other rare causes include mycotic aneurysms and Marfan's or Behcet's syndrome [24]. MR angiography is an accurate noninvasive tool in the diagnosis of aneurysm and of its most frequent complication, thrombosis.

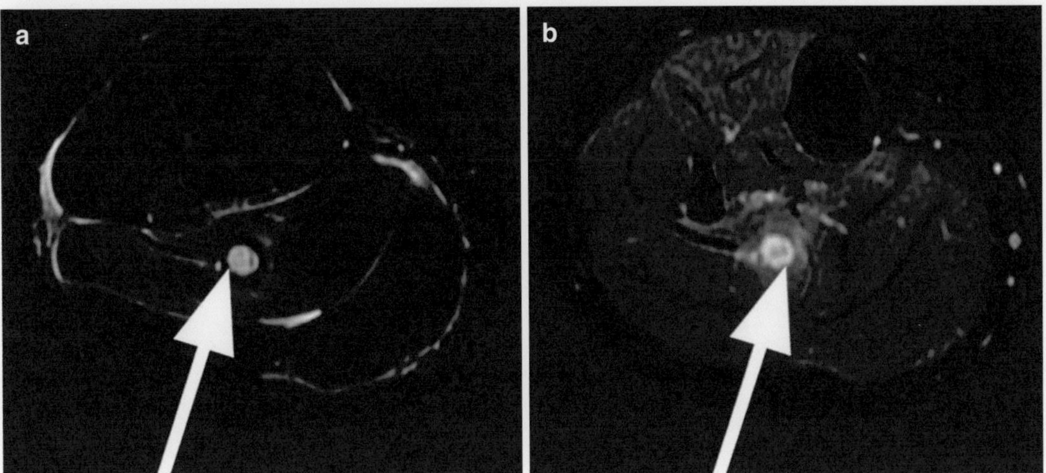

Fig. 10.6 Acute thrombophlebitis in a 27 year old female. Axial T2-weighted fat-suppressed image (**a**) and axial T1-weighted fat-suppressed postcontrast image (**b**) show the enlargement of the posterior tibial vein and edema around the vessel (*arrow* in **a**, **b**)

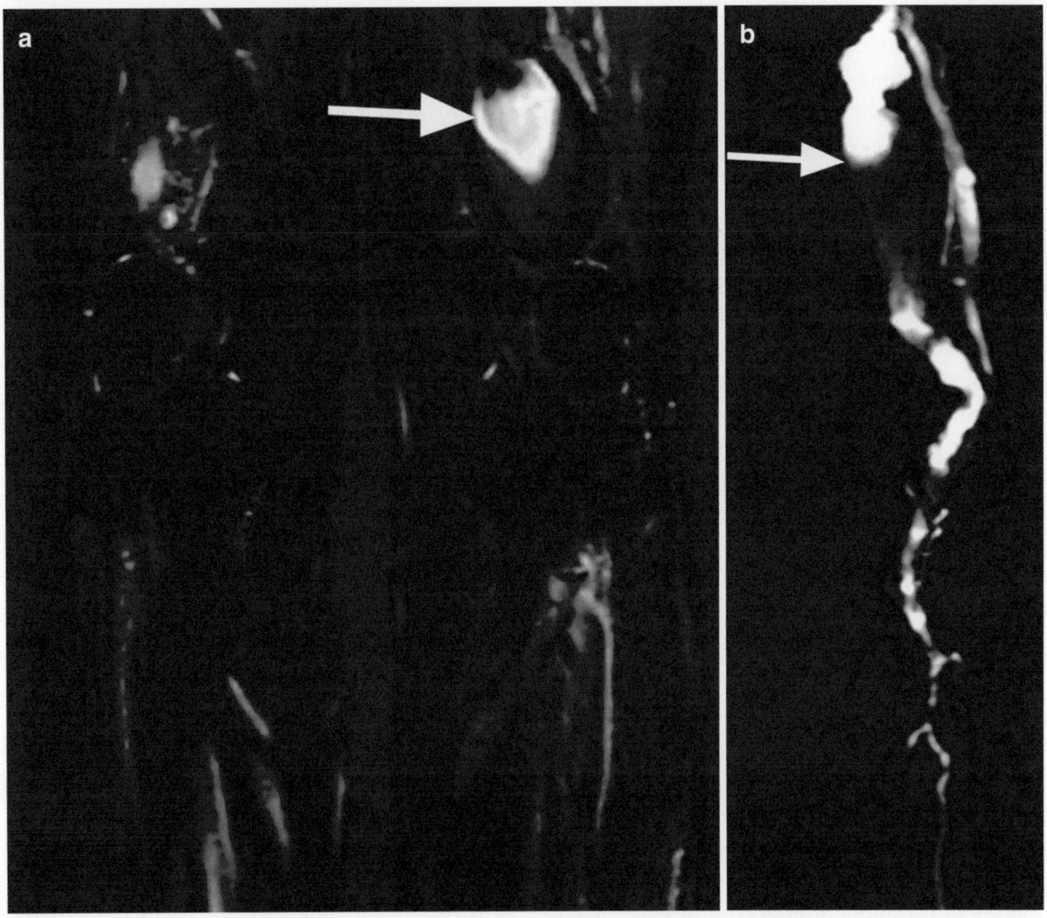

Fig. 10.7 Popliteal aneurysm in a 74 year old male. MR angiography (**a**) and MR subtraction angiography (**b**) show a true aneurysm (>2 cm) of the proximal popliteal artery (*large arrow* in **a**, **b**) in this patient with atherosclerosis

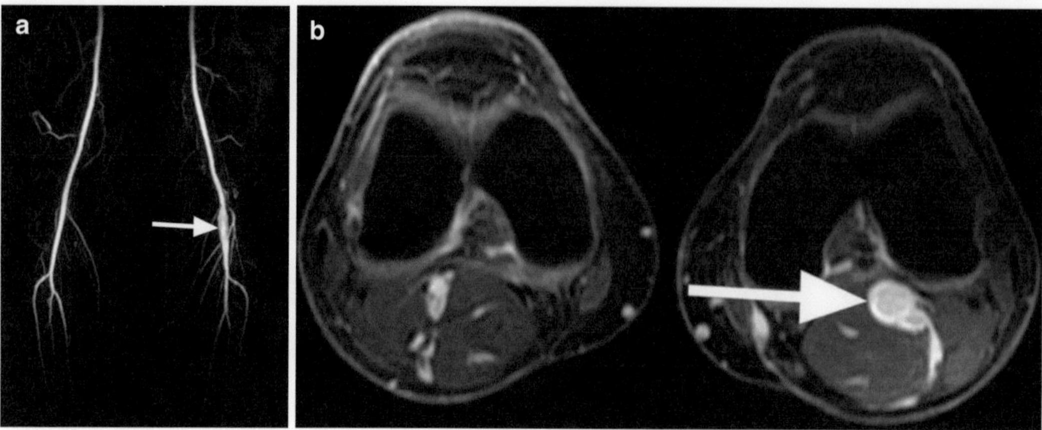

Fig. 10.8 Iatrogenic popliteal pseudoaneurysm in a 33 year old male. MR angiography (**a**, **b**) shows a fusiform pseudoaneurysm of the left popliteal artery (*large arrow* in **a**, **b**) after endarterectomy

10.2.3 Traumatic and Iatrogenic Injuries

Severe trauma to the knee including penetrating and blunt trauma, knee dislocations, and bone fractures may lead to injuries of the knee arteries and veins such as occlusion, penetration, dissection, and pseudoaneurysm formation [10]. However, a successful management of traumatic occlusion or disruption of the popliteal artery depends on a prompt diagnosis and repair, and therefore, the role of MR imaging and MR angiography is limited in these patients.

Popliteal pseudoaneurysm or false popliteal aneurysm may appear after knee trauma or postoperatively, and the popliteal artery is considered aneurysmal if its diameter exceeds 7 mm in diameter (Fig. 10.8) [10]. Almost any type of arthroscopy or open surgery may have pseudoaneurysms as one of the possible complications (cruciate ligament repair, total knee arthroplasty, tibial osteotomy). An extremely rare entity is nontraumatic pseudoaneurysm secondary to a located osteochondroma closely compressing the artery.

10.2.4 Artery Entrapment Syndrome

Arterial entrapment syndrome is defined as a permanent or transitory arterial compression by normal or anomalous gastrocnemius or popliteus muscles. The condition is underestimated and may be overlooked since the clinical manifestations are nonspecific. The latter vary from minor claudication and paresthesia to more severe symptoms of arterial ischemia. A chronic compression may lead in time to arterial stenosis, aneurysm, and thrombosis. There is no uniformly agreed classification of popliteal entrapment syndrome. There are essentially five types of compressions that refer to anatomic compressions and a "functional" type of compression secondary to gastrocnemius hypertrophy (Table 10.4) [10, 25]. MR imaging combined with MR angiography is the ideal imaging method for diagnosing arterial compression. It enables to locate the arterial stenosis as well as the anatomical relations between the artery and the adjacent muscle [26]. It has been demonstrated that stress MR imaging can improve the diagnosis of popliteal entrapment syndrome [27]. Therefore, the knee is imaged during active plantar flexion against resistance, which increases the ability to detect a signal loss in the artery due to muscular compression [27]. However, stress MR angiography is clinically difficult to perform and images frequently suffer from motion artifacts.

10.2.5 Hemangiomas

Soft tissue hemangiomas are distinct soft tissue vascular masses with enlarged feeding arteries and draining veins [17]. Frequently, there is confusion regarding the terminology and the diagnosis of hemangiomas and vascular malformations. Although both pathologies are included in the same large group of vascular anomalies, they are different pathological entities with

Table 10.4 Classification of popliteal entrapment syndrome [10]

Type of entrapment	Anatomical abnormality
1	Abnormal medial course of the popliteal artery around the normal medial head of the gastrocnemius
2	Medial displacement of the popliteal artery due to anomalous lateral insertion of the medial head of the gastrocnemius muscle
3	Medial displacement of the popliteal artery due to anomalous third head of the gastrocnemius muscle
4	Popliteal artery compression due to fibrous band of popliteus muscle, the popliteus muscle or the accessory popliteus muscle
5	Any 1–4 type that involves the popliteal vein as well
6	Compression due to hypertrophied gastrocnemius muscle

different diagnosis criteria. Hemangiomas are benign vascular tumors that originate from the proliferation of the endothelial cells. In comparison to vascular malformations, hemangiomas may have a rapid evolution and later involution [14, 17, 28]. Hemangiomas may be extra-articular in the soft tissues and muscles around the knee or intra-articular as hemangioma of the synovial membrane.

Extra-articular hemangiomas are well-defined lobulated lesions with a hyperintense or intermediate signal intensity on T2-weighted images and with intermediate signal intensity on T1-weighted images. There is no adjacent edema or soft tissue reaction (Fig. 10.9) [28]. On gradient-echo and spin-echo sequences, flow voids may be identified within the feeding arteries and draining veins [29]. The lesion enhances uniformly after contrast administration (Fig. 10.9). The involuting hemangiomas may display areas of fat and a reduced contrast enhancement [29].

Intra-articular synovial hemangiomas occur most frequently at the knee joint and are rare benign tumors. They may cause pain and spontaneous hemarthrosis in children and young adults [30, 31]. The MR imaging appearance is similar to

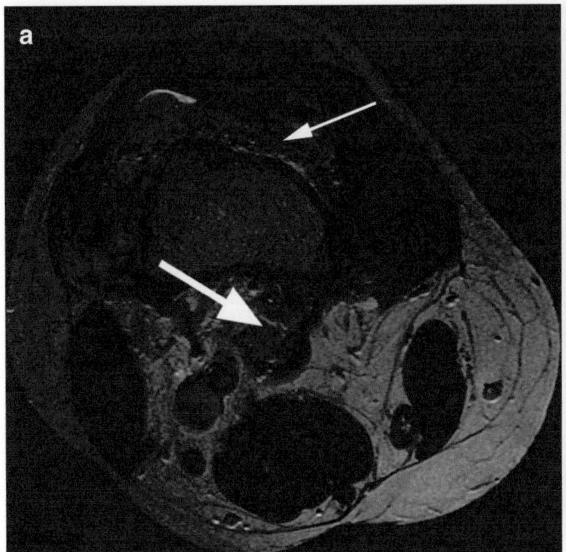
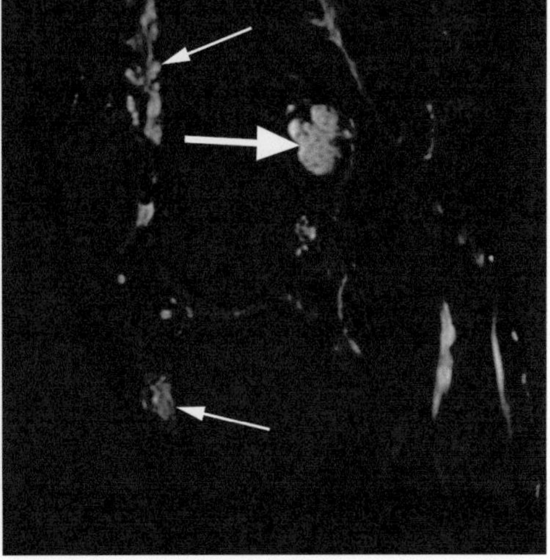

Fig. 10.9 Intra-articular and extra-articular hemangioma. Axial T2-weighted image (**a**) and sagittal T1-weighted fat-suppressed postcontrast image (**b**) show well-defined lobulated lesions with intermediate signal intensity on T2-weighted images without adjacent edema or soft tissue reaction. The MR imaging appearance is similar for the intra-articular hemangioma (*small arrows* in **a**, **b**) and for the extra-articular form (*large arrows* in **a**, **b**). The lesion enhances uniformly after contrast administration (*arrows* in **b**)

Table 10.5 Classification of vascular malformations [14, 29]

	Histological characteristics and subtypes
Low-flow malformations	Venous, lymphatic, capillary, capillary-venous, capillary-lymphatic-venous
High-flow malformations	Arteriovenous malformations, arteriovenous fistulas

that of hemangiomas in other locations (Fig. 10.9). The intra-articular lesion is lobulated with high-signal-intensity convoluted vessels without bone involvement. The presence of hemarthrosis may hinder the diagnosis and mimic a hemophiliac arthritis or a pigmented villonodular synovitis [30]. Early degenerative changes to the cartilage with early onset of osteoarthritis represent a complication of intra-articular hemangiomas.

10.2.6 Vascular Malformations

Vascular malformations are formed by dysplastic vessels with normal endothelial turnover. Contrary to the hemangiomas, vascular malformations usually grow without regression [14, 17, 28]. The classification of the vascular malformations is based on their flow dynamics (Table 10.5).

At the knee joint, vascular malformations can involve all structures such as muscles, ligaments, capsule, and even bones. Pain is a leading symptom [32]. The differentiation of the flow dynamics of the vascular malformations is very important for choosing the best treatment option (surgical excision or image-guided procedure) [29, 33]. MR imaging offers a complete anatomical and functional description of the lesion when combined with MR angiography. Anatomically, MR imaging defines the location and extent of the lesion. Functionally, MR angiography has become essential in differentiating between low-flow and high-flow malformations (Fig. 10.10). The modality of choice is dynamic time-resolved MR angiography (see description above) which enables a rapid acquisition with high temporal resolution showing the contrast material arriving in the malformation. A clear delineation of the arterial

inflow and subsequent arteriovenous or venous filling is possible. Time-resolved MR angiography also shows early venous shunting and the abnormally enlarged draining channels [29]. As a thumb of, low-flow vascular malformations have a contrast arrival time of more than 50 s after injection, whereas high-flow malformations have a rise time of less than 20 s after injection [34]. Despite measuring the time, it is also feasible and simple to compare the filling time of a vascular malformation with nearby normal arteries and veins. If the malformation fills at approximately the same time as the nearby artery, the lesion is more likely a high-flow malformation. If the lesion fills at approximately the same time as the nearby vein, the lesion is more likely a low-flow malformation. MR imaging has proved to be also a safe technique for guiding percutaneous sclerotherapy of low-flow malformations with high degree of technical success [33].

10.3 MRI Pathological Findings: Nerves

The nerves around the knee can be the subject of different pathologies including trauma, inflammation, and tumors. Although the diagnosis is traditionally based on clinical examination and electrodiagnostic tests, MR imaging plays an increasing role in the definition of the type, site, and extent of the lesions [35]. A complete MR examination, also called MR neurography, of the peripheral nerves includes sequences for "anatomical" as well as for "functional" MR imaging.

Standard MR sequences (T1 weighted and T2 weighted) provide anatomical information regarding the nerve signal intensity, the nerve diameter, and the relationship with the surrounding structures (Fig. 10.11). MR imaging also enables an accurate assessment of the muscles affected by denervation and, indirectly, provides information about the affected nerve and the severity of the lesion. In acute and subacute denervation, muscles show diffuse high signal intensity on T2-weighted images and low signal intensity on T1-weighted images due to intramuscular edema (Fig. 10.11) [36, 37]. This situation

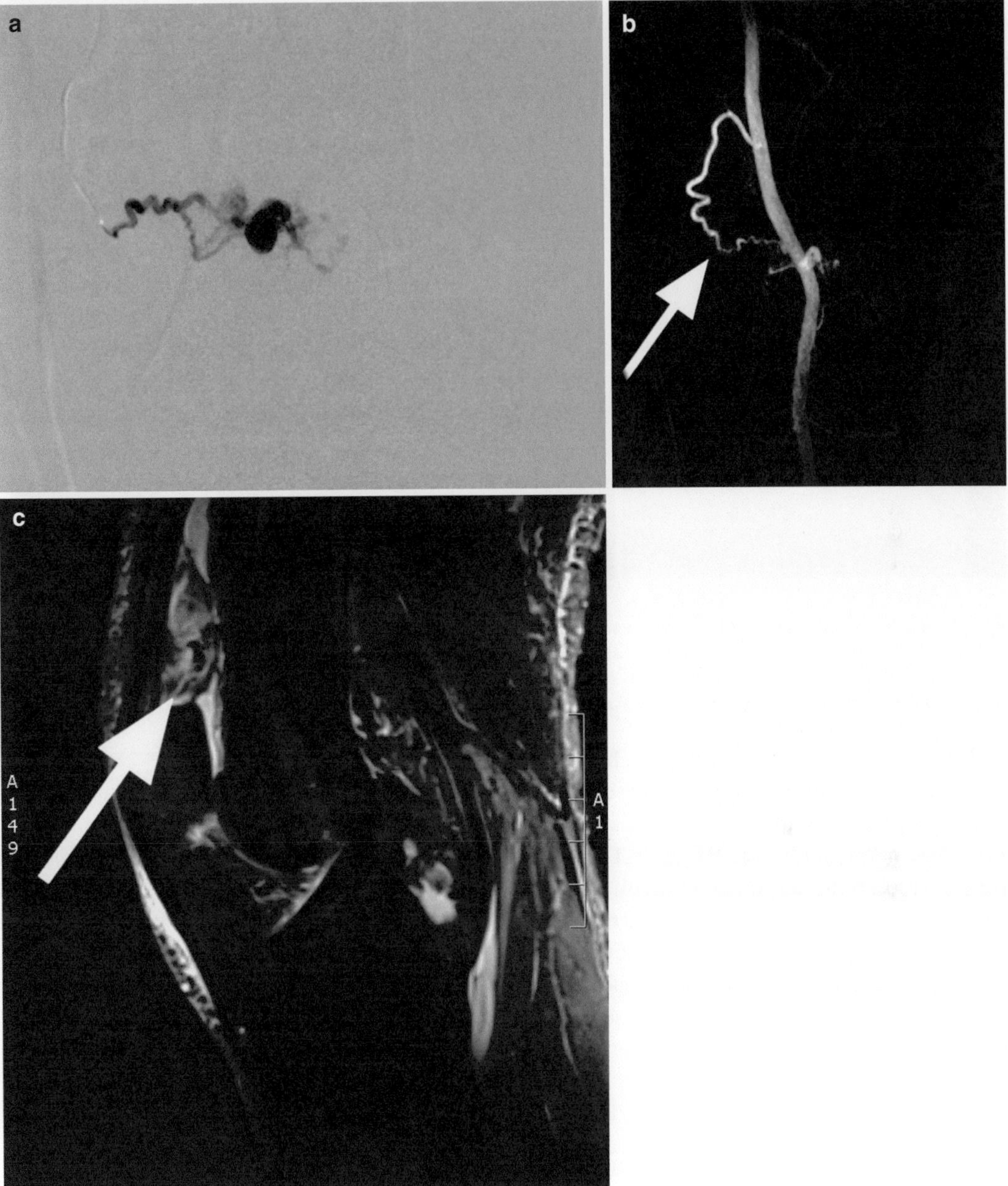

Fig. 10.10 Arteriovenous malformations in the suprapatellar recess just above the patella in a 59 year old female. The supraselective catheterization (**a**) was performed after the MR diagnosis. Time-resolved MR angiography (**b**) shows the feeding artery (*arrow* in **b**) and the T1-weighted fat-suppressed image after angiography (**c**) shows the exact location and dimension (*arrow* in **c**) of this high-flow malformation

is usually referred to as "neurogenic edema" or "denervation edema." In chronic denervation, there is a decreased muscle volume and an increased signal on T1-weighted images because of fatty infiltration [36]. The presence of fatty changes within the muscle is suggestive of irreversible chronic atrophy of the affected muscle [38]. It needs to be noted that in subacute phases, "neurogenic edema" and muscle atrophy can be present at the same time.

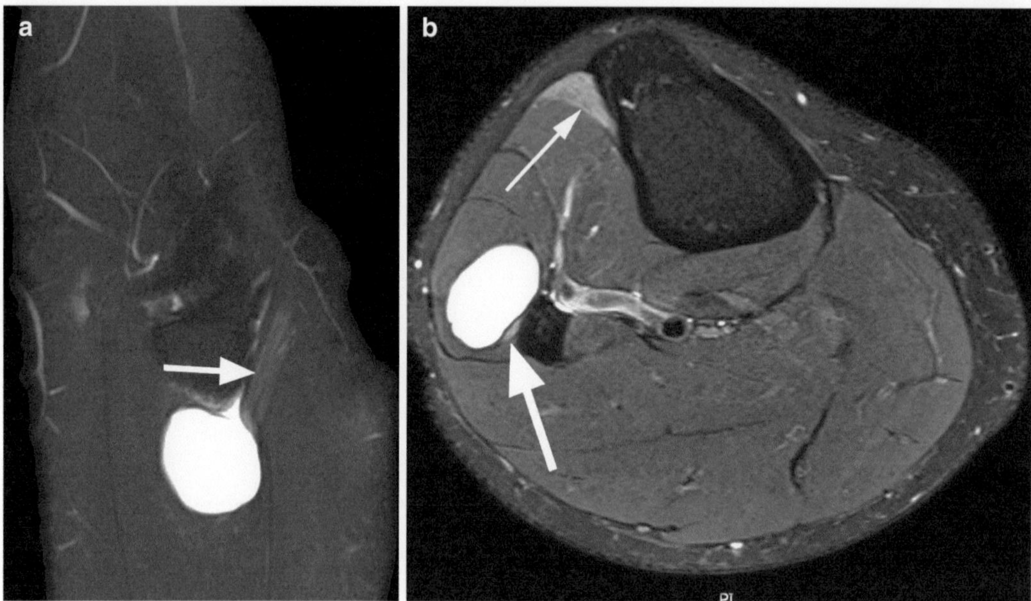

Fig. 10.11 Common peroneal nerve compression. Sagittal T2-weighted fat-suppressed image (**a**) and axial proton-density (PD) fat-suppressed image (**b**) show a cystic mass which compresses the common peroneal nerve which appears with high signal intensity and enlarged (*large arrow* in **a**, **b**). Note the diffuse high-signal-intensity edema of the tibialis anterior muscle (*small arrow* in **b**) which is an indirect sign of subacute denervation

MR imaging at 1.5 T can depict changes in diameter and signal intensity, but there is often poor conspicuity of the surrounding structures [39]. MR neurography (MRN) at 3 T with its higher resolution, its thinner slices, and its superior contrast-to-noise ratio is currently the preferred MR imaging technique for evaluation of the peripheral nerves. Besides standard T1- and T2-weighted sequences, new MR sequences can be used for anatomical MR neurography. These new sequences include 3D isotropic sequences (3D SPACE (Siemens), CUBE (GE), VISTA (Philips)), 3D T1 gradient-echo with SPAIR fat suppression, and 3D STIR or T2-weighted fat-suppressed images. Normally, the nerves around the knee display isointense signal intensity on T1-weighted images and isointense to slightly hyperintense signal intensity on T2-weighted images. The common peroneal nerve is usually thinner than the tibial nerve (Fig. 10.12) [35].

"Functional" MR neurography is based on diffusion tensor imaging (DTI), which provides information regarding the apparent diffusion coefficient of the nerve and the fractional anisotropy, and can be used to obtain fiber tractography

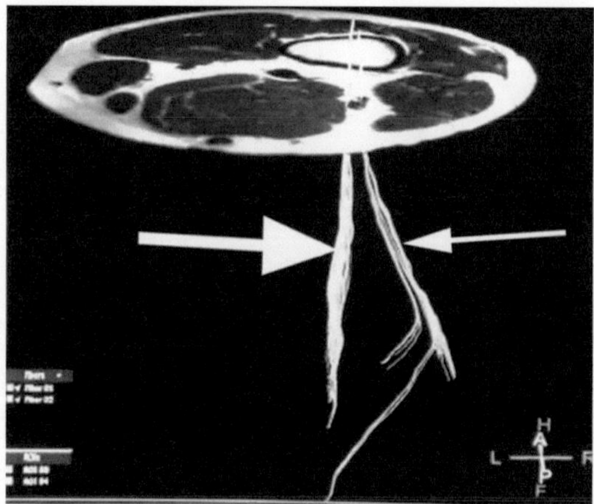

Fig. 10.12 Example of fiber tractography showing the tibial nerve (*large arrow*) and common peroneal nerve (*small arrow*) at the level of the distal thigh just above the knee. The fibers are reconstructed from a diffusion tensor imaging data set which was acquired using a standard echo planar imaging (EPI) sequence on a standard clinical 3.0 T MR scanner. The fibers represent the intact diffusion along the individual nerves and thus are biomarkers for normal microanatomy and thus nerve function. Note that the common peroneal nerve is usually thinner than the tibial nerve

(Fig. 10.12) [39]. However, the technique is currently only used in dedicated imaging centers because of technical challenges [39].

10.3.1 Habitual, Traumatic, and Iatrogenic Nerve Disorders

The habitual disorders refer to functional anatomical changes that can result in stretch injuries to the tibial or common peroneal nerve [35]. The common peroneal nerve, due to its superficial location, is more frequently involved, being the most common injured peripheral nerve in the lower extremity [35]. Habitual leg crossing, repetitive exercises involving inversion and pronation, and improper footwear may cause stretch injuries to the nerves [35].

Nerve stretching, nerve discontinuity, or amputation neuromas are the most frequent lesions encountered after trauma or after surgery.

On MR neurography, the pathological nerves may show disruption or enlargement, course deviation, and edema. The use of contrast media is indicated in cases of suspected tumors and in postoperative cases for a better visualization of the perineural inflammation or for the differentiation between traumatic neuroma or perineuroma, which do not enhance from enhancing peripheral nerve tumor [40]. Enhancement represents a sign of disruption of the normal blood-nerve barrier.

10.3.2 Entrapment Neuropathies

The tibial nerve may be compressed by a thickened fibromuscular sling of the soleus muscle, ganglion cysts, Baker's cyst, popliteal aneurysm, and popliteal tumors. In the soleus sling syndrome, MR imaging demonstrated a thickened soleus sling (>2 mm) with T2 hyperintensity of the tibial nerve at the level of the sling and denervation changes in muscles of the posterior compartment of the leg [41].

The common site of *peroneal common nerve* compression is at the level of the peroneal tunnel, which is formed by the neck of the fibula and the two heads of the peroneus longus muscles. Repeated peroneal muscle contraction related to plantar flexion or ankle inversion determines nerve compression in the tunnel against the fibular neck. On MR imaging the nerve shows thickening from perineural fibrosis as well as abnormally high signal intensity on T2-weighted

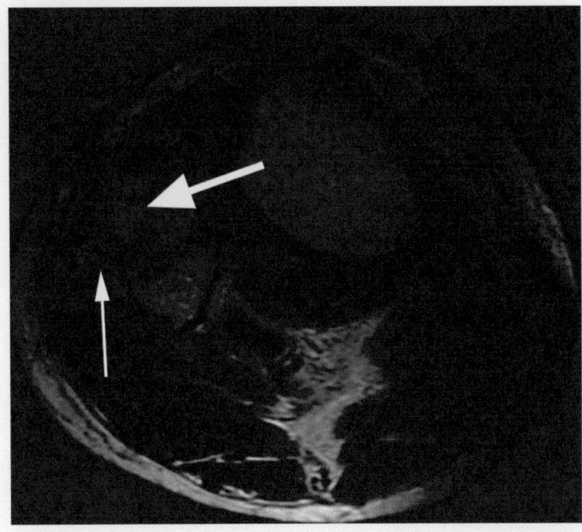

Fig. 10.13 Peroneal nerve damage after complex fracture of the proximal fibula. Axial proton-density (PD) image shows a displaced fracture fragment of the head of the fibula (*large arrow*) and the signal intensity changes of the peroneal nerve due to secondary nerve entrapment (*small arrow*)

images at or just proximal to the tunnel (Fig. 10.13) [35]. Nerve flattening at the compression site may be also seen (Fig. 10.11) [35]. Less commonly, entrapment of both the tibial nerve at the soleal sling site and common peroneal nerve at the peroneal tunnel may occur [35].

10.3.3 Tumors and Tumorlike Lesions

The most common tumors of the nerves around the knee joint including the tibial and the common peroneal nerve are neurofibromas and schwannomas. On MR imaging they appear as well-defined nodular lesions that display contrast enhancement (Fig. 10.14).

In contrast to the enhancement pattern of the nerve tumors, the so-called intraneural ganglion cyst is a nodular cystic non-enhancing lesion that commonly arises on the peroneal nerve near the head of fibula [38].

10.3.4 Systemic Diseases That Involve the Peripheral Nerves

Systemic diseases that may involve the peripheral nerves, including the tibial and common peroneal nerves, are rare. Amyloidosis, sarcoidosis,

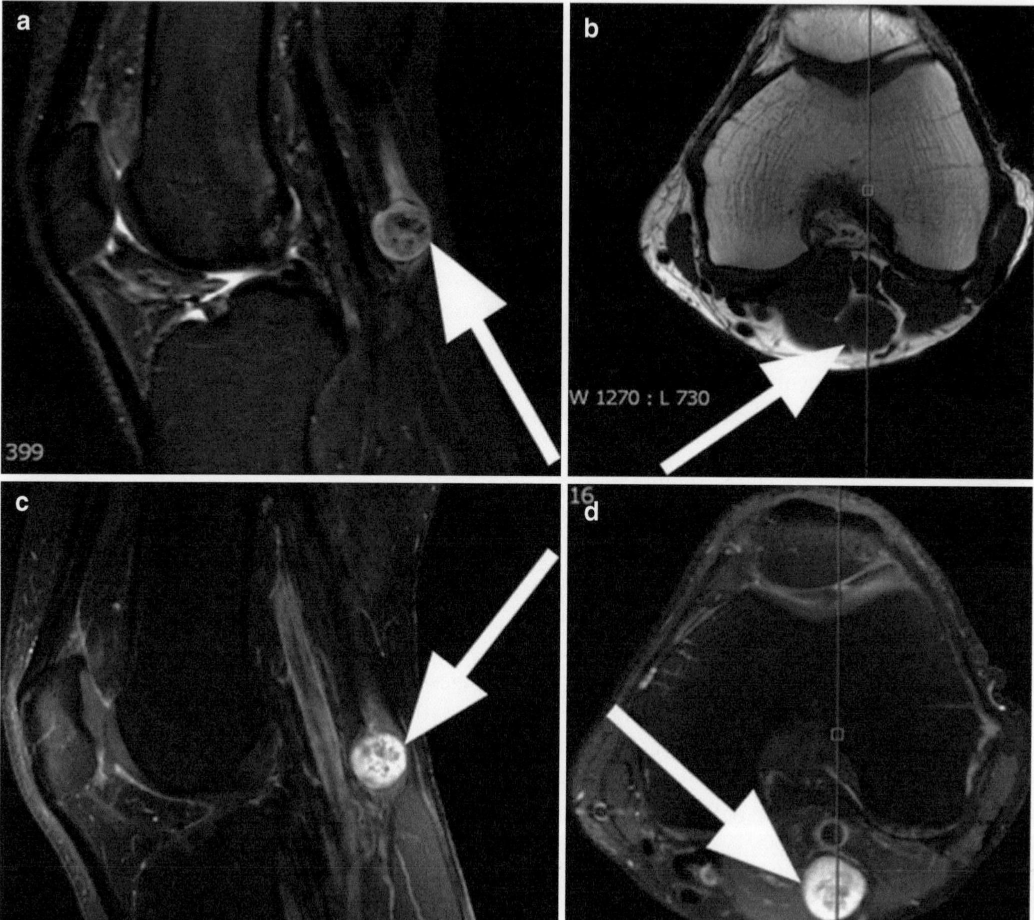

Fig. 10.14 Benign peripheral nerve sheath tumor (schwannoma) of the tibial nerve. Sagittal T2-weighted fat-suppressed image (**a**), axial T1-weighted image (**b**), and sagittal (**c**) and axial (**d**) T1-weighted fat-suppressed post-contrast images show a well-defined nodular lesion of the tibial nerve that displays contrast enhancement (*arrows*)

leprosy, lymphoma, Charcot-Marie-Tooth disease, or Dejerine-Sottas disease were reported [38, 42, 43]. The role of MRI is to identify the pathological changes of the nerve and to distinguish them from other more common lesions such as tumors or traumatic lesions.

10.4   MRI Impression

10.4.1 Arteries and Veins

1. Arterial atherosclerosis with stenosis (low-grade stenosis <50 % narrowing or high-grade stenosis >50 % narrowing); location and length of the stenosis

2. Popliteal aneurysm (focal enlargement >2 cm diameter); with or without thrombosis; with or without perivascular inflammation

3. Aneurysmal dilation (>7 mm)

4. Arterial stenosis due to the anatomical relations between the artery and the adjacent muscle = entrapment syndrome; may indicate further examination: "functional" MR angiography of the knee during active plantar flexion against resistance

5. Hemangioma of the knee: size and location (synovial or extra-articular); with or without hemarthrosis

6. Vascular malformation: size, location, and type (low flow or high flow based on the contrast rise time of more than 50 s or less than 20 s)

10.4.2 Nerves

1. Pathological MRI appearance (enlargement, disruption, edema): location and size; unilateral or bilateral
2. Thickened nerve and/or flattening of the nerve with abnormal high signal intensity on T2-weighted images at and just proximal to an anatomical tunnel; suggestive of entrapment syndrome (soleal sling, peroneal tunnel) or compressive pathology (secondary to cysts, tumors, osteochondromas)
3. Focal nodular lesion; enhancing lesion (schwannoma or neurofibroma); non-enhancing lesion (probably intraneural ganglion cyst)
4. Diffuse bilateral pathological nerve appearance that may orient the diagnosis to a systemic peripheral nerve disease

References

1. Arnoczky SP. Anatomy of the anterior cruciate ligament. Clin Orthop Relat Res. 1983;172:19–25.
2. Gray JC. Neural and vascular anatomy of the menisci of the human knee. J Orthop Sports Phys Ther. 1999;29(1):23–30.
3. Nemschak G, Pretterklieber ML. The patellar arterial supply via the infrapatellar fat pad (of Hoffa): a combined anatomical and angiographical analysis. Anat Res Int. 2012;2012:713838.
4. Day CP, Orme R. Popliteal artery branching patterns – an angiographic study. Clin Radiol. 2006;61(8):696–9.
5. Ozgur Z, Ucerler H, Aktan Ikiz ZA. Branching patterns of the popliteal artery and its clinical importance. Surg Radiol Anat. 2009;31(5):357–62.
6. Klecker RJ, et al. The aberrant anterior tibial artery: magnetic resonance appearance, prevalence, and surgical implications. Am J Sports Med. 2008;36(4):720–7.
7. Vohra S, et al. Normal MR imaging anatomy of the knee. Magn Reson Imaging Clin N Am. 2011;19(3):637–53, ix–x.
8. Salaria H, Atkinson R. Anatomic study of the middle genicular artery. J Orthop Surg (Hong Kong). 2008;16(1):47–9.
9. Gray H. Anatomy of the human body. New York: Bartleby.com; 2000. http://www.bartleby.com/107/159.html.
10. Wright LB, et al. Popliteal artery disease: diagnosis and treatment. Radiographics. 2004;24(2):467–79.
11. Tocci SL, et al. Magnetic resonance angiography for the evaluation of vascular injury in knee dislocations. J Knee Surg. 2010;23(4):201–7.
12. Atkins HJ, Key JA. A case of myxomatous tumour arising in the adventitia of the left external iliac artery; case report. Br J Surg. 1947;34(136):426.
13. Love JW, Whelan TJ. Popliteal artery entrapment syndrome. Am J Surg. 1965;109:620–4.
14. Mulliken JB, Glowacki J. Hemangiomas and vascular malformations in infants and children: a classification based on endothelial characteristics. Plast Reconstr Surg. 1982;69(3):412–22.
15. Erdoes LS, et al. Popliteal vascular compression in a normal population. J Vasc Surg. 1994;20(6):978–86.
16. Frykberg ER. Popliteal vascular injuries. Surg Clin North Am. 2002;82(1):67–89.
17. Moukaddam H, Pollak J, Haims AH. MRI characteristics and classification of peripheral vascular malformations and tumors. Skeletal Radiol. 2009;38(6):535–47.
18. Rofsky NM, Adelman MA. MR angiography in the evaluation of atherosclerotic peripheral vascular disease. Radiology. 2000;214(2):325–38.
19. Dawson I, Sie RB, van Bockel JH. Atherosclerotic popliteal aneurysm. Br J Surg. 1997;84(3):293–9.
20. Henke PK. Popliteal artery aneurysms: tried, true, and new approaches to therapy. Semin Vasc Surg. 2005;18(4):224–30.
21. Galland RB. Popliteal aneurysms: from John Hunter to the 21st century. Ann R Coll Surg Engl. 2007;89(5):466–71.
22. Szilagyi DE, Schwartz RL, Reddy DJ. Popliteal arterial aneurysms. Their natural history and management. Arch Surg. 1981;116(5):724–8.
23. Hollier LH, et al. Arteriomegaly: classification and morbid implications of diffuse aneurysmal disease. Surgery. 1983;93(5):700–8.
24. Galland RB. Popliteal aneurysms: controversies in their management. Am J Surg. 2005;190(2):314–8.
25. Eliahou R, Sosna J, Bloom AI. Between a rock and a hard place: clinical and imaging features of vascular compression syndromes. Radiographics. 2012;32(1):E33–49.
26. Atilla S, et al. MR imaging and MR angiography in popliteal artery entrapment syndrome. Eur Radiol. 1998;8(6):1025–9.
27. Di Cesare E, et al. Stress MR imaging for evaluation of popliteal artery entrapment. J Magn Reson Imaging. 1994;4(4):617–22.
28. Dubois J, Alison M. Vascular anomalies: what a radiologist needs to know. Pediatr Radiol. 2010;40(6):895–905.
29. Flors L, et al. MR imaging of soft-tissue vascular malformations: diagnosis, classification, and therapy follow-up. Radiographics. 2011;31(5):1321–40; discussion 1340–1.
30. Bruns J, Eggers-Stroeder G, von Torklus D. Synovial hemangioma–a rare benign synovial tumor. Report of four cases. Knee Surg Sports Traumatol Arthrosc. 1994;2(3):186–9.
31. Akgun I, et al. Intra-articular hemangioma of the knee. Arthroscopy. 2003;19(3):E17.
32. Theruvil B, et al. Vascular malformations in muscles around the knee presenting as knee pain. Knee. 2004;11(2):155–8.

33. Andreisek G, et al. MR imaging-guided percutaneous sclerotherapy of peripheral venous malformations with a clinical 1.5-T unit: a pilot study. J Vasc Interv Radiol. 2009;20(7):879–87.
34. Ohgiya Y, et al. Dynamic MRI for distinguishing high-flow from low-flow peripheral vascular malformations. AJR Am J Roentgenol. 2005;185(5):1131–7.
35. Chhabra A, et al. High-resolution 3-T MR neurography of peroneal neuropathy. Skeletal Radiol. 2012;41(3):257–71.
36. Fleckenstein JL, et al. Denervated human skeletal muscle: MR imaging evaluation. Radiology. 1993; 187(1):213–8.
37. Andreisek G, et al. MRI of the intrinsic muscles of the hand: spectrum of imaging findings and clinical correlation. AJR Am J Roentgenol. 2005;185(4):930–9.
38. Lacour-Petit MC, Lozeron P, Ducreux D. MRI of peripheral nerve lesions of the lower limbs. Neuroradiology. 2003;45(3):166–70.
39. Chhabra A, et al. 3-T high-resolution MR neurography of sciatic neuropathy. AJR Am J Roentgenol. 2012;198(4):W357–64.
40. Chhabra A, et al. MR neurography of neuromas related to nerve injury and entrapment with surgical correlation. AJNR Am J Neuroradiol. 2010;31(8): 1363–8.
41. Ladak A, et al. MRI findings in patients with tibial nerve compression near the knee. Skeletal Radiol. 2013;42(4):553–9.
42. Tachi N, et al. MRI of peripheral nerves and pathology of sural nerves in hereditary motor and sensory neuropathy type III. Neuroradiology. 1995;37(6): 496–9.
43. Wadhwa V, et al. Sciatic nerve tumor and tumor-like lesions – uncommon pathologies. Skeletal Radiol. 2012;41(7):763–74.

Bones

Nicolae Bolog, Gustav Andreisek,
and Erika Ulbrich

11.1 Anatomy and Normal MRI Appearance

The performance of MR imaging regarding the evaluation of bone structures varies from the poorly detailed information regarding the cortical bone to its unique capability of bone marrow assessment. Although some MR sequences (also called "black-bone" MRI) based on a partial flip angle technique or new ultrashort echo (UTE) techniques have been used for providing images of the cortical bone, computed tomography (CT) remains the imaging method of choice for cortical bone evaluation in the clinical routine (Fig. 11.1) [1].

MR imaging is the only practical imaging technique and the most sensitive technique that enables direct visualization of the bone marrow (Fig. 11.2) [2], despite recent developments in CT using dual-energy acquisitions. The bone

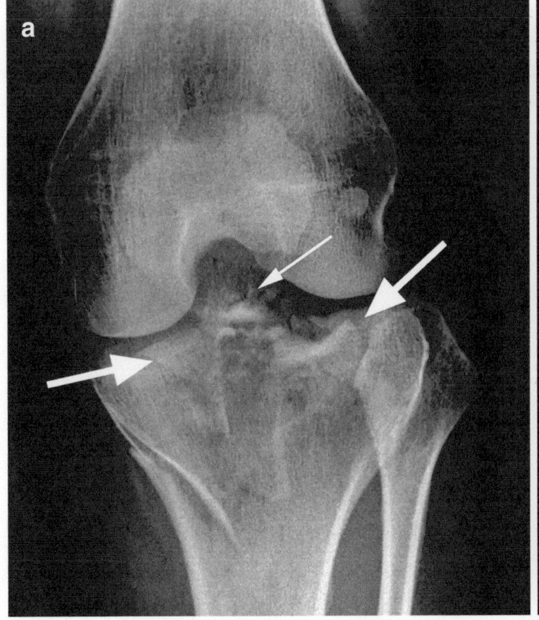
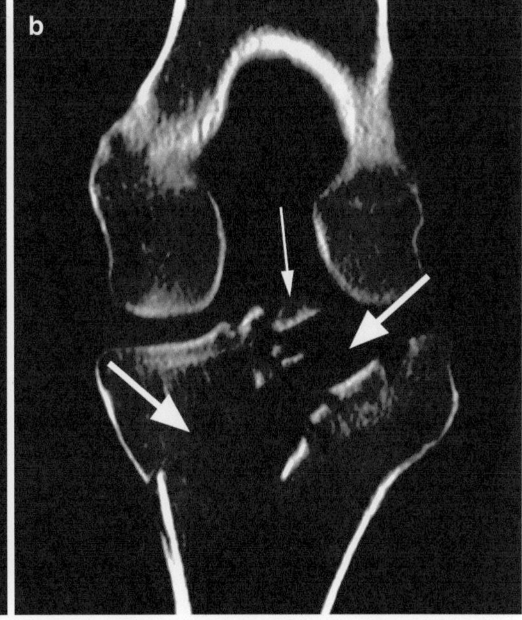

Fig. 11.1 Complex fracture of the tibial plateau (type Schatzker V). Radiography (**a**) and coronal reconstructed CT image (**b**) show a complex fracture of the tibial plateau which implies both the medial and lateral tibial plateau (*large arrows* in **a**, **b**). Note the small intra-articular fragments (*small arrow* in **a**, **b**)

N.V. Bolog et al., *MRI of the Knee: A Guide to Evaluation and Reporting*,
DOI 10.1007/978-3-319-08165-6_11, © Springer International Publishing Switzerland 2015

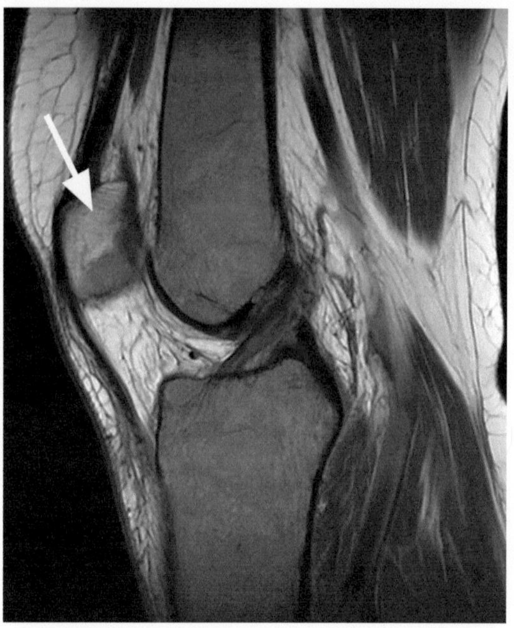

Fig. 11.2 Leukemia in a 27 year old female. Sagittal proton-density (PD) image demonstrates the diffuse abnormality of the bone marrow which is low signal intensity with the exception of the superior part of the patella which has a normal MR imaging appearance (*arrow*)

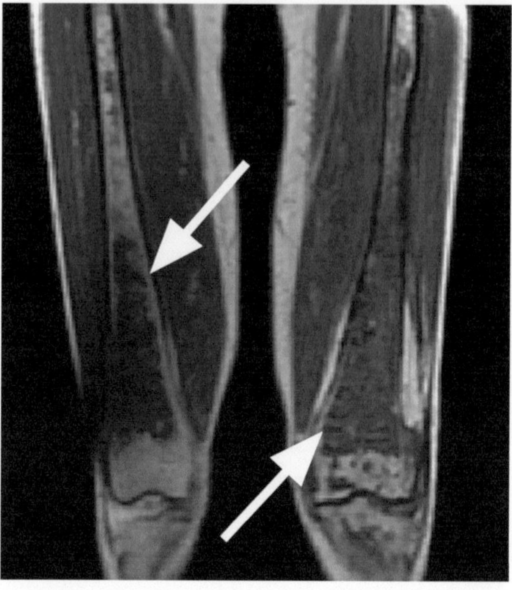

Fig. 11.3 Gaucher's disease. Coronal T1-weighted image shows bilateral femoral low-signal-intensity bone marrow replacement and bone infarction (*arrows*) indicating severe involvement

Table 11.1 Ossification centers around the knee and the approximate age of fusion [5, 6]

Bone	Number of ossification centers	Age of fusion (years)
Femur – distal epiphysis	1	19–22
Tibia		
Proximal epiphysis	1	18–23
Tuberosity	1	12–13
Fibula – proximal epiphysis	1	21–24

marrow contains yellow and red marrow with different percentages of fat and water (80 % fat in yellow marrow and 40 % fat in red marrow) [3]. The cellular component is complex and is comprised of stem cells as well as supportive cellular environment [4]. On T1-weighted images, the normal bone marrow displays an intermediate-signal-intensity appearance higher than the skeletal muscles. Decreased signal intensity on T1-weighted images (lower signal intensity than muscles) may be diffuse or focal and is the result of replacement of fatty marrow with cellular tissue or edema (Fig. 11.3) [4]. The fat-suppressed T2-weighted images are particularly useful in increasing the conspicuity of the high-signal-intensity lesions from the adjacent normal bone marrow, which has low signal intensity due to fat suppression. The MRI appearance of the femur, tibia, and patella as well as fabella depends on the bone marrow distribution and the presence of the synchondroses and ossification centers. Knowing the ossification

centers and their age of fusion is useful in avoiding misinterpretations of particular fractures or avulsion fractures (Table 11.1).

11.2 MRI Pathological Findings

MR imaging is very sensitive in diagnosing the entire spectrum of bone pathology including bone marrow diseases, fractures, and tumors. The role of MR imaging in the evaluation of patients with radiographically recognized

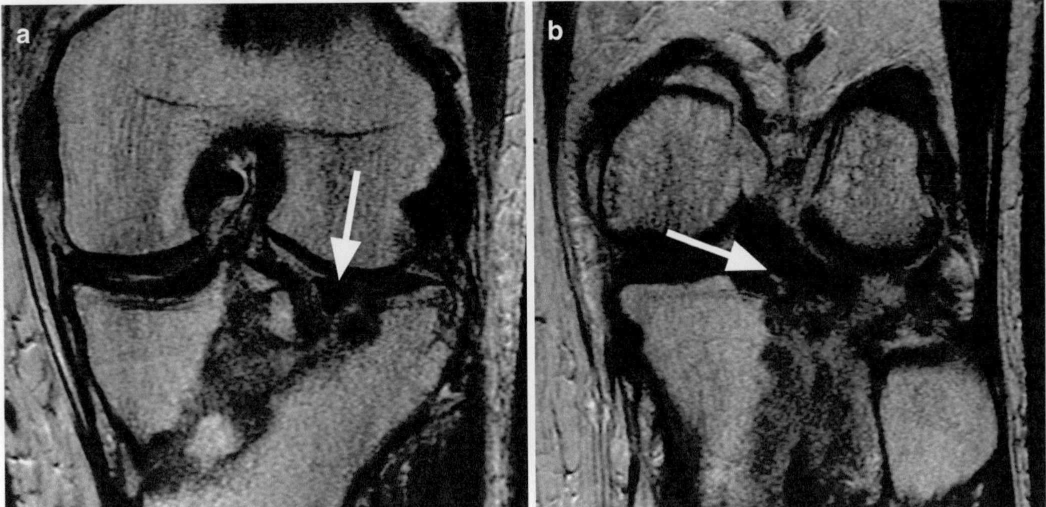

Fig. 11.4 Complex tibial fracture in a 43 year old male. Coronal proton-density (PD) images (**a**, **b**) show a completely dislocated lateral meniscus (*arrow* in **a**) and bony avulsion of the posterior root of the lateral meniscus (*arrow* in **b**)

traumatic fractures of the distal end of the femur or proximal part of the tibia is, however, equivocal and is limited to the cases in which a complete assessment of the associated soft tissue lesions is necessary (Fig. 11.4). Radiography and CT are the most used imaging methods for diagnosis, classification, and management of bone fractures. On the other hand, MR imaging plays a crucial role and is superior to other imaging techniques in the diagnosis of subtle bone marrow changes (bone marrow edema; bone contusions; occult, pathologic, insufficiency and stress fractures; synchondrosis lesions; avulsion fractures).

11.2.1 Transient Bone Marrow Edema

Diffuse bone marrow edema is present in different pathological conditions including osteoporosis, fractures, osteonecrosis, and tumors. The MR imaging appearance is nonspecific in the absence of additional bone changes such as line fractures or cortical defects. Transient bone marrow edema is a syndrome that refers to any patient with reversible bone marrow edema on MR images [7]. The most frequently affected bones are the femoral head and neck and the

distal femur where the bone marrow edema involves commonly the medial condyle. Usually, the patients do not remember a traumatic event. The etiology is unclear, but transient osteoporosis, neuromuscular dysfunctions, and transient ischemia are the probable causes for the presence of pain and edema [7]. However, some authors prefer the term of transient bone marrow edema to be used only in patients in whom osteopenia is not demonstrated on radiographs [7]. Clinically, the patients complain of pain, and the MR imaging shows a diffuse high-signal-intensity edema on T2-weighted images without any additional bone pathological changes (Fig. 11.5). A small amount of synovial fluid may be present. The diagnosis is based on the clinical findings, the absence of the previous trauma, the evolution of the pain, and the observation in MR imaging that the edema disappears spontaneously after a while.

11.2.2 Disuse Osteopenia and Epiphyseal Growth Arrest Lines

Disuse osteopenia is a diffuse bone marrow change that appears after immobilization probably due to bone resorbtion and compromised

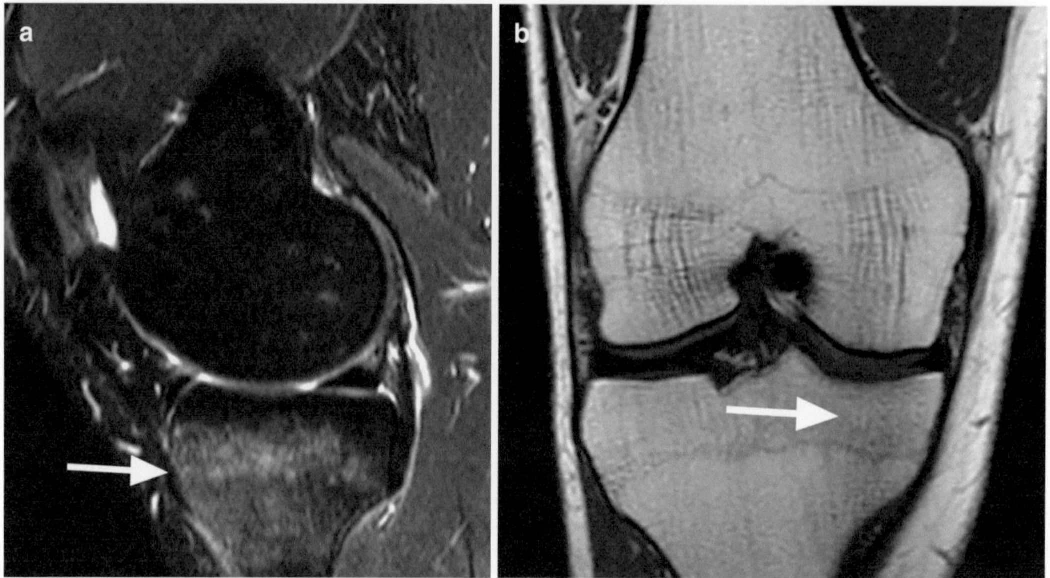

Fig. 11.5 Transient bone marrow edema in a 39 year old male with pain and no history of trauma. Sagittal T2-weighted image (**a**) and coronal T1-weighted image (**b**) show a diffuse edema of the lateral tibial plateau without any other pathological changes (*arrows*)

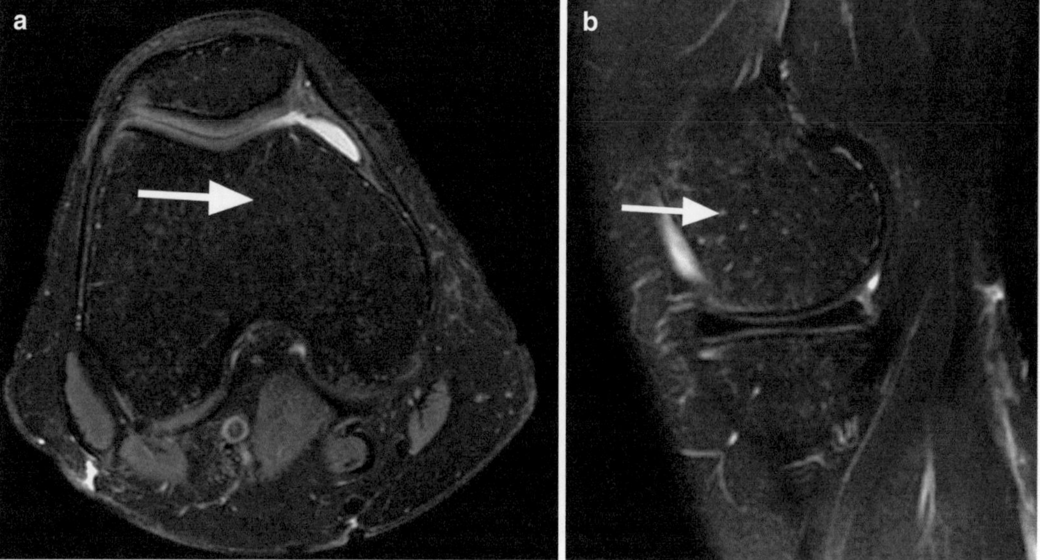

Fig. 11.6 Disuse osteopenia in a 30 year old female after immobilization. Axial proton-density (PD) fat-suppressed image (**a**) and sagittal T2-weighted fat-suppressed image (**b**) show small high-signal-intensity lesions of the bone marrow with a "spotty" distribution (*arrows*)

architecture [8–10]. The changes are best seen on T2-weighted fat-suppressed images and may have different patterns from a generalized and diffuse high signal intensity relative to the hyaline cartilage lesions to a more "spotty" distribution of the lesions (Fig. 11.6) [8, 11]. The peak of the signal intensity changes is between 10 and 25 weeks after injury with the abnormalities

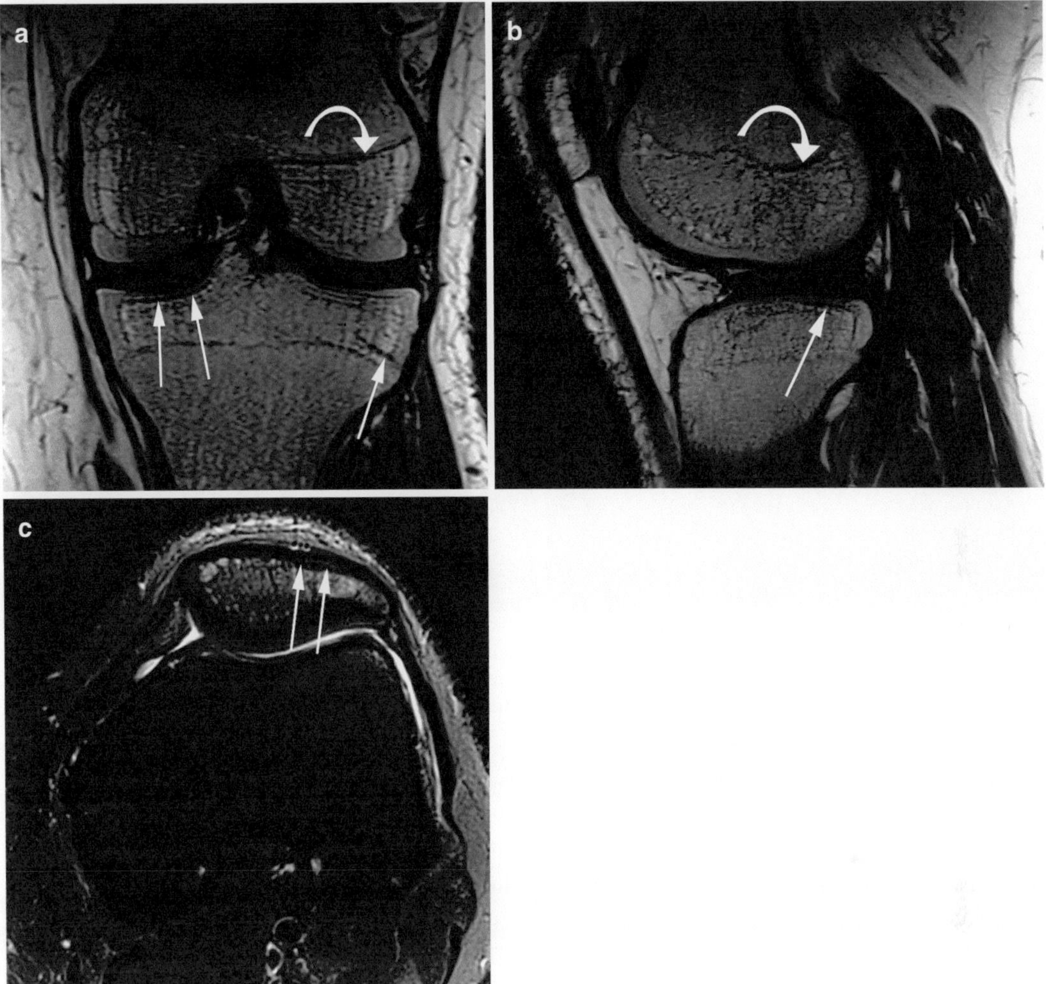

Fig. 11.7 Epiphyseal growth arrest lines in a 31 year old male after immobilization when he was 5 years old. Coronal T1-weighted image (**a**), sagittal proton-density (PD) image (**b**), and axial proton-density (PD) fat-suppressed image (**c**) show low-signal-intensity lines of bone parallel with the subchondral bone of the femur and patella (*arrows* in **a–c**). Note also the presence of metaphyseal femoral growth arrest line (*curved arrow* in **a, b**)

disappearing after 65 weeks [11]. To recognize these changes is clinically important since the original bone strength is decreased during the presence of the bone marrow changes and there is an increased risk of fractures [12]. Although, on radiography, the disuse changes may mimic more aggressive pathologies as bone necrosis, multiple myeloma, or other malignant lesions, on MR imaging, the diagnosis is straightforward especially when correlated with the patient's history.

The epiphyseal growth arrest lines represent low-signal-intensity linear changes of the subchondral bone and long bone metaphyses [13–15] (Fig. 11.7). They may be caused by immobilization during childhood, infection, or malnutrition [13–15]. MR imaging enables a better visualization of this bone-within-bone appearance compared to radiography [15].

11.2.3 Avascular Necrosis and Bone Marrow Infarction

The necrosis that involves the subchondral bone usually is referred to as avascular osteonecrosis, whereas necrosis of metaphyseal regions is

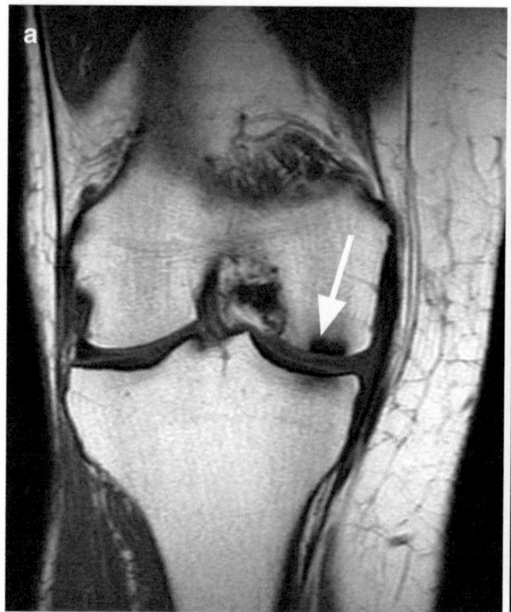
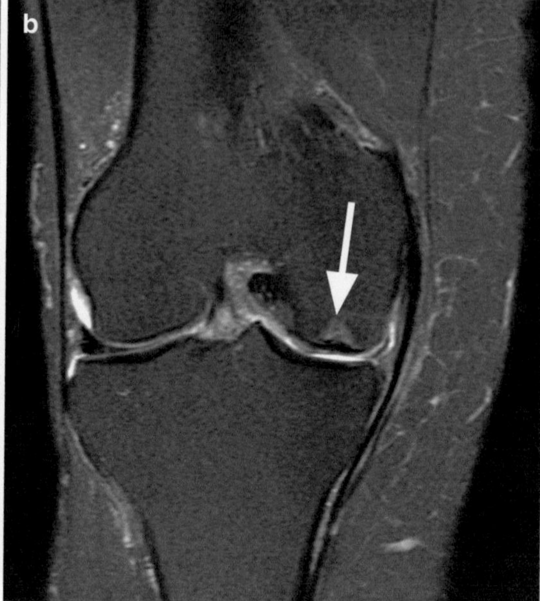

Fig. 11.8 Avascular osteonecrosis of an osteochondral fragment in a 76 year old woman. Coronal T1-weighted image (**a**) and coronal proton-density (PD) fat-suppressed image (**b**) show a subchondral fragment of low signal intensity on both sequences with surrounding edema (*arrows*)

referred to as bone infarction [16]. Spontaneous avascular osteonecrosis of the knee (SONK) is the second most common localization for osteonecrosis after the hip and affects mainly the medial condyle of elderly women over 55 years (Fig. 11.8) [17, 18]. Necrosis may be primary or secondary due to a variety of factors such as trauma (e.g., osteochondral fractures), systemic steroid therapy, alcoholism, or after arthroscopy. The secondary form of necrosis affects younger patients and may be bilateral [17]. In the early stage of osteonecrosis, MR imaging may show only presence of diffuse bone marrow edema within the medial condyle. In later stages, MR imaging demonstrates a serpiginous low-signal-intensity line in the medial condyle. The subchondral fragment may have similar signal intensity to the bone marrow or may display a hypointense signal on both T2-weighted and T1-weighted images with bone depression (Fig. 11.8).

Bone marrow infarction is usually asymptomatic and occurs predominantly in fatty marrow within metaphysis and diaphysis because of poor blood supply in comparison with the hematopoietic marrow which has a higher blood supply. The risk factors for bone infarction are sickle-cell disease, Gaucher's disease, Hodgkin lymphoma, HIV infection, renal transplantation, myeloproliferative disorders, and chemotherapeutic and corticosteroid therapy (Figs. 11.3 and 11.9) [16, 18–21]. On T2-weighted images, the lesion is heterogeneously hyperintense and usually surrounded by an outer rim of low signal intensity with an inner rim of high signal intensity ("the double-line sign") (Fig. 11.10) [16]. The outer rim is thought to represent sclerotic bone and the inner rim vascularized granulation tissue [16]. Very rarely, cyst formation in infarcted bones occurs [22].

11.2.4 Subchondral Bone Contusions (Bone Bruises)

The bone bruises or bone contusions are the result of direct or indirect trauma to the knee and are seen on MR images as subchondral, focal,

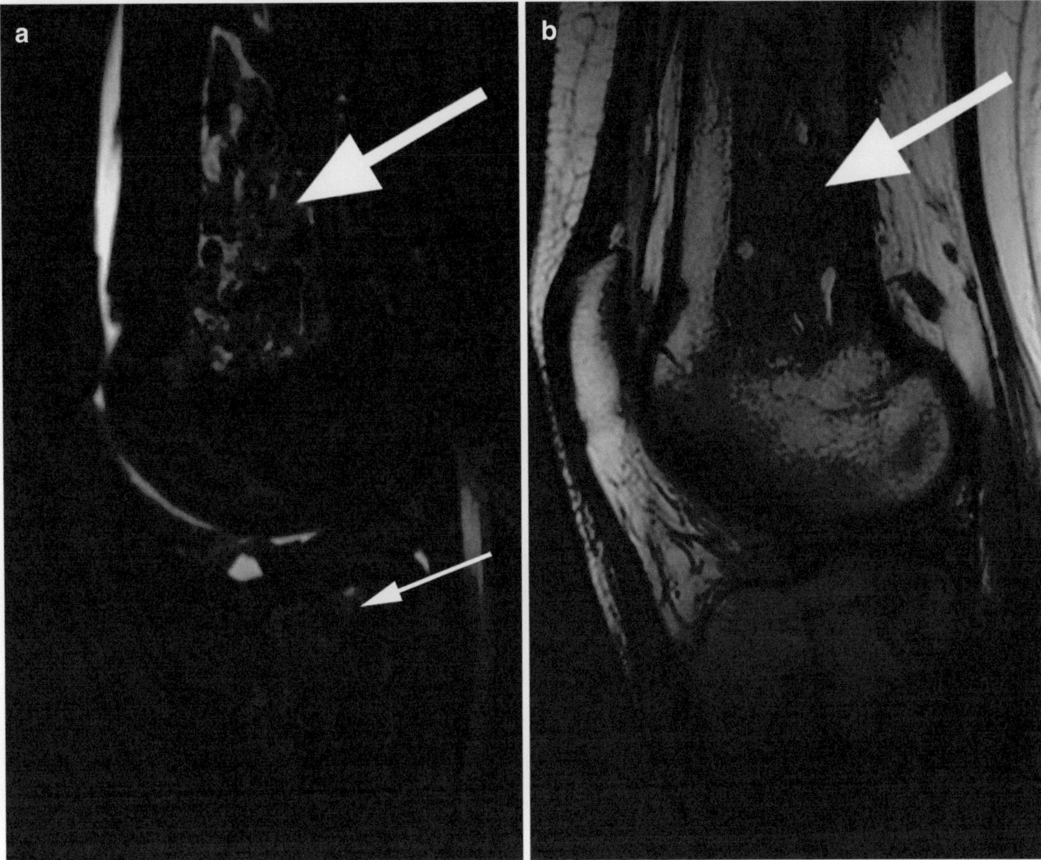

Fig. 11.9 Bone marrow infarction in an 18 year old female with leukemia. Sagittal T2-weighted fat-suppressed image (**a**) and sagittal proton-density (PD) image (**b**) show heterogeneous hyperintense bone infarction of the femoral metaphysis (*large arrow* in **a**, **b**) and tibial plateau. Note the "the double-line sign" represented by an outer rim of low signal intensity with an inner rim of high signal intensity (*small arrow* in **a**)

ill-defined lesions of high signal intensity on T2-weighted images and low signal intensity on T1-weighted images. Usually, the adjacent bone contour is unaffected or may be discretely deepened. Pathologically, in the areas of contusions, edema, trabecular microfractures, and hemorrhage are present. In most of the cases, the bone bruises are secondary signs that accompany more severe lesions of the knee structures. Bone contusions may be single or multiple and are detected in 14–80 % of the patients with knee injuries [23]. The lateral tibial condyle is the most frequently involved area that is diagnosed on MR imaging (Fig. 11.11). When the bone contusions occur on both surfaces of the femoral and tibial articular surfaces, they are known as kissing contusions [24]. There are different injury patterns, and knowing the distribution of the lesions brings important information regarding the mechanism of the knee injury (Table 11.2). Moreover, the location of the bone bruise is an important information and may focus the attention to injuries that could be expected based on specific contusion patterns (Table 11.2). The strongest correlation between bone and ligamentous injuries is the correlation between the anterior cruciate ligament tear and the posterolateral tibial contusion alone or together with lateral femoral contusion (Fig. 11.12) [25].

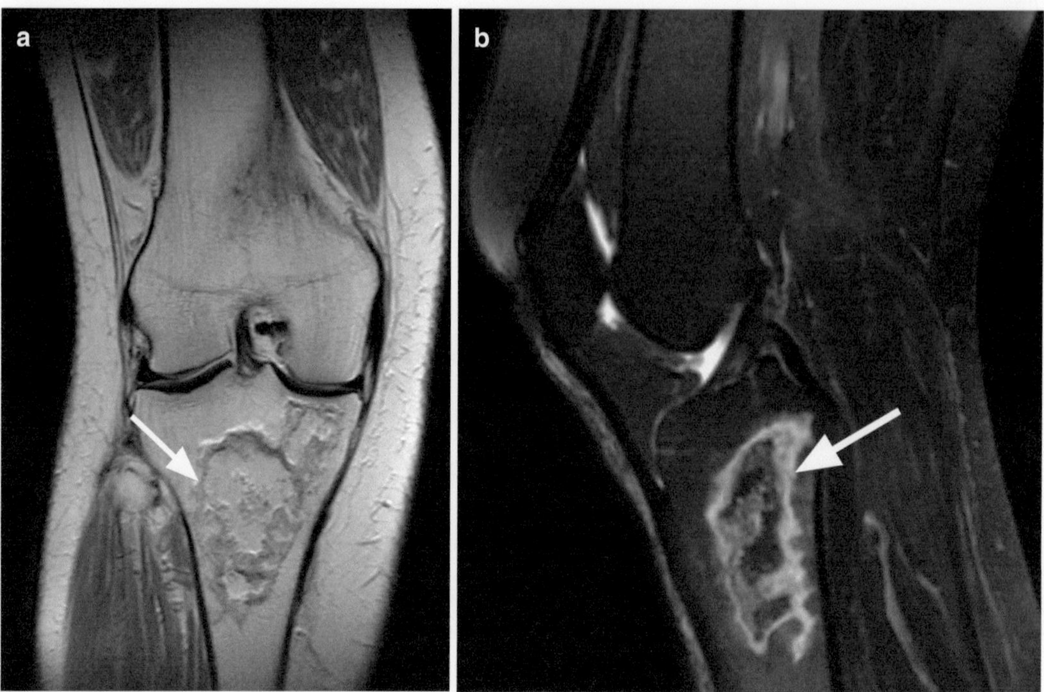

Fig. 11.10 Bone marrow infarction in a 65 year old female. Coronal proton-density (PD) image (**a**) and sagittal T2-weighted fat-suppressed image (**b**) show an area of bone marrow necrosis of the tibial metaphysis with an outer rim of sclerotic bone (*arrows*)

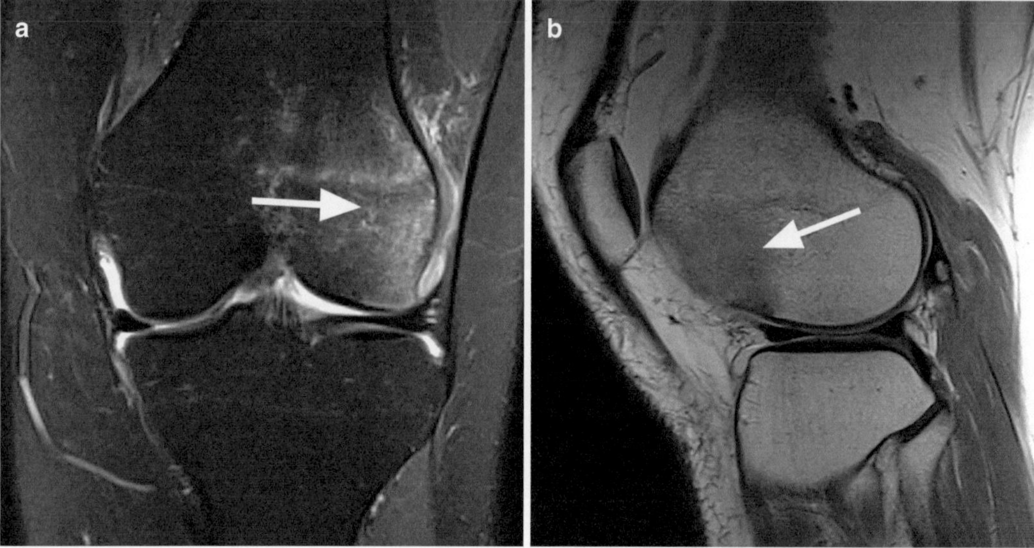

Fig. 11.11 Direct blow injury to the lateral femoral condyle in a 30 year old female. Coronal proton-density (PD) fat-suppressed image (**a**) and sagittal proton-density (PD) image (**b**) show a diffuse area of anterolateral femoral bone contusion (*arrows*)

Table 11.2 The pattern of bone contusions in relation with the mechanism of injury and the expected associated lesions [24, 26]

Contusion pattern	Mechanism of injury	Expected injured structures
Single contusion		
Patellar contusion (Fig. 11.13)	Hyperextension injury[a]	Cartilage contusions
	Direct blow to the patella	Cartilage fracture
	Patellar dislocation[b]	Medial patellar retinaculum
Lateral tibial condyle		
Posterior	Pivot shift injury[c]	Anterior cruciate ligament
	Clip injury[d]	Lateral collateral ligament
		Posterior cruciate ligament
		Lateral meniscus
Central	Pivot injury[c]	Posterior cruciate ligament
	Dashboard injury[e]	
Anterior	Dashboard injury[e]	Posterior cruciate ligament
Medial tibial condyle (Fig. 11.14)		
Posterior	Pivot shift injury[c]	Posterior cruciate ligament
	Clip injury[d]	Lateral meniscus
Central	Clip injury[d]	Lateral collateral ligament
Anterior	Dashboard injury[e]	Lateral collateral ligament
Lateral femoral condyle (Fig. 11.11)		
Posterior	Pivot injury[c]	Posterior cruciate ligament
	Lateral patellar dislocation[b]	Medial retinaculum
Central	Pivot injury[c]	Lateral collateral ligament
	Dashboard injury[e]	Medial retinaculum
Anterior	Lateral patellar dislocation[b]	Medial retinaculum
Medial femoral condyle		
Posterior	Dashboard injury[e]	Rarely medial retinaculum
Central	Dashboard injury[e]	Rarely medial retinaculum
	Hyperextension[a]	
Anterior	Hyperextension[a]	Lateral collateral ligament
Kissing contusions		
Lateral femoral condyle and lateral tibial condyle (Fig. 11.12)	Pivot shift injury[c]	Anterior cruciate ligament
		Medial collateral ligament
		Meniscal tears
Anterior femoral condyle and anterior tibial condyle	Hyperextension injury[a]	Anterior cruciate ligament
		Posterior cruciate ligament
		Meniscal injury
Lateral femoral condyle and medial tibial condyle	Pivot shift injury[c]	Anterior cruciate ligament
		Medial collateral ligament
Anterior tibia and posterior patella	Dashboard injury[e]	Posterior cruciate ligament
Anterolateral femoral condyle and inferomedial patella (Fig. 11.15)	Lateral patellar dislocation[b]	Medial retinaculum

[a]Hyperextension injury: direct force to the anterior tibia or indirect force, such as kicking motion; common in pedestrians hit by a car bumper [26]

[b]Lateral patellar dislocation: transient dislocation of the patella after minor effort in knee flexion or direct medial blow to patella; appears usually in young adults

[c]Pivot shift injury: noncontact injury with a valgus load applied to the knee in various stages of flexion; common in skiers and American football players [26]

[d]Clip injury: direct injury with pure valgus force to the flexed knee; common in American football, soccer, and rugby players

[e]Dashboard injury: force applied to the anterior aspect of the tibia with the knee in flexion; common in car accidents [26]

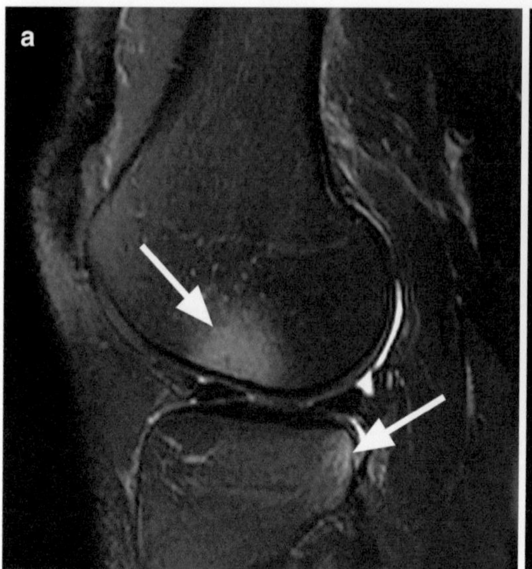 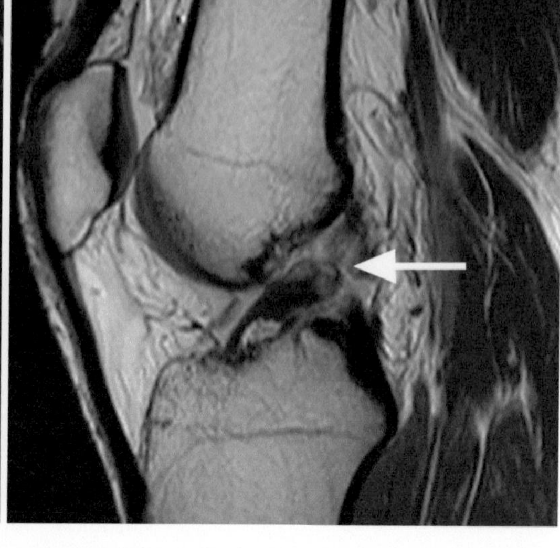

Fig. 11.12 Kissing contusions in a 28 year old male associated with anterior cruciate ligament (ACL) tear. Sagittal T2-weighted fat-suppressed image (**a**) shows contusions of the anterolateral femoral condyle and postero- lateral tibial condyle (*arrows*). Sagittal proton-density (PD) image (**b**) shows the complete tear of the anterior cruciate ligament (ACL) (*arrow*)

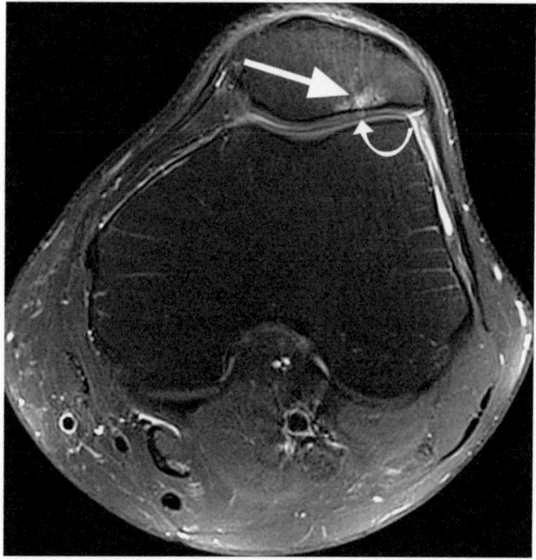

Fig. 11.13 Direct blow to the patella in a 50 year old male. Axial proton-density (PD) fat-suppressed image shows the diffuse edema of the lateral patellar facet (*large arrow*). Note the small acute cartilage lesion (*curved arrow*)

11.2.5 Trauma to Synchondroses

The distal synchondroses of the tibia is the third most common synchondrosis involved in trauma after the distal end of radius and the distal end of the humerus [6]. Knowledge of this type of lesions is important since 25–30 % of patients develop some degree of deformity [6]. According to the Salter-Harris classification, there are five types of synchondrosis injuries from a simple epiphyseal separation to more complex growth plate fractures associated with epiphyseal or metaphyseal fractures [27]. MR imaging is superior to conventional unilateral radiography in the diagnosis of these lesions especially in the cases of pure epiphyseal separation or in cases of discrete associated fractures (Fig. 11.16).

11.2.6 Avulsion Fractures

An avulsion fracture is a detachment of a bone fragment that results from a pulling away mechanism of tendons, ligaments, or capsule from the bone [28]. The young adults and adolescents are particularly vulnerable to avulsion fractures due to the weakness of their apophyses [28]. The most common mechanisms of injury are a single, violent contraction or repeated contractions of a

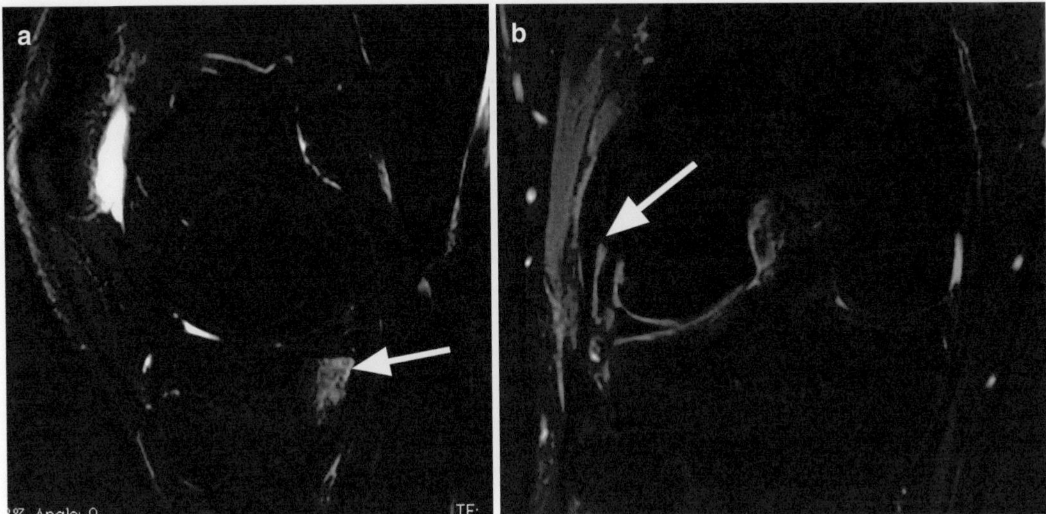

Fig. 11.14 Single contusion in a 27 year old male associated with lateral collateral ligament (LCL) injury. Sagittal T2-weighted fat-suppressed image (**a**) shows contusion of the posteromedial tibial condyle (*arrow*). Coronal proton-density (PD) fat-suppressed image (**b**) shows edema at the insertion of the lateral collateral ligament (LCL) (*arrow*) indicating a sprain of the ligament without fiber discontinuity

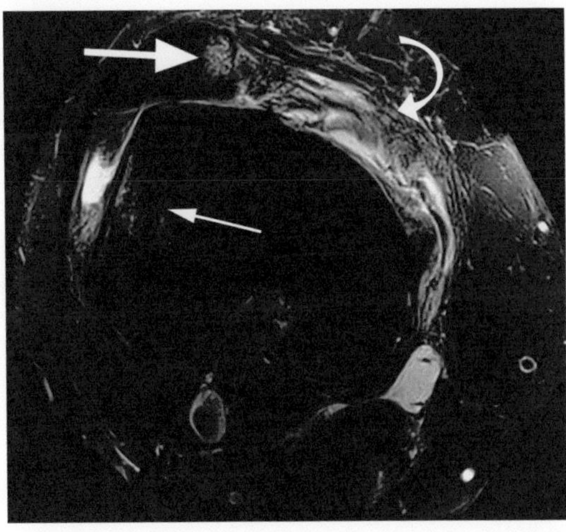

Fig. 11.15 Patellar dislocation in a 26 year old male. Axial proton-density (PD) fat-suppressed image shows kissing contusions of the medial patella (*large arrow*) and lateral femoral condyle (*small arrow*). Note the complete tear of the medial retinaculum (*curved arrow*)

muscle transmitted through its tendon [5]. The first diagnostic choice is radiography, but these fractures may be easily missed because of their subtle appearance with often only minimal cortical breaching. The best diagnostic approach is a correlation of radiography and MR imaging findings that enables the visualization of the bone fragment as well as the associated tendinous and/or ligamentous injuries. Without having a radiograph, pure MR imaging visualization of the bone fragment depends on the size of the fragment. Small fragments are difficult to be demonstrated on MRI especially when the avulsed fragment is entirely low signal intensity on T1-weighted and high signal intensity on T2-weighted images due to bone marrow edema. In these cases, the fragment may be indistinct from the surrounding soft tissue edema and hemorrhage. However, the bone marrow edema and the cortical defect at the site of the avulsed fragment together with the pathological changes of the tendons or ligaments are reliable MR imaging findings for diagnosis. The knee is one of the most frequently involved joint in such injuries due to its numerous tendinous, ligamentous, and capsular attachments (Table 11.3) [28].

11.2.7 Stress Injuries/Fractures

Stress fractures are bone lesions encountered in patients with rapid increase or alteration in physical loading magnitude or intensity of

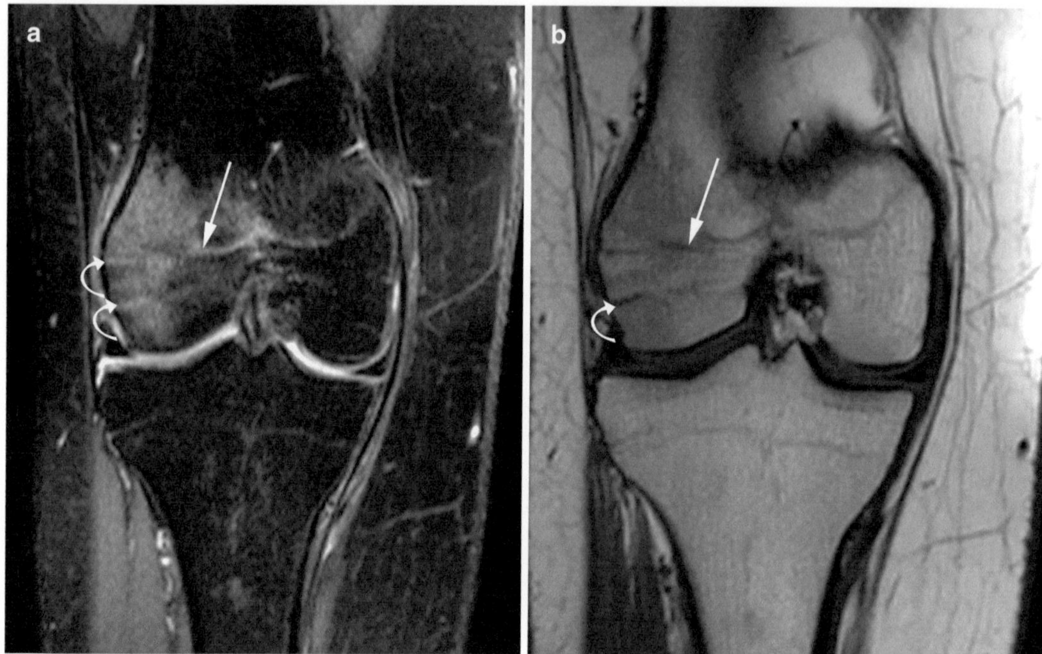

Fig. 11.16 Trauma to femoral syncondroses in a 18 year old female. Coronal proton-density (PD) fat-suppressed image (**a**) and coronal T1-weighted image (**b**) show syn-condoroses injury (*arrow* in **a** and **b**) and discrete lines of fractures (*curved arrows* in **a** and **b**)

Table 11.3 Avulsion injuries to the knee – mechanism and involvement of specific tendons or ligaments [5, 28–33]

Avulsion injury	Mechanism of injury	Tendons/ligaments involved
Tibial spine avulsion (intercondylar eminence) (Fig. 11.17)	Pivot shift injury Clip injury Hyperextension/hyperflexion	Anterior cruciate ligament or posterior cruciate ligament at the tibial insertion
Lateral tibial cortical plateau – Segond fracture (see Fig. 4.20)	Internal rotation and varus stress	Lateral capsule and iliotibial band
Medial tibial cortical plateau – reverse Segond fracture (see Fig. 3.17)	External rotation and valgus stress	Deep component of medial collateral ligament
Gerdy's tibial tubercle avulsion (iliotibial band avulsion) (Fig. 11.18)	Varus force with knee in flexion and internal rotation	Iliotibial band
Tibial tuberosity avulsion (Osgood-Schlatter disease) (Fig. 11.19)	Violent extension or severe hyperflexion of the knee Microavulsions with repeated fractures of the tibial tubercle (Osgood-Schlatter disease)	Patellar tendon
Posteromedial tibia – semimembranosus avulsion	External rotation and abduction of knee in flexion	Semimembranosus tendon
Superior pole of the patella	Hyperflexion or hyperextension with traction from the quadriceps tendon Patella baja	Quadriceps tendon
Inferior pole of the patella (Sinding-Larsen-Johansson syndrome) or Cartilaginous inferior patellar sleeve avulsion	Traction of patellar tendon	Patellar tendon
Proximal head of fibula – the "arcuate" sign (see Figs. 4.18 and 4.19)	Direct varus force to the anteromedial aspect of the hyperextended knee	Lateral collateral ligament, biceps tendon, arcuate ligament, popliteofibular ligament, or fabellofibular ligament

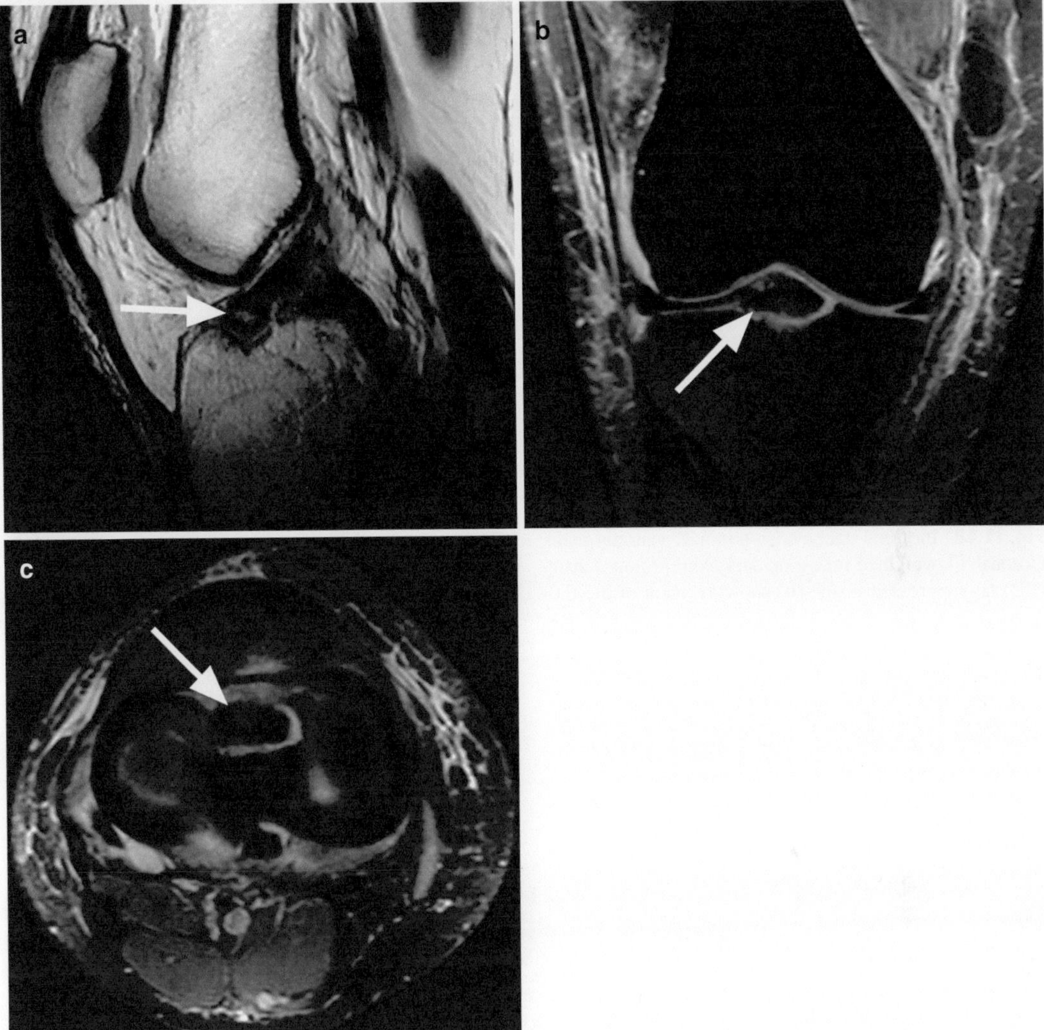

Fig. 11.17 Tibial spine avulsion in a 53 year old male. Sagittal proton-density (PD) image (**a**), coronal proton-density (PD) fat-suppressed image (**b**), and axial proton-density (PD) fat-suppressed image (**c**) show the avulsion of a bone fragment from the intercondylareminence (*arrows*) without tear of the anterior cruciate ligament (ACL)

physical activities [34]. In a large series of 1,330 patients with exercise-induced knee pain who underwent MR imaging, it was been shown that 25 % of the patients had bilateral bone stress injuries and 28 % had unilateral stress injuries to the knee [35]. The stress injuries may be classified into five grades as follows: grade I, endosteal marrow edema; grade II, periosteal edema and endosteal marrow edema; grade III, muscle edema, periosteal edema, and endosteal marrow edema; grade IV, fracture line; and grade V, callus in cortical bone [34]. Even in the cases in which the stress fracture is located at the weight-bearing surfaces, depression of the articular surface of the bone might not be present, and radiography does not enable the diagnosis [36]. MR imaging is the method of choice, being able to identify all the abovementioned pathological changes. Thus, it is recommended as a routine examination in patients with regular physical activities associated with the onset of pain symptoms [35]. The MR findings include the bone marrow edema as localized ill-defined high signal intensity on fat-suppressed T2-weighted images and low signal intensity on T1-weighted images and the presence of fine fractures visible as low-signal-intensity lines in the underlying medullary portion of the bone.

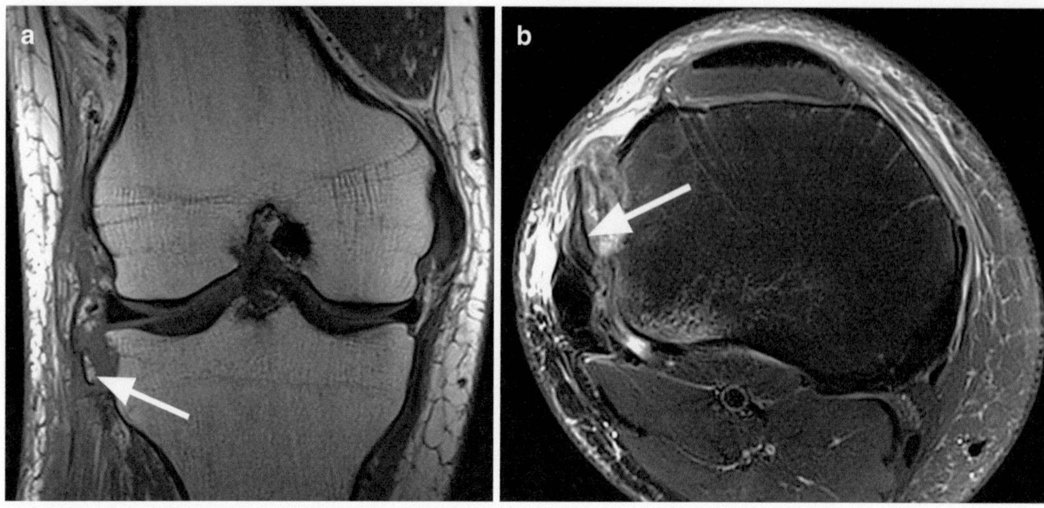

Fig. 11.18 Iliotibial tract avulsion in a 37 year old male. Coronal T1-weighted image (**a**) and axial proton-density (PD) fat-suppressed image (**b**) show avulsion of the ilio-tibial tract from its attachment on the Gerdy's tibial tubercle (*arrow*)

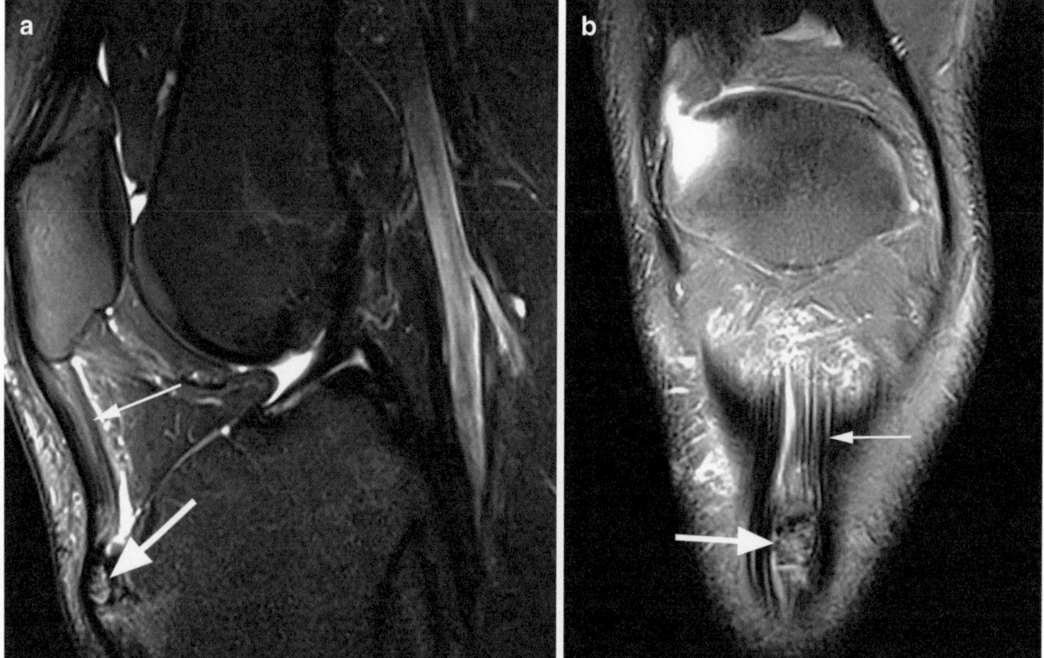

Fig. 11.19 Osgood-Schlatter disease in a 22 year old male. Sagittal T2-weighted fat-suppressed image (**a**) and coronal proton-density (PD) fat-suppressed image (**b**) show a small fragment of bone detached from the attachment's site of patellar tendon (*large arrow* in **a, b**). Note the longitudinal tear of the patellar tendon (*small arrow* in **a, b**)

Diffuse periosteal edema is usually identified on MR imaging in patients with the stress injuries (Fig. 11.20). Around the knee, the most commonly involved sites are the medial tibial plateau, the tibial shaft, and the subchondral femoral condyles.

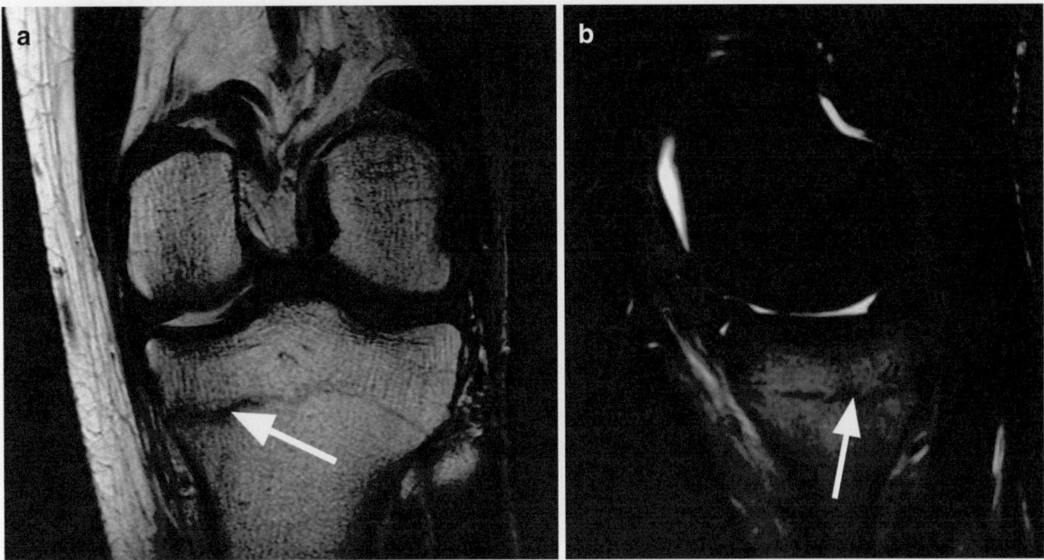

Fig. 11.20 Grade IV stress fracture in a 32 year old male with medial knee pain after running. Coronal proton-density (PD) image (**a**) and sagittal T2-weighted fat- suppressed image (**b**) show extensive bone marrow edema and a fracture line of the medial tibial plateau (*arrows*)

11.2.8 Bone Tumors Around the Knee

The most common bone tumors and tumorlike lesions are detailed in Table 11.4. In the majority of the cases, the benign bone lesions are discovered incidentally during routine MRI examinations, and the most frequent lesions are enchondroma and osteochondroma.

Enchondroma is a common, benign, cartilage-forming tumor that occurs in most of the cases as a single, asymptomatic lesion [37]. On MR images the lesion is of variable size, well delineated but with irregular contour, and inhomogeneous signal intensity. The non-mineralized component of the tumor is always low to intermediate signal intensity on T1-weighted images and intermediate to high signal intensity on T2-weighted images (Fig. 11.21) [38]. Rarely, patients present with multiple lesions which is defined as enchondromatosis (Fig. 11.22) [37]. Sometimes the differentiation between enchondroma and low-grade chondrosarcoma is difficult, but recently, it has been shown that the dynamic contrast-enhanced MR imaging may

Table 11.4 The most common bone tumors and tumor-like lesions affecting the knee [43, 44]

	Most common sites	Peak age (years)
Benign tumors		
Enchondroma (Figs. 11.21 and 11.22)	Distal femur, proximal tibia	10–40
Osteochondroma (Fig. 11.23)	Distal femur, proximal tibia	10–30
Periosteal chondroma	Distal femur	10–40
Chondroblastoma	Distal femur, proximal tibia, patella	10–30
Chodromixoid fibroma	Proximal tibia, distal femur	10–30
Giant cell tumor (Fig. 11.24)	Distal femur, proximal tibia	20–45
Lipoma	Femur	Adults
Malignant tumors		
Primary chondrosarcoma	Distal femur	50–80
Osteosarcoma (Fig. 11.25)	Distal femur, proximal tibia	10–30
Low-grade central osteosarcoma	Distal femur, proximal tibia	20–40
Parosteal osteosarcoma	Posterior distal femur	20–50
Periosteal osteosarcoma	Femur, tibia	10–30
Fibrosarcoma	Knee region	40–70

(continued)

Table 11.4 (continued)

	Most common sites	Peak age (years)
Malignant giant cell tumor	Knee region	20–60
Metastases (Fig. 11.26)	Knee region	>40
Tumorlike lesions		
Paget disease	Tibia, femur	>50

play a complementary role in differentiating these two entities [39].

Osteochondroma is an easy diagnosis on radiography as well as on MR images. It appears as a bone abnormality growing in the wrong direction having the cortex in continuity with that of the normal bone of origin (Fig. 11.23) [40]. The role of imaging is to differentiate between a

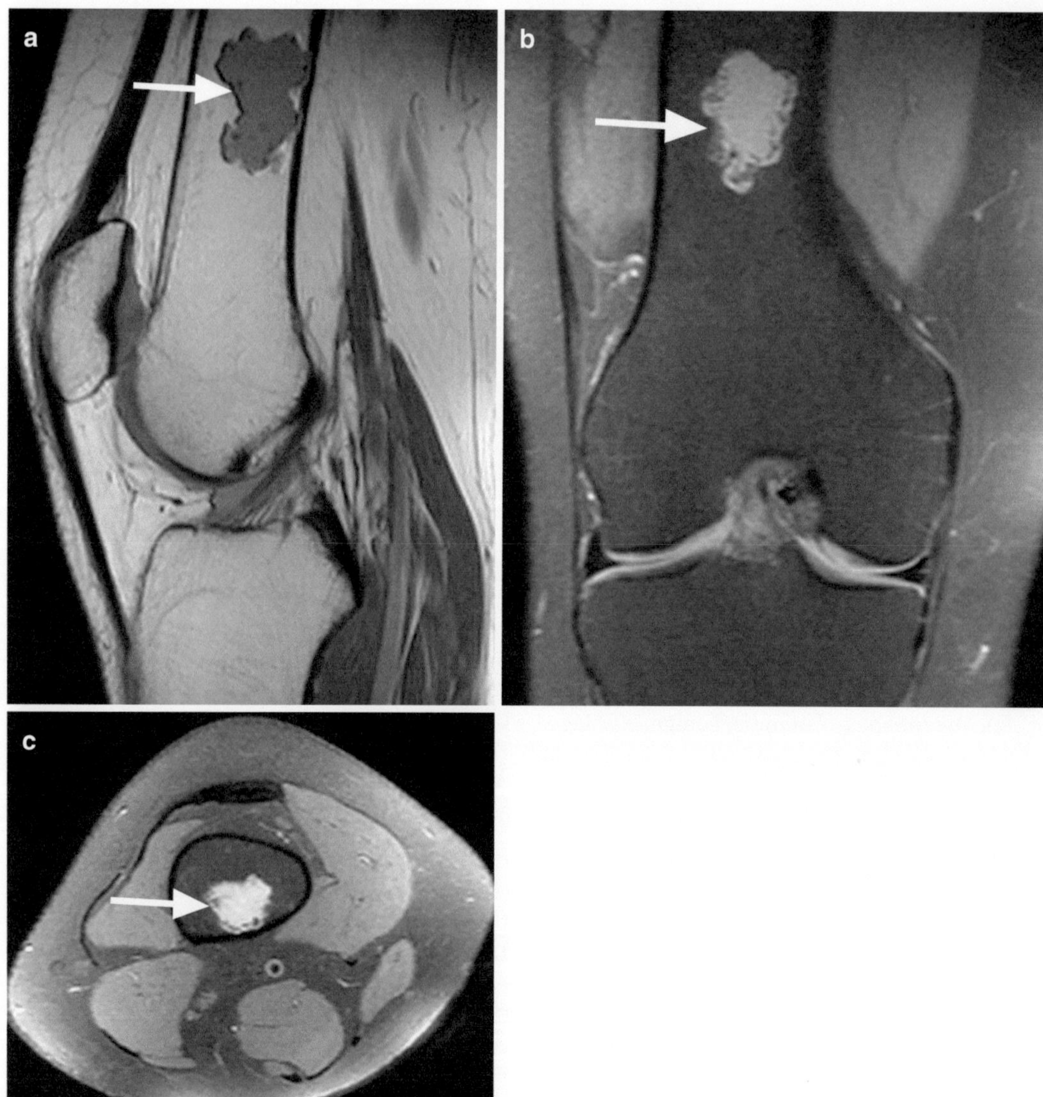

Fig. 11.21 Enchondroma in a 40 year old female. Sagittal proton-density (PD) image (**a**), coronal proton-density (PD) fat-suppressed image (**b**) and axial proton-density (PD) fat-suppressed image (**c**) show a well delineated lesion with irregular margins (*arrows*) indicating an enchondroma

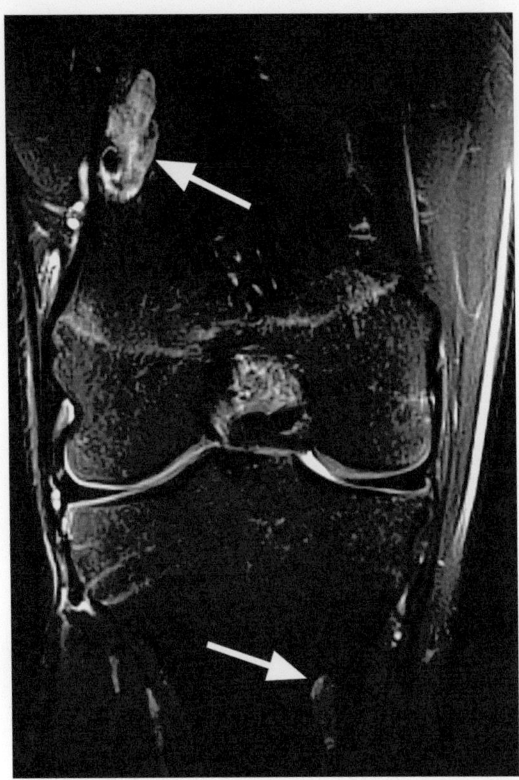

Fig. 11.22 Enchondromatosis in a 20 year old male. Coronal proton-density (PD) fat-suppressed image shows a femoral and a tibial lesion (*arrows*) with typical appearance of enchondromas

benign lesion and a possible chondrosarcoma. The growth of the lesion in an adult, a cartilage thicker than 3 cm, and the presence of adjacent infiltrative soft tissue changes suggest a malignant lesion [41].

The diagnosis of malignant bone tumors is based on a multimodality imaging approach in which the classic radiograph remains the basis of the evaluation [42]. Computed tomography provides complimentary information on the bone cortex and on tumor matrix calcifications. MR imaging, however, due to its superior tissue contrast capabilities, is useful for staging purposes and treatment follow-up. MR imaging may also give valuable information regarding the tumor structure, including the presence of various intratumoral changes such as fat, necrosis, or hemorrhage. A complete description of a bone tumor should refer to its intra- or extra-compartmental extent, the intra-articular invasion, the degree of the bone marrow involvement, the presence of possible intramedullary skip lesions, and the relation (invasion or not) of the neurovascular structures (Fig. 11.24).

11.3 MRI Impression

1. Transient bone marrow edema (absence of trauma)
2. Disuse osteopenia (correlated with the patient's history)
3. Avascular necrosis (subchondral bone)
4. Bone marrow infarction
5. Bone contusions or bone bruises – specify distribution
6. Synchondrosis injury – Salter-Harris classification
7. Stress fracture – grade I–V
8. Bone tumor
   - Benign
   - Malignant: intra- or extra-compartmental extent, the intra-articular invasion, intramedullary skip lesions, and invasion or not of the neurovascular structures

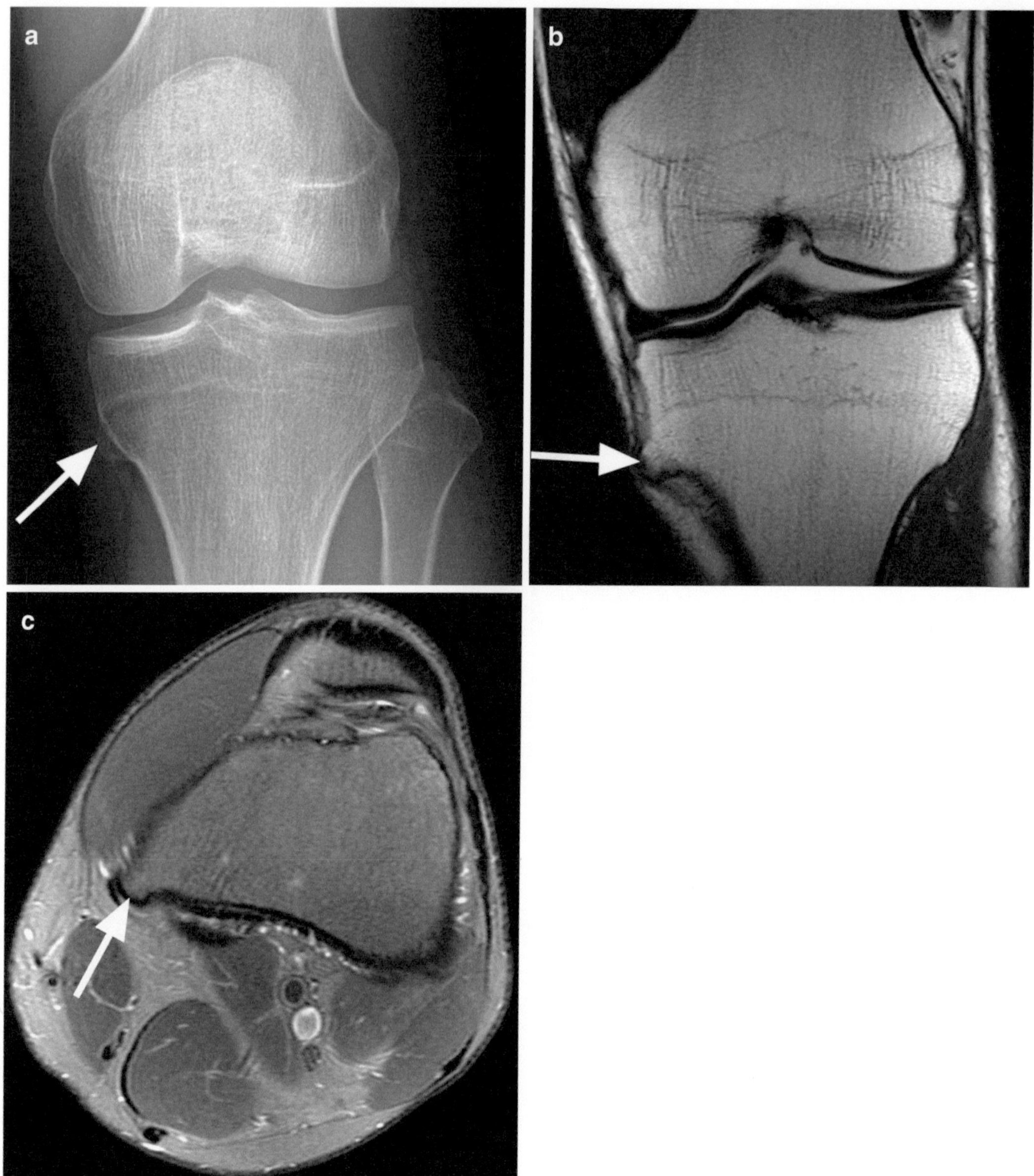

Fig. 11.23 Osteochondroma in a 24 year old male. Radiography (**a**), coronal proton-density (PD) MR image (**b**), and axial proton-density (PD) fat-suppressed MR image (**c**) show a sessile small solitary exostosis of the posteromedial tibial metaphysis (*arrow*)

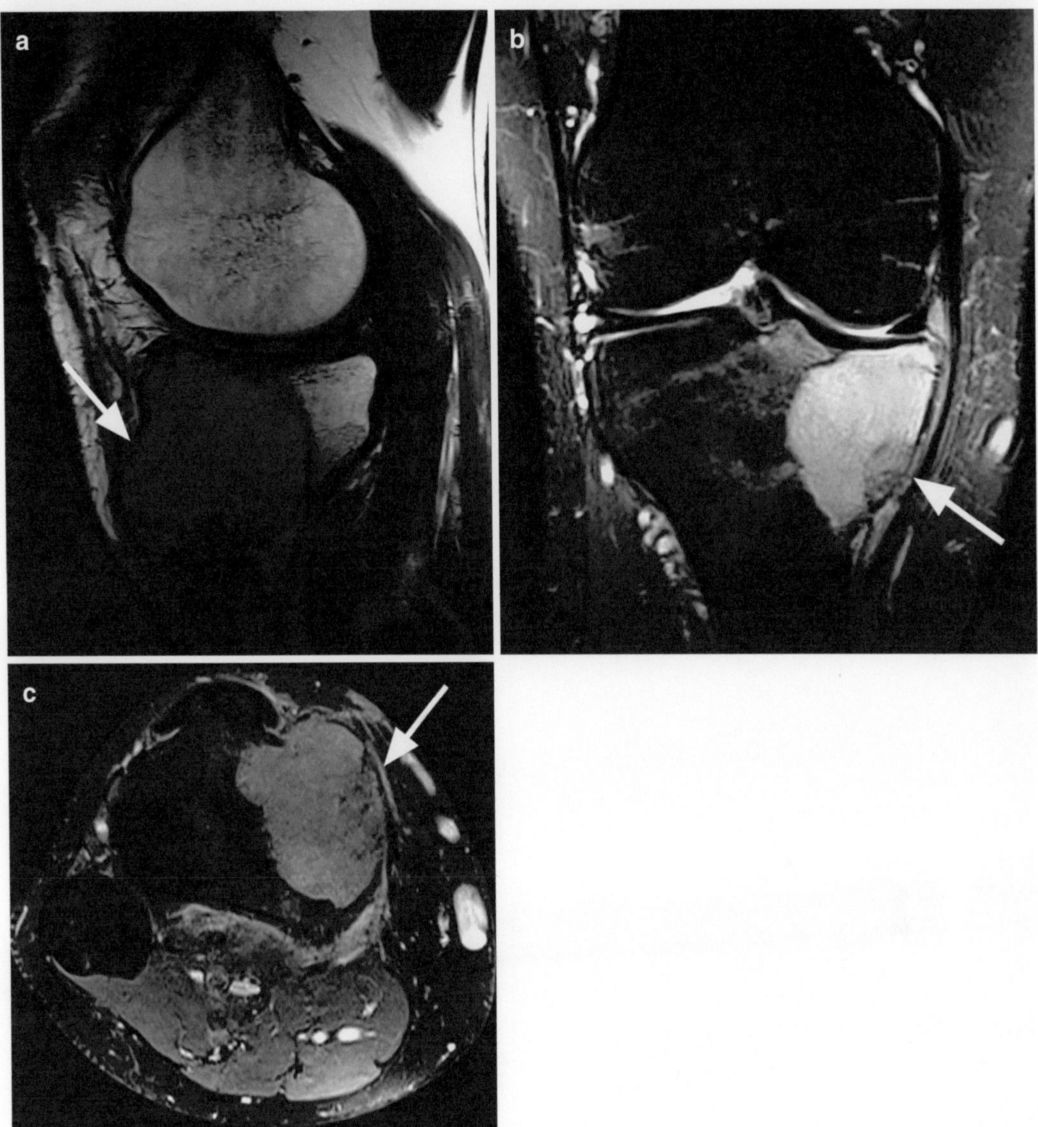

Fig. 11.24 Giant cell tumor in a 26 year old male. *S*agittal proton-density (PD) image (**a**), coronal proton-density (PD) fat-suppressed image (**b**), and axial T1-weighted fat-suppressed postcontrast image (**c**) show an expansile cystic mass, delineated by a thin band of low signal intensity with moderate enhancement. Note the soft tissue extension (*arrow* in **a–c**) which is common in this types of tumors

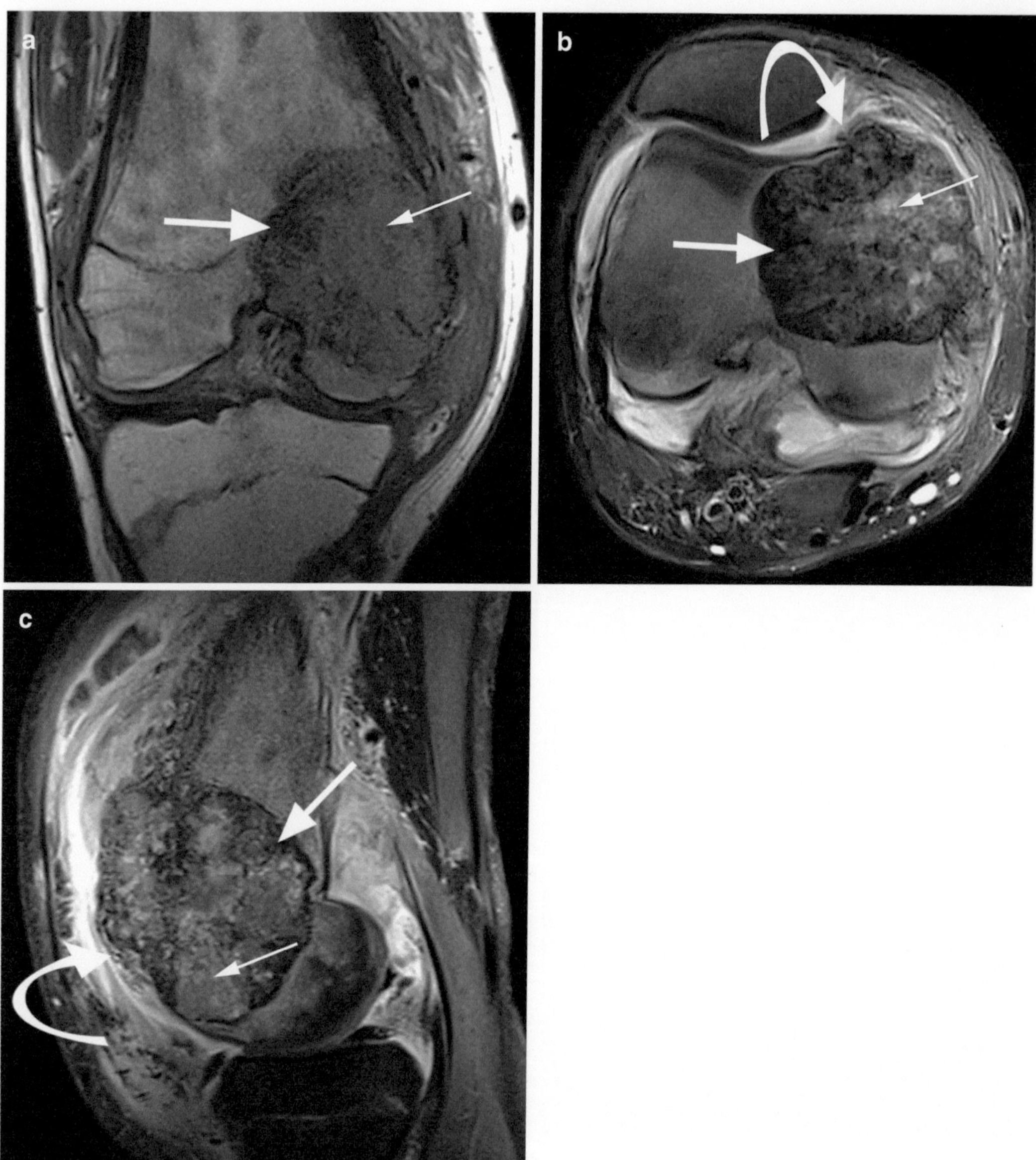

Fig. 11.25 Osteosarcoma in a 17 year old male. Coronal T1-weighted image (**a**), axial proton-density (PD) fat-suppressed image (**b**), and sagittal T1-weighted fat-suppressed postcontrast image (**c**) show an inhomogeneous epiphyseal tumor of the distal femur with an osteoid portion which appears low signal intensity (*large arrow* in **a**, **b**, and **c**). The non-osteoid portion is intermediate signal intensity (*small arrow* in **a** and **b**)and enhances after contrast administration (*small arrow* in **c**). The lesion is eccentrically located and invades the adjacent soft tissue and the femoropatellar joint (*curved arrow* in **b** and **c**)

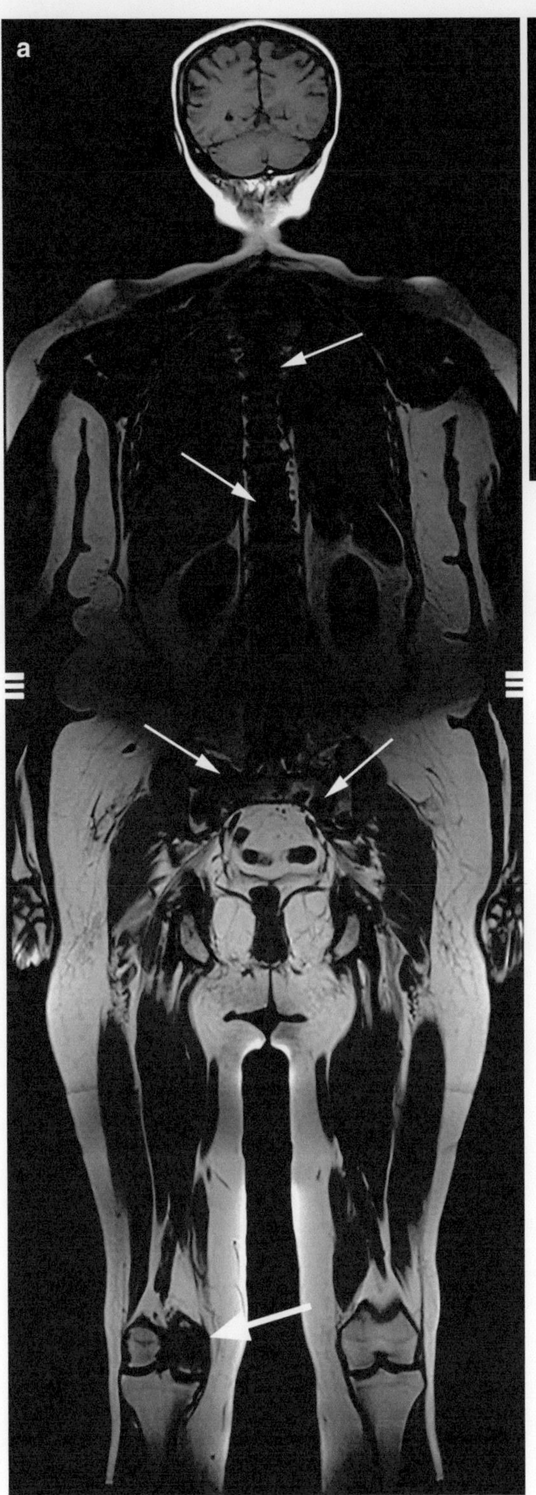

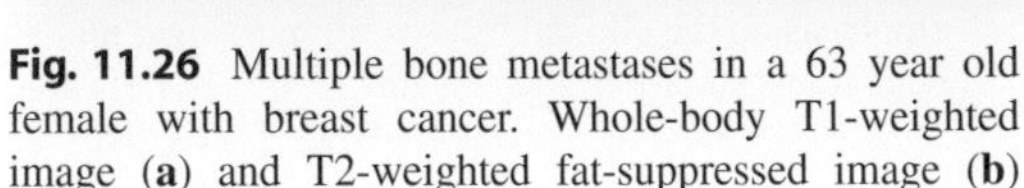

Fig. 11.26 Multiple bone metastases in a 63 year old female with breast cancer. Whole-body T1-weighted image (**a**) and T2-weighted fat-suppressed image (**b**) show multiple bone lesions (*small arrows* in **a**) including metastases of the distal femur (*large arrows* in **a**, **b**)

References

1. Eley KA, et al. "Black bone" MRI: a partial flip angle technique for radiation reduction in craniofacial imaging. Br J Radiol. 2012;85(1011):272–8.
2. Hanna SL, et al. Magnetic resonance imaging of disseminated bone marrow disease in patients treated for malignancy. Skeletal Radiol. 1991;20(2):79–84.
3. Vanel D. MRI of bone metastases: the choice of the sequence. Cancer Imaging. 2004;4(1):30–5.
4. Shah LM, Hanrahan CJ. MRI of spinal bone marrow: part I, techniques and normal age-related appearances. AJR Am J Roentgenol. 2011;197(6):1298–308.
5. Tehranzadeh J. The spectrum of avulsion and avulsion-like injuries of the musculoskeletal system. Radiographics. 1987;7(5):945–74.
6. Taylor J, Hughes TH, Resnick D. Chapter 1. In: Taylor J, Hughes TH, Resnick D, editors. Skeletal imaging: atlas of the spine and extremities. Maryland Heights: Saunders; 2010. ISBN-10: 1-4160-5623-8.
7. Hayes CW, Conway WF, Daniel WW. MR imaging of bone marrow edema pattern: transient osteoporosis, transient bone marrow edema syndrome, or osteonecrosis. Radiographics. 1993;13(5):1001–11; discussion 1012.
8. Joyce JM, Keats TE. Disuse osteoporosis: mimic of neoplastic disease. Skeletal Radiol. 1986;15(2):129–32.
9. Poole KE, Warburton EA, Reeve J. Rapid long-term bone loss following stroke in a man with osteoporosis and atherosclerosis. Osteoporos Int. 2005;16(3):302–5.
10. Lang TF, et al. Adaptation of the proximal femur to skeletal reloading after long-duration spaceflight. J Bone Miner Res. 2006;21(8):1224–30.
11. Nardo L, et al. Bone marrow changes related to disuse. Eur Radiol. 2013;23(12):3422–31.
12. Loomer PM. The impact of microgravity on bone metabolism in vitro and in vivo. Crit Rev Oral Biol Med. 2001;12(3):252–61.
13. Park EA. The imprinting of nutritional disturbances on the growing bone. Pediatrics. 1964;33(SUPPL): 815–62.
14. Ogden JA. Growth slowdown and arrest lines. J Pediatr Orthop. 1984;4(4):409–15.
15. Yao L, Seeger LL. Epiphyseal growth arrest lines. MR findings. Clin Imaging. 1997;21(4):237–40.
16. Saini A, Saifuddin A. MRI of osteonecrosis. Clin Radiol. 2004;59(12):1079–93.
17. Mont MA, et al. Atraumatic osteonecrosis of the knee. J Bone Joint Surg Am. 2000;82(9):1279–90.
18. Breer S, et al. Spontaneous osteonecrosis of the knee (SONK). Knee Surg Sports Traumatol Arthrosc. 2013;21(2):340–5.
19. Rowe CW, Haggard ME. Bone infarcts in sickle-cell anemia. Radiology. 1957;68(5):661–8.
20. Jensen KE, et al. Magnetic resonance imaging of the bone marrow following treatment with recombinant human erythropoietin in patients with end-stage renal disease. Int J Artif Organs. 1990;13(8):477–81.
21. Umans H, Haramati N, Flusser G. The diagnostic role of gadolinium enhanced MRI in distinguishing between acute medullary bone infarct and osteomyelitis. Magn Reson Imaging. 2000;18(3):255–62.
22. Norman A, Steiner GC. Radiographic and morphological features of cyst formation in idiopathic bone infarction. Radiology. 1983;146(2):335–8.
23. Adalberth T, et al. Magnetic resonance imaging, scintigraphy, and arthroscopic evaluation of traumatic hemarthrosis of the knee. Am J Sports Med. 1997; 25(2):231–7.
24. Terzidis IP, et al. The appearance of kissing contusion in the acutely injured knee in the athletes. Br J Sports Med. 2004;38(5):592–6.
25. Zeiss J, et al. Comparison of bone contusion seen by MRI in partial and complete tears of the anterior cruciate ligament. J Comput Assist Tomogr. 1995;19(5): 773–6.
26. Sanders TG, et al. Bone contusion patterns of the knee at MR imaging: footprint of the mechanism of injury. Radiographics. 2000;20(Spec No):S135–51.
27. Brown JH, DeLuca SA. Growth plate injuries: Salter-Harris classification. Am Fam Physician. 1992;46(4): 1180–4.
28. Gottsegen CJ, et al. Avulsion fractures of the knee: imaging findings and clinical significance. Radiographics. 2008;28(6):1755–70.
29. Capps GW, Hayes CW. Easily missed injuries around the knee. Radiographics. 1994;14(6):1191–210.
30. Hall FM, Hochman MG. Medial Segond-type fracture: cortical avulsion off the medial tibial plateau associated with tears of the posterior cruciate ligament and medial meniscus. Skeletal Radiol. 1997;26(9):553–5.
31. Stevens MA, et al. Imaging features of avulsion injuries. Radiographics. 1999;19(3):655–72.
32. Hayes CW, et al. Mechanism-based pattern approach to classification of complex injuries of the knee depicted at MR imaging. Radiographics. 2000; 20(Spec No):S121–34.
33. Bolog N, Hodler J. MR imaging of the posterolateral corner of the knee. Skeletal Radiol. 2007;36(8): 715–28.
34. Niva MH, et al. Bone stress injuries are common in female military trainees: a preliminary study. Clin Orthop Relat Res. 2009;467(11):2962–9.
35. Niva MH, et al. Bone stress injuries causing exercise-induced knee pain. Am J Sports Med. 2006;34(1): 78–83.
36. Rosenthal MD, Moore JH, DeBerardino TM. Diagnosis of medial knee pain: atypical stress fracture about the knee joint. J Orthop Sports Phys Ther. 2006;36(7):526–34.
37. Herget GW, et al. Insights into Enchondroma, Enchondromatosis and the risk of secondary Chondrosarcoma. Review of the literature with an emphasis on the clinical behaviour, radiology, malignant transformation and the follow up. Neoplasma. 2014;61(4):365–78. doi: 10.4149/neo_2014_046.

38. Murphey MD, et al. Enchondroma versus chondrosarcoma in the appendicular skeleton: differentiating features. Radiographics. 1998;18(5):1213–37; quiz 1244–5.
39. De Coninck T, et al. Dynamic contrast-enhanced MR imaging for differentiation between enchondroma and chondrosarcoma. Eur Radiol. 2013;23(11):3140–52.
40. Vanel D, et al. The incidental skeletal lesion: ignore or explore? Cancer Imaging. 2009;9(Spec No A):S38–43.
41. Masciocchi C, Sparvoli L, Barile A. Diagnostic imaging of malignant cartilage tumors. Eur J Radiol. 1998;27 Suppl 1:S86–90.
42. Nomikos GC, et al. Primary bone tumors of the lower extremities. Radiol Clin North Am. 2002;40(5): 971–90.
43. Kindblom L. Bone tumors: epidemiology, classification, pathology. In: Davies AS, James M, editors. Bone tumors and tumor-like lesions. Berlin/Heidelberg/Leipzig: Springer; 2010. p. 1–17.
44. Taylor J, Hughes TH, Resnick D. Chapter 9. In: Taylor J, Hughes TH, Resnick D, editors. Skeletal imaging: atlas of the spine and extremities. Maryland Heights: Saunders; 2010. ISBN-10: 1-4160-5623-8.

Index

A

Achilles allograft, 45

ACL. *See* Anterior cruciate ligament (ACL)

Amyloidosis, 153

Anterior cruciate ligament (ACL), 66, 71, 133, 152, 159, 214

  acute tear

    primary signs, 3–5

    secondary signs, 3–4, 6–7

  anatomy, 1, 2

  avulsion fracture, 5–6, 8

  chronic tear

    diffuse/focal midsubstance intermediate signal changes, 8, 9

    diffuse/focal midsubstance low signal changes, 8, 9

    focal fibrotic changes, 8, 10

    with knee instability, 8, 11

    without trauma, 8, 11

  fixation devices, 16

  ganglion cyst, 8–9, 11

  iliotibial band friction syndrome, 16

  infections, 16, 18

  mucoid degeneration, 9–10, 12

  nonsurgical ACL, 17

  partial tear, 4–5, 7–8

  postoperative ACL

    arthrofibrosis, 15–17

    femoral and tibial tunnels, 11, 13

    graft's signal intensity, 12, 14

    MRI impression, 17–18

    partial graft tear, 13, 15

    tunnel cysts and enlargement, 13, 15, 16

    tunnels misplacement, 12, 14–15

  unilateral congenital absence, 1, 3

Anterior oblique band (AOB), 49, 51

Anterior transverse ligament, 67–69

Anterolateral ligament (ALL), 49

  complete tears, 55, 58

  knee arthroplasty, 50

  reinforcement, 50

  thin hypointense linear structure, 51, 53

Arcuate ligament (AL)

  complete tears, 55, 58

  lateral limb, 54

  origin, 51

  sign, 59, 60

  Y-shaped thickening capsule, 51

Arteries

  inferior lateral genicular artery, 191

  inferior medial genicular artery, 191

  medial and lateral sural arteries, 191

  middle genicular artery, 189

  MRI impression, 202

  MRI pathological findings

    aneurysms, 194–195

    artery entrapment syndrome, 196

    atherosclerosis and thrombosis, 194

    embolism, 194

    hemangiomas, 196–198

    traumatic and iatrogenic injuries, 196

    vascular malformations, 198

  popliteal artery, 189

  superior lateral genicular artery, 191

  superior medial genicular artery, 191

Arthrofibrosis, 33, 132, 133

  large cyclopoid lesions, 15, 17

  Small cyclopoid lesions, 15, 16

Articular cartilage

  calcified cartilage zone, 95

  cartilage thickness and signal intensity, 95–97

  compositional MRI techniques, 96, 97

  deep/radial zone, 95

  functional unit, 95

  impression, 110–111

  morphological evaluation, 95–97

  nontraumatic cartilage changes

    degenerative changes, 98, 99

    delamination, 99

    denuded areas, 100

    thickness changes and signal-intensity alteration, 98

  osteochondritis dissecans

    grade II lesion (stable), 105, 107, 108

    grade I lesion (stable), 105, 106, 108

    grade IV lesion (unstable), 105, 106, 108

  superficial zone, 95

  transitional zone, 95

  traumatic cartilage injuries

N.V. Bolog et al., *MRI of the Knee: A Guide to Evaluation and Reporting,*
DOI 10.1007/978-3-319-08165-6, © Springer International Publishing Switzerland 2015

Articular cartilage (*cont.*)
    acute cartilage contusion, 104
    acute cartilage fracture, 104, 105
    acute cartilage lesion, 104
    avascular osteonecrosis, 103, 104
    classification, 104, 106
    delamination, 98, 99, 104
    patellar cartilage fissure, 104
    severe acute cartilage injury, 104, 105

B
Biceps tendon (BT), 49–51, 174, 192
    arcuate signs, 59
    avulsion fractures, 183
    and lateral collateral ligament, 51
    posterolateral muscle group, 172
    subtotal biceps tendon, 186
Bones
    anatomy and normal MRI appearance,
        205–206
    attrition of, 102
    avascular necrosis and bone marrow infarction,
        209–210
    avulsion fractures, 214–216
    bone attachment (*see* Lateral meniscus;
        Medial meniscus)
    bone fragment, 60
    bone marrow edema, 18, 26, 27
    bone-patellar tendon-bone grafts, 32
    and capsular attachments, 70–71
    diatal synchondroses, 214
    disuse osteopenia, 207–209
    enchondroma, 219–220
    epiphyseal growth arrest, 209
    multiple bone metastases, 225
    myositis ossificans, 178
    osteochondroma, 220–223
    patella (*see* Patella)
    stress injuries/fractures
        classification, 217
        diffuse periosteal edema, 218
        grade IV stress fracture, 219
        MR findings, 217
    subchondral bone (*see* Subchondral bone)
    subchondral bone contusions
        bone contusions, 211, 213
        kissing contusions, 214
        lateral femoral condyle, 212
        T2-weighted images, 211
    transient bone marrow edema, 206, 208
Boston-Leeds osteoarthritis knee score
        (BLOKS), 96
Bursitis, 35, 147, 181
    acute suprapatellar bursitis, 154
    adventitial bursitis, 155
    chronic medial collateral bursitis, 151, 155
    pes anserinus bursitis, 155, 156
    prepatellar bursitis and deep infrapatellar
        bursitis, 154
    superficial pretibial bursitis, 154, 155

C
Calcium pyrophosphate dihydrate crystal
        deposition (CPPD), 153
Cleft sign, 80, 81
Coronary ligament, 70, 76

D
Deep infrapatellar bursa, 116, 126, 140, 154
Delayed gadolinium-enhanced magnetic resonance
        imaging of cartilage (dGEMRIC), 97

E
Extra-articular ganglion cyst, 158

F
Fabellofibular ligament (FFL), 52, 54, 55, 58
Floating meniscus, 73–76

G
Ganglion cysts, 8, 28
    extra-articular ganglion cyst, 158
    intra-articular ganglion cyst, 156–158, 160
    intratendinous ganglion cyst, 184, 186
    MR imaging, 156
    mucoid cystic degeneration, 155
    periosteal ganglion cyst, 158–159
Genicular veins, 191
Geniculate ligament. *See* Anterior transverse ligament
Giant cell tumor, 162–163, 223
Gout, 142, 148, 153, 180

H
Hamstring allograft, 45
Hamstring autograft, 12, 45
Humphrey ligament, 23, 70
Hydroxyapatite, 153

I
Iliotibial band friction syndrome, 16, 181–183, 185
Iliotibial tract avulsion, 218
Inferior lateral genicular artery, 191
Inferior medial genicular artery, 191
Intra-articular ganglion cysts
    clinical symptoms, 156
    intraosseous ganglion cyst, 157, 160
    lateral meniscus, 157
    mucoid degeneration, 156, 159
    prevalence, 156

J
Joint effusions
    hemarthrosis, 141–142
    lipohemarthrosis, 142, 145
    synovial fluid, 139–141

K
Knee arteries, 191, 202
Knee osteoarthritis scoring system (KOSS), 96

L
Lateral collateral ligament (LCL)
    arcuate sign, 59, 60
    complete tears, 55, 57
    impression, 63
    partial tear, 53, 55, 56
    preoperative MRI, 60–61
    Segond fracture, 59, 60
    sprain, 53, 55
Lateral meniscotibial ligament, 70
Lateral meniscus
    bone and capsular attachments
        anterior cruciate ligament, 71
        anterior lateral root ligament, 71
        anterior meniscofemoral ligament, 70
        lateral meniscotibial ligament, 70
        meniscofibular ligament, 71
        posterior lateral root ligament, 71
        posterior meniscofemoral ligament, 70
    intermeniscal connections
        anterior transverse ligament, 67–69
        lateral oblique ligament, 69
        medial oblique ligament, 68–69
        posterior transverse ligament, 68
    PMF, 69
LCL. *See* Lateral collateral ligament (LCL)
Leukemia, 206
Lipoma arborescens, 163
Localized nodular synovitis, 162–163

M
MCL. *See* Medial collateral ligament (MCL)
Medial collateral ligament (MCL)
    acute tear
        avulsed bone fragment, 41, 42
        meniscocapsular separation, 41, 43
        partial/incomplete tear, 39, 40
        POL injury, 41–43
        reverse segond fracture, 41, 44
        sprain, 39, 40
    anatomy
        deep layer, 35, 37
        layer 1/medial supporting structures, 35, 36
        medial patellar retinaculum, 35, 37
        meniscofemoral ligament, 35, 36, 38
        meniscotibial ligament, 35–36, 38
        outer margin, 36, 39
        patellomeniscal ligament, 36, 39
        POL, 35, 37
        posteromedial corner, 35, 37
        superficial layer, 35, 37
    chronic injury, 41–42, 45
    healing stages, 42–43, 45–46
    impression, 46
    reattachment, 44–45, 47
Medial gastrocnemius bursa, 65
Medial meniscus
    bone attachments
        ACL attachment, 66, 67
        anterior medial root ligament, 66, 68
        medial anterior meniscofemoral ligament,
            66–67
        posterior cruciate ligament, 66, 67
        posterior lateral root ligament, 66, 67
        posterior medial root ligament, 66–68
    capsular attachments
        meniscofemoral ligament, 65, 67
        meniscotibial ligament, 65, 67
        patellomeniscal ligament, 65, 67
    intermeniscal connections
        anterior transverse ligament, 67–69
        lateral oblique ligament, 69
        medial oblique ligament, 68–69
        posterior transverse ligament, 68
Medial posterior femoral recess, 65
Meniscocapsular ligament, 70
Meniscofemoral ligaments
    anterior, 21–23
    characteristic localization, 22
    orientation, 22
    posterior, 21–23
Meniscus
    calcifications
        chondrocalcinosis, 89
        meniscal ossicles, 88–90
    degenerative changes, 77, 78
    homogeneous low-signal intensity structures, 65
    impression, 92
    lateral discoid meniscus
        abnormal width meniscus, 73, 74
        complete variants, 72–73
        degenerative changes, 73, 75
        diagnosis, 73
        incomplete variants, 72–73
        intercondylar notch, 73, 74
        3 mm slice thickness, 73–74
        multiple tears, 73, 75
        Wrisberg type, 73
    lateral meniscus (*see* Lateral meniscus)
    medial (*see* Medial meniscus)
    medial meniscal flounce, 71–72
    medial meniscus (*see* Medial meniscus)
    meniscal avulsion, 73–76
    meniscal contusion, 77–78
    meniscal extrusion, 75, 76
    meniscal root ligaments, 65
    meniscal tear
        bucket-handle tear, 82–83, 85
        classifications, 79
        free meniscal fragment, 84–85, 87
        ghost meniscus sign, 81, 82
        horizontal meniscal tear, 82, 84
        inferior articular surface, 80
        lateral meniscal roots injuries, 81, 82
        location, 80
        parrot-beak tear, 84, 87

Meniscus (*cont.*)
    posterior lateral meniscus root tear, 81, 82
    radial root tears, 81
    size, 80
    superior articular surface, 80
    vertical longitudinal tears, 77, 80
    vertical radial tears, 80–82
  meniscocapsular separation, 76, 77
  parameniscal cysts, 85–88
  postoperative findings
    autologous meniscal transplantation, 92
    complications, 92
    intrameniscal changes, 90–91
    medial meniscus, 90, 91
    meniscectomy, 79, 90
    meniscus repair, 90
Muscles and tendons
  anomalous knee muscles
    accessory popliteus muscle, 176
    anomalous gastrocnemius variation, 173–175
    tensor fascia suralis muscle, 176
  anterior muscle group, 169–170
  intratendinous and peritendinous ganglion cyst,
    184, 185
  MRI impression, 186
  MRI pathological findings
    muscular contusions, 178–179
    strains/tears, 179
    tendinous avulsions, 179, 184
    traumatic injuries, 176–178
  normal MRI appearance, 169, 170
  posterolateral muscle group
    biceps muscle, 172, 174
    iliotibial band/iliotibial tract, 172, 173
    plantaris muscle, 173, 177
    popliteus muscle, 172–173, 175–176
  posterolateral muscle group injuries
    iliotibial band syndrome, 181–182
    mechanism of injury, 182
    MR imaging finding, 182
    plantaris muscle, 183–184
    popliteus muscle, 183, 186–187
    subtotal biceps tendon tear, 182, 186
  posteromedial muscle group
    medial head, gastrocnemius muscle, 171–172
    sartorius muscle, 170, 171
    semimembranosus muscle, 170, 171
  posteromedial muscle group injuries, 181

N
Nerves
  common peroneal nerve, 192
  deep peroneal nerve, 192
  MRI impression, 203
  MRI pathological findings
    chronic denervation, 199
    entrapment neuropathies, 201
    functional MR neurography, 200

    habitual disorders, 201
    standard MR sequences, 198
    systemic diseases, 201–202
    traumatic and iatrogenic nerve disorder, 201
    tumors and tumorlike lesions, 201
  superficial perineal nerve, 192
  tibial nerve, 192

O
Osgood-Schlatter disease, 218
Osteochondroma, 220, 222
Osteosarcoma, 224

P
Patella
  bipartite, 117
  femoropatellar joint, 114–116
  infrapatellar fat pad, 116
    Hoffa disease, 129
    intra-articular nodular synovitis, 129–130
    intracapsular chondroma, 129
    lipoma arborescens, 131–132
    postoperative fibrosis/arthrofibrosis, 132
    shear injury, 130–131
  instability of, 120–122
  intra-articular surface, 113
  lateral retinaculum, 113, 114
  medial retinacula, 113, 114
  MRI postoperative findings
  nonoperative findings, 134
  patella alta and patella baja, 118–120
  patellar calcar, 116–117
  patellar dislocation
    chronic patellar instability, 123
    definition, 122
    free osteochondral fragment, 123, 126
    joint effusion, 123
    "kissing contusions," 123, 125
    lateral patellar dislocation, 123
    medial retinaculum, 124
    musculotendinous junction lesion, 125
    osteochondral injuries, 123
    soft tissue injuries, 123
    treatment of, 132
  patellar dysplasias, 117–118
  patellar tendon, 113
    Osgood-Schlatter syndrome, 126, 129
    partial/complete tendon tears, 126, 127
    Sinding-Larsen-Johansson syndrome, 126,
      128–129
    tendinosis and tendon tears, 125–126
  postoperative findings, 134
  prepatellar bursa, 113
  quadriceps muscle, 113
  rectus femoris tendons, 113
  suprapatellar fat pad, 116
  vastus intermedius, 113

PCL. *See* Posterior cruciate ligament (PCL)
Pellegrini-Stieda disease, 41–42, 45
Periosteal ganglion cyst, 158–159
Pigmented villonodular synovitis (PVNS), 162
Plica syndrome, 159–160
Popliteal (Baker's) cyst, 155
Popliteal tendon (PT)
    anterior deep bundle, 49–50
    partial tear, 53–54, 56
    popliteal bursa, 50, 52
    posterior superficial bundle, 49–50
    well-defined and well-delineated structures, 53, 63
Popliteal vein, 191
Popliteofibular ligament (PFL), 51, 54
Popliteomeniscal fascicles (PMF), 51, 53, 55, 58, 69
Posterior cruciate ligament (PCL)
    acute tear
        complete tear, 24–25
        partial interstitial tear, 25–26
    anterolateral bundle, 21
    avulsion fracture, 26–27
    axial, sagittal, and coronal images, 21, 22
    chronic tear, 28
    ganglion cyst, 28, 30
    MRI pathological findings
        arthrofibrosis, 33
        infection, 33
        intraarticular loose bodies, 33
        tear, 33
        tunnel cysts and enlargement, 33
        tunnels misplacement, 32–33
    mucoid degeneration, 28, 29
    nonsurgical PCL, 33
    posteromedial bundle, 21
    postoperative graft
        femoral and tibial tunnels, 30–32
        graft's signal intensity, 32
        MRI impression, 33
    retrocruciate fat pad, 24, 28, 31
Posterior oblique ligament (POL), 35, 37, 41–43
Posterolateral corner (PLC), 76, 90, 182, 184
    ALL, 50–51, 53, 55, 58
    AOB, 49, 51
    arcuate ligament, 51–52, 54, 55, 58
    diagnosis, 61
    FFL, 52, 54, 55, 58
    impression, 63
    indications, 61
    operative *vs.* nonoperative management, 61–62
    PFL, 51, 54
    PMF, 51, 53, 55, 58
    popliteal tendon, 49–50, 52–54, 56
    postoperative MRI, 62–63
    surgical repair, 62
    surgical techniques, 62
    two-tailed reconstruction, 62
Prepatellar bursa, 140, 154
Primary synovial osteochondromatosis, 160
Pseudogout, 89, 153

Q
Quadriceps tendon autograft, 45

S
Salter-Harris classification, 214
Subchondral bone
    bone attrition, 101, 102
    bone contusion, 106
    cyst formation, 99
    cysts, 100, 101
    degenerative and inflammatory diseases, 99
    denuded areas, 99
    functional unit, 95
    impression, 110–11
    intracartilaginous osteophyte, 101, 102
    osteoarthritis, 99
    osteonecrosis
        avascular osteonecrosis, 102, 103
        double-line sign, 102, 103
        secondary osteonecrosis, 102
        spontaneous idiopathic osteonecrosis, 102
    postoperative findings
        autologous chondrocyte implantation, 109
        autologous osteochondral transplants,
            107–110
        bone marrow edema, 110
        compositional MR techniques, 110
        delamination, 109
        3-dimensional (3D) T1 gradient-echo (GRE)
            sequences, 108
        indication, 107
        marrow-stimulating techniques, 107, 108
        proliferative phase, 109
        T2-weighted turbo-spin echo sequences, 108
        weighted sequences, 108
    subchondral fracture, 106–107
    tibial and femoral edema, 100, 101
Superior lateral genicular artery, 191
Superior medial genicular artery, 191
Sural veins, 191
Synovitis
    acute synovitis, 145, 150
    arthridities and metabolic diseases, 153
    chronic synovitis, 145, 149
    hemosiderotic synovitis, 151–153
    Hoffa's fat pad, 145
    infectious synovitis, 151
    inflammatory synovitis, in rheumatological
        disorders, 145–146, 150
    MR imaging diagnosis, 145
    in osteoarthritis, 150–151
    synovial hypertrophy, 145
Synovium
    medial and lateral femorotibial compartments, 137
    MRI impression, 164
    MRI pathological findings
        bursitis, 153–155
        ganglion cysts, 155–160

Synovium (*cont.*)
    intra-articular bodies, 143–144, 149
    joint effusions, 139–143
    synovial cysts, 155
    synovial tumor-like lesions and synovial
      tumors, 160–164
    synovitis, 145–153
  synovial bursae and recesses, 137
    central synovial recess, 138, 141
    deep infrapatellar bursa, 138, 140
    gastrocnemius-semimembranosus bursa, 138, 142
    lateral collateral ligament-biceps femoris bursa,
      138, 143
    lateral gastrocnemius bursa, 138, 141
    medial gastrocnemius bursa, 138, 141
    parameniscal recesses, 138, 143
    posterior capsular recess, 138, 143
    prepatellar bursa, 138, 140
    subpopliteus bursa, 138, 142
    suprahoffatic and infrahoffatic recesses, 138, 141
    suprapatellar bursa, 138, 140
  synovial chondrosarcoma, 164
  synovial cysts, 155
  synovial hemangioma, 163
  synovial plicae, 139
  synovial sarcoma, 163–164
  synoviocytes, 137

T
Tibial spine avulsion, 217

Tibial tubercle transfer technique, 133
Traumatic osteochondral lesions
  cartilage injuries
    acute cartilage contusion, 104
    acute cartilage fracture, 104, 105
    acute cartilage lesion, 104
    avascular osteonecrosis, 103, 104
    classification, 104, 106
    delamination, 98, 99, 104
    patellar cartilage fissure, 104
    severe acute cartilage injury, 104, 105
  osteochondritis dissecans
    grade II lesion (stable), 105, 107, 108
    grade I lesion (stable), 105, 106, 108
    grade IV lesion (unstable), 105, 106, 108
Trochleoplasty, 133

V
Veins
  genicular veins, 191
  great saphenous vein, 191
  MRI impression, 202
  popliteal vein, 191
  sural veins, 191

W
Whole-organ MR imaging score (WORMS), 96
Wrisberg ligament, 21, 23, 70, 159

MIX
Papier aus verantwortungsvollen Quellen
Paper from responsible sources
FSC® C105338

If you have any concerns about our products,
you can contact us on
ProductSafety@springernature.com

In case Publisher is established outside the EU,
the EU authorized representative is:
Springer Nature Customer Service Center GmbH
Europaplatz 3, 69115 Heidelberg, Germany

Printed by Libri Plureos GmbH
in Hamburg, Germany